Medical Terminology

3rd Edition

by Beverley Henderson, CMT-R, HRT
and Jennifer L. Dorsey, PhD

for dummies®
A Wiley Brand

Medical Terminology For Dummies®, 3rd Edition

Published by: **John Wiley & Sons, Inc.**, 111 River Street, Hoboken, NJ 07030-5774, www.wiley.com

Copyright © 2020 by John Wiley & Sons, Inc., Hoboken, New Jersey

Published simultaneously in Canada

No part of this publication may be reproduced, stored in a retrieval system or transmitted in any form or by any means, electronic, mechanical, photocopying, recording, scanning or otherwise, except as permitted under Sections 107 or 108 of the 1976 United States Copyright Act, without the prior written permission of the Publisher. Requests to the Publisher for permission should be addressed to the Permissions Department, John Wiley & Sons, Inc., 111 River Street, Hoboken, NJ 07030, (201) 748-6011, fax (201) 748-6008, or online at http://www.wiley.com/go/permissions.

Trademarks: Wiley, For Dummies, the Dummies Man logo, Dummies.com, Making Everything Easier, and related trade dress are trademarks or registered trademarks of John Wiley & Sons, Inc., and may not be used without written permission. All other trademarks are the property of their respective owners. John Wiley & Sons, Inc., is not associated with any product or vendor mentioned in this book.

LIMIT OF LIABILITY/DISCLAIMER OF WARRANTY: THE CONTENTS OF THIS WORK ARE INTENDED TO FURTHER GENERAL SCIENTIFIC RESEARCH, UNDERSTANDING, AND DISCUSSION ONLY AND ARE NOT INTENDED AND SHOULD NOT BE RELIED UPON AS RECOMMENDING OR PROMOTING A SPECIFIC METHOD, DIAGNOSIS, OR TREATMENT BY PHYSICIANS FOR ANY PARTICULAR PATIENT. THE PUBLISHER AND THE AUTHOR MAKE NO REPRESENTATIONS OR WARRANTIES WITH RESPECT TO THE ACCURACY OR COMPLETENESS OF THE CONTENTS OF THIS WORK AND SPECIFICALLY DISCLAIM ALL WARRANTIES, INCLUDING WITHOUT LIMITATION ANY IMPLIED WARRANTIES OF FITNESS FOR A PARTICULAR PURPOSE. IN VIEW OF ONGOING RESEARCH, EQUIPMENT MODIFICATIONS, CHANGES IN GOVERNMENTAL REGULATIONS, AND THE CONSTANT FLOW OF INFORMATION, THE READER IS URGED TO REVIEW AND EVALUATE THE INFORMATION PROVIDED IN THE PACKAGE INSERT OR INSTRUCTIONS FOR EACH MEDICINE, EQUIPMENT, OR DEVICE FOR, AMONG OTHER THINGS, ANY CHANGES IN THE INSTRUCTIONS OR INDICATION OF USAGE AND FOR ADDED WARNINGS AND PRECAUTIONS. READERS SHOULD CONSULT WITH A SPECIALIST WHERE APPROPRIATE. NEITHER THE PUBLISHER NOR THE AUTHOR SHALL BE LIABLE FOR ANY DAMAGES ARISING HEREFROM.

For general information on our other products and services, please contact our Customer Care Department within the U.S. at 877-762-2974, outside the U.S. at 317-572-3993, or fax 317-572-4002. For technical support, please visit https://hub.wiley.com/community/support/dummies.

Wiley publishes in a variety of print and electronic formats and by print-on-demand. Some material included with standard print versions of this book may not be included in e-books or in print-on-demand. If this book refers to media such as a CD or DVD that is not included in the version you purchased, you may download this material at http://booksupport.wiley.com. For more information about Wiley products, visit www.wiley.com.

Library of Congress Control Number: 2019953066

ISBN 978-1-119-62547-6 (pbk); ISBN 978-1-119-62548-3 (ebk); ISBN 978-1-119-62551-3 (ebk)

Manufactured in the United States of America

SKY10077836_061824

Contents at a Glance

Introduction 1

Part 1: Living for Linguistics 5

CHAPTER 1: Scrubbing In to Master Medical Terminology 7
CHAPTER 2: Medical Terminology: The How and Why 15
CHAPTER 3: Introducing the Big Three: Prefixes, Roots, and Suffixes 23
CHAPTER 4: Acronyms, Eponyms, Homonyms, Multiples, and Plurals — Oh My! 37
CHAPTER 5: Say What? Pronunciation and Usage 53

Part 2: Mapping Words and Bodies 63

CHAPTER 6: As It Was in the Beginning: Prefixes 65
CHAPTER 7: So It Shall Be in the End: Suffixes 79
CHAPTER 8: Hey, I Know You: Word Recognition 87
CHAPTER 9: Deconstruction Junction: Breaking Down Words 95
CHAPTER 10: An Org Chart to Live By: Organization of the Body 105
CHAPTER 11: All Systems Go: When Systems Combine 119

Part 3: In Terms of Anatomy 129

CHAPTER 12: Boning Up on the Skeletal System 131
CHAPTER 13: Getting Ripped: The Muscular System 149
CHAPTER 14: Skin Deep: Skin, Glands, Nails, and Hair 163
CHAPTER 15: It Depends on Your Perception: The Sensory Systems 179

Part 4: Let's Get Some Physiology Terminology 197

CHAPTER 16: The Heart of the Matter: The Cardiovascular and Lymphatic Systems 199
CHAPTER 17: Just Breathe: The Respiratory System 223
CHAPTER 18: Feeding Time: The Gastrointestinal System 241
CHAPTER 19: Gatekeepers of Health: The Endocrine System 261
CHAPTER 20: Calming Down: The Nervous System 279

Part 5: Name That Plumbing 295

CHAPTER 21: When You Gotta Go: The Urinary System 297
CHAPTER 22: Check the Plumbing: The Male Reproductive System 311
CHAPTER 23: A Life Force: The Female Reproductive System 325

Part 6: The Part of Tens 347
CHAPTER 24: Ten Essential Medical Terminology References 349
CHAPTER 25: Ten or So Useful Mnemonic Devices 353
CHAPTER 26: Ten Sets of Terminology Tongue-Twisting Diseases 357
CHAPTER 27: Top Ten Crazy-Hard-to-Spell Medical Terms 363

Appendix: Handy Study Guide 365

Index 375

Table of Contents

INTRODUCTION 1

About This Book 1
Foolish Assumptions 2
Icons Used in This Book 3
Beyond the Book 4
Where to Go from Here 4

PART 1: LIVING FOR LINGUISTICS 5

CHAPTER 1: **Scrubbing In to Master Medical Terminology** 7

The Tale behind the Terms 7
Making Terminology Work for You 8
Building a Foundation of Vocabulary 9
In Terms of Anatomy 9
All Systems Go 10
Down-Under Details 12
The Ultimate Resource: You 13

CHAPTER 2: **Medical Terminology: The How and Why** 15

Defining Medical Terminology 15
Medical Terminology in the Real World 16
In theory and practice 16
Writing it down 17
Changes in Medical Terminology 18
It's Greek and Latin to Me 19
Modernizing Medicine 19

CHAPTER 3: **Introducing the Big Three: Prefixes, Roots, and Suffixes** 23

Rooting Around for Answers 24
Exterior root words 24
Interior root words 27
Prefix as Precursor 33
Common Prefixes 33
Suffixes: Final Thoughts 34

CHAPTER 4: **Acronyms, Eponyms, Homonyms, Multiples, and Plurals — Oh My!** 37
Acronyms 38
Eponyms 40
Homonyms 42
Deriving a Plural the Medical Way 43
Medical rules for forming plurals 43
English rules of forming plurals 46
Welcome to the Peanut Gallery: More Exceptions to the Plural Rules 48

CHAPTER 5: **Say What? Pronunciation and Usage** 53
Hooked on Phonics 53
Pronouncing Common Prefixes and Beginning Sounds 54
The sound of silence 54
From your ear to the dictionary 55
Pronouncing Common Suffixes and Endings 56
Pronouncing Common Combinations 57
Putting It All Together 58
What Condition Your Condition Is In 60
Suffering Suffixes 60

PART 2: MAPPING WORDS AND BODIES 63

CHAPTER 6: **As It Was in the Beginning: Prefixes** 65
Common Prefixes 65
A–E prefixes 66
F–J prefixes 67
K–O prefixes 68
P–Z prefixes 69
Matching Prefixes to Situations 69
In your body 70
In the doctor's office and hospital 71
In the pharmacy and research lab 72
Retro Root Rewind A–M 72
Retro Root Rewind N–Z 76

CHAPTER 7: **So It Shall Be in the End: Suffixes** 79
Common Suffixes 79
-itis 80
-oma 80
-pathy 80
And lots more suffixes 81

Matching Suffixes to Situations 83
In your body 83
In the doctor's office and hospital 84
In the pharmacy and research lab 85

CHAPTER 8: **Hey, I Know You: Word Recognition** 87
The Inside Story: Terms for Your Interior 87
Terms for the Outside of Your Body 92
Pathological Conditions 93

CHAPTER 9: **Deconstruction Junction: Breaking Down Words** 95
Finding Parts of Words 96
Identifying word elements 96
Defining the prefix 96
Defining the root word 97
Identifying the combining vowel 98
Defining the suffix 98
Going Deeper into Suffixes 99
Adding Up Individual Word Meanings 101

CHAPTER 10: **An Org Chart to Live By: Organization of the Body** 105
Looking at the Big Picture 105
Cells 106
Tissues 107
Organs and Systems 108
Cavities of the Body 109
Directional Terms and Anatomical Planes 110
Regions of the Body 113

CHAPTER 11: **All Systems Go: When Systems Combine** 119
Anatomical Systems Working Together 119
The musculoskeletal system 120
The integumentary system 120
The sensory system 121
Physiology Systems Working Together 121
The cardiovascular and lymphatic systems 121
The respiratory system 123
The gastrointestinal system 124
The endocrine system 125
The nervous system 126
The urinary and reproductive systems 127

PART 3: IN TERMS OF ANATOMY 129

CHAPTER 12: **Boning Up on the Skeletal System** 131
How the Skeletal System Works 132
Bones and osteology 132
Axial skeleton 134
Appendicular skeleton 137
Joints 138
Skeletal Root Words 139
More Anatomical Terms 141
Common Skeletal Conditions 143
Finding the Culprit: Skeletal Diseases and Pathology 145
Testing, Testing: Skeletal Radiology and Diagnostic Tests 146
Paging Dr. Terminology: Skeletal Surgeries and Procedures 147

CHAPTER 13: **Getting Ripped: The Muscular System** 149
How the Muscular System Works 149
Classes of muscles 150
Types of muscles 151
Muscles and tendons 151
Roundup of the superficial muscles 152
Muscular Roots and Suffixes 156
Action Item: The Movement of Your Muscles 157
Common Muscular Conditions 158
Finding the Culprit: Muscular Diseases and Pathology 159
Testing, Testing: Muscular Radiology and Diagnostic Tests 160
Paging Dr. Terminology: Muscular Surgeries and Procedures 161
It's All Related: More Muscular Terms 161

CHAPTER 14: **Skin Deep: Skin, Glands, Nails, and Hair** 163
Layers of Skin 163
Epidermis 165
Dermis 166
Subcutaneous layer 166
Glands, Both Sebaceous and Sudoriferous 166
Hair and Nails 168
Integumentary Root Words 169
Common Integumentary Conditions 171
Finding the Culprit: Integumentary Diseases and Pathology 172
Testing, Testing: Integumentary Radiology and Diagnostic Tests 175
Paging Dr. Terminology: Integumentary Surgeries and Procedures 175
More Integumentary Terms 177

CHAPTER 15: **It Depends on Your Perception: The Sensory Systems** 179
The Eye 179
Inner eye 180
Outer eye 182
The Ear 182
Outer ear 184
Middle ear 184
Inner ear 184
The Nose 185
The Mouth 186
The Touch Receptor 186
Sensory Root Words 186
It's All Related: More Anatomical Terms 190
Common Sensory Conditions 192
Finding the Culprit: Sensory Diseases and Pathology 193
Testing, Testing: Sensory Radiology and Diagnostic Tests 194
Paging Dr. Terminology: Surgeries and Procedures 195
Terminology RX: Sensory Pharmacology 196

PART 4: LET'S GET SOME PHYSIOLOGY TERMINOLOGY 197

CHAPTER 16: **The Heart of the Matter: The Cardiovascular and Lymphatic Systems** 199
How the Cardiovascular System Works 200
The heart 201
Blood vessels 202
Blood 203
How the Lymphatic System Works 206
Cardiovascular and Lymphatic Root Words 207
Common Cardiovascular and Lymphatic Conditions 212
Finding the Culprit: Cardiovascular and Lymphatic Diseases and Pathology 213
Testing, Testing: Cardiovascular and Lymphatic Radiology and Diagnostic Tests 217
Paging Dr. Terminology: Cardiovascular and Lymphatic Surgeries and Procedures 219
Terminology Rx: Cardiovascular and Lymphatic Pharmacology 221

CHAPTER 17: **Just Breathe: The Respiratory System** 223
How the Respiratory System Works 223
Nose 225
Pharynx and larynx 225
Trachea 225
Bronchi 226
Lungs 226
Respiratory Root Words 228
It's All Related: More Anatomical Terms 230
Common Respiratory Conditions 233
Finding the Culprit: Respiratory Diseases and Pathology 235
Testing, Testing: Respiratory Radiology and Diagnostic Tests 236
Paging Dr. Terminology: Respiratory Surgeries and Procedures 238
Terminology RX: Respiratory Pharmacology 239

CHAPTER 18: **Feeding Time: The Gastrointestinal System** 241
How the Gastrointestinal System Works 242
Mouth and pharynx 242
Esophagus 244
Stomach 244
Liver 245
Pancreas 245
Gallbladder 245
Intestines 245
Gastrointestinal Root Words 246
Common Gastrointestinal Conditions 250
Finding the Culprit: Gastrointestinal Diseases and Pathology 253
Testing, Testing: Gastrointestinal Radiology and Diagnostic Tests 254
Gastrointestinal Surgeries and Procedures 257
Terminology RX: Gastrointestinal Pharmacology 258

CHAPTER 19: **Gatekeepers of Health: The Endocrine System** 261
How the Endocrine System Works 262
Hormones 263
Pituitary and hypothalamus 263
Thyroid 265
Pancreas 266
Adrenals 266
Gonads 267
Endocrine Root Words 268
It's All Related: More Endocrine Anatomical Terms 270
Common Endocrine Conditions 271

Finding the Culprit: Endocrine Diseases and Pathology 274
Testing, Testing: Endocrine Radiology and Diagnostic Tests 275
Paging Dr. Terminology: Endocrine Surgeries and Procedures 276
Terminology RX: Endocrine Pharmacology 277

CHAPTER 20: **Calming Down: The Nervous System** 279
How the Nervous System Works 279
The Central Nervous System 280
Brain 280
Spinal cord 283
Peripheral Nervous System 284
Nervous Root Words 285
It's All Related: More Nerve-Wracking Terms 287
Common Nervous Conditions 288
Finding the Culprit: Nervous Diseases and Pathology 290
Testing, Testing: Nervous Radiology and Diagnostic Tests 292
Paging Dr. Terminology: Nervous Surgeries and Procedures 293
Terminology RX: Nervous Pharmacology 294

PART 5: NAME THAT PLUMBING 295

CHAPTER 21: **When You Gotta Go: The Urinary System** 297
How the Urinary System Works 298
Kidneys 299
Ureters 300
Urinary bladder 300
Urethra 300
Urinary Root Words 302
Common Urinary Conditions 304
Finding the Culprit: Urinary Diseases and Pathology 304
Testing, Testing: Urinary Radiology and Diagnostic Tests 306
Paging Dr. Terminology: Urinary Surgeries and Procedures 308
Terminology RX: Urinary Pharmacology 309

CHAPTER 22: **Check the Plumbing: The Male Reproductive System** 311
How the Male Reproductive System Works 312
Testes 313
Ducts 313
Urethra 314
Prostate 314
Penis 314

Male Reproductive Root Words....315
Pathological Male Reproductive Conditions....316
Finding the Culprit: Male Reproductive Diseases and Pathology....318
Testing, Testing: Male Reproductive Radiology and Diagnostic Tests....319
Paging Dr. Terminology: Male Reproductive Surgeries and Procedures....321
Terminology RX: Male Reproductive Pharmacology....322
Say What? Male Terminology Tongue Twisters....323

CHAPTER 23: **A Life Force: The Female Reproductive System**....325
How the Female Reproductive System Works....325
Ovaries....326
Fallopian tubes....327
Uterus....327
Vagina....328
Female Reproductive Root Words....330
It's All Related: More Female Reproductive Anatomical Terms....334
Common Female Reproductive Conditions....337
Finding the Culprit: Female Reproductive Diseases and Pathology....339
Testing, Testing: Female Reproductive Radiology and Diagnostic Tests....341
Paging Dr. Terminology: Female Reproductive Surgeries and Procedures....341
Terminology RX: Female Reproductive Pharmacology....346

PART 6: THE PART OF TENS....347

CHAPTER 24: **Ten Essential Medical Terminology References**....349
Medterms.com....349
Medilexicon.com....350
webMD.com....350
Dorland's Illustrated Medical Dictionary, 32nd Edition....350
Mosby's Medical Dictionary, 10th Edition....350
Stedman's Medical Dictionary and Flashcards for Health Professionals and Nursing Illustrated, 7th Edition....351
Taber's Cyclopedic Medical Dictionary, 23rd Edition....351
Sloane's Medical Word Book, 5th Edition....351
Medicalmnemonics.com....352
Medical Terminology Systems Quick Study Guide....352

CHAPTER 25: **Ten or So Useful Mnemonic Devices** 353
Cranial Nerves 353
Lung Lobe Numbers 354
The Size of a Thyroid 354
Scalp Layers 354
Muscles of the Rotator Cuff 354
Radial Nerve 355
Face Nerves 355
Perineal versus Peroneal 355
Sperm Path through Male Reproductive Tract 355
Carpal Bone Locations 356
Cranial Bones 356

CHAPTER 26: **Ten Sets of Terminology Tongue-Twisting Diseases** 357
Skeletal 357
Muscular 358
Integumentary 358
Sensory 359
Cardiovascular and Lymphatic 359
Respiratory 359
Gastrointestinal 360
Endocrine 360
Nervous 360
Urinary and Reproductive 361

CHAPTER 27: **Top Ten Crazy-Hard-to-Spell Medical Terms** 363
Crazy-Hard-to-Spell Terms 363

APPENDIX: HANDY STUDY GUIDE 365

INDEX 375

Introduction

Welcome to *Medical Terminology For Dummies!* Consider this your personal, private course in the study of the medical terms used every day in doctor's offices, hospitals, clinics, billing and insurance companies, labs, and even pharmacies. This is a personal grand tour through not only the world of medical terminology, but also through your own body.

You'll find as you read this book that learning medical terms is a two-part proposition. First, you've got to master the landscape of language itself. Don't worry, though — there will be no quiz. We just want you to better understand how to both create and break down words. Once you get to know more about prefixes, suffixes, and root words, you can do darn near anything with the terminology. For example, you can go inside the body to discover the terms that match up with different systems, diseases, procedures, and pharmaceutical products.

Mastering medical terminology involves more than just memorizing. Exploring these terms and how they can be created will unlock not only medical mysteries for you, but great opportunities as well.

About This Book

Getting to know the world of medical terminology can get a bit repetitive at times. That's why we decided to break the book down into several parts about all kinds of different things. You start by getting the backstory of terminology — the history and the players involved with bringing this "language" to the masses. Then you get into the nitty-gritty of how words are formed and all about word parts, usage, pronunciation, and recognition. Finally, you take a gander at all the different body systems and the words associated with them. We even throw in some bonus top ten lists at the end that we hope you find useful.

There's a lot to learn about medical terminology, we admit, but we'll be right there with you for the whole wild, crazy ride. Keep in mind that you don't have to read this book cover to cover, nor do you have to remember all the details from chapter to chapter. Read out of order, skip what you don't need. It will all be there for you should you choose to revisit the sections, tips, or sidebars at another time.

Keep in mind that this is not a giant textbook of terms, nor is it a dictionary. Those are both great resources, and we recommend you pick up both if you are a medical professional. This is a friendly take on the topic, and our main goal is to show you the basics of how these words are made so that you can go out in the big, bad world and master the creation and use of medical terms on your own terms. We're not giving you a fish; we're teaching you to fish.

We do rely on some conventions within this book that you may not see elsewhere in an attempt to keep the tone fun and conversational. So, please be prepared to see a lot of the following:

We have included chapters about language and medical terminology's place in it. You will notice we also make extensive use of lists in this book. We do this for your sanity. Be honest: Wouldn't you rather be able to study these terms in organized, easy-to-find lists and tables rather than picking through long, boring paragraphs trying to find the words you need to learn? We thought so.

Major chapters are divided by systems of the body. Each system chapter tells you a bit about how that particular body system works, to give you some context for its words.

We aren't doctors, so we try our best to explain things using simple language. That means you might see words like *pee* and *poo* from time to time. We figure you're knee-deep in official-sounding terms here, so it doesn't hurt to lighten up once in a while.

New terms are in italics to make them easier to spot.

Many of the body system chapters include artistic renderings. Don't be alarmed by those little pictures you see peppering the pages of this book. Feel free to be distracted, however — that's the point. We want you to stop and look at these great kernels of knowledge as you go through the book.

Foolish Assumptions

We are assuming you fall into one of these categories:

- A medical student hoping to get a jump-start on general terminology before that first big quiz.

- A medical professional looking to brush up on terms if you're a bit out of practice or just want to know more about how these terms are made.
- A curious adult interested in speaking your doctor's language and learning more about the terms that describe how your body functions.

No matter what possessed you to pick up this book, we hope it gives you the terminology boost you need for your particular circumstances. The human body has hundreds and hundreds of working parts, and they all have names. Moreover, there are names for all kinds of associated terms relating to functions, conditions, diseases, pathology, and even pharmacology. It's a whole lot, we grant you. But you are eager, right? And no amount of 50-cent words frighten you away from your goal: to become a medical terminology Zen master. You can do it, Grasshopper.

Icons Used in This Book

This book makes extensive use of icons — those little pictures that denote an important tidbit of information. Be on the lookout for these, as they provide even more tools for your terminology toolbox:

TIP

Points out concrete tips and tricks that you can put to use as you are studying medical terminology.

REMEMBER

Highlights passages that are good to keep in mind when mastering medical terminology.

WARNING

Alerts you to common mistakes that can trip you up in your medical terminology studies.

TECHNICAL STUFF

This icon indicates something cool and perhaps a little offbeat from the discussion at hand.

Beyond the Book

In addition to the material in the print or e-book you're reading right now, this product also comes with some access-anywhere goodies on the web. No matter how hard you study for your medical terminology exams, you'll likely come across a few questions where you don't have a clue. To check out the free Cheat Sheet, go to `www.dummies.com` and type "Medical Terminology For Dummies Cheat Sheet" in the search box. The Cheat Sheet gives you more helpful medical terminology roots, prefixes, suffixes, and tongue-twisting terms.

Where to Go from Here

By all means, if you're feeling spunky you can jump right into this book at any point and start working on your terminology savvy. Mastering the how and why of medical terms is sometimes as important as learning the terms themselves, which is why we put those chapters first. But by all means, feel free to hunt and peck the sections that are most useful to you.

Be bold. Be brave. And, most importantly, proceed through this book with confidence. Once you get the hang of how these words are made, you'll have no problem committing them to memory and to your daily life.

1 Living for Linguistics

IN THIS PART . . .

An overview of the basic building blocks of learning terminology

A background dossier on terminology and its history

An introduction to root words

A trip through the world of multiples and plurals

Tips and tricks on pronunciation and usage

IN THIS CHAPTER

- Getting to know the history of medical terminology
- Mastering the basics of word building and pronunciation
- Familiarizing yourself with basic parts of your anatomy
- Discovering the wide range of systems in the body

Chapter 1

Scrubbing In to Master Medical Terminology

Did you realize that when you picked up this book, you were beginning a journey into a whole new language? Don't worry — you haven't grabbed *Greek For Dummies* by mistake — it's all English, or at least "English." But once you get deep into the world of medical terms, you will find that it is a whole new way of speaking. Your journey will indeed take you to ancient Greece as well as to Rome. You will meet some of the pioneers of the medical world. You will gain entrance into a whole new world: the body.

The Tale behind the Terms

Medical terminology is made up of the terms that describe human anatomy and physiology (body organs, systems, and their functions), body locations, diseases, clinical, diagnostic imaging, and laboratory testing, together with clinical procedures, surgeries, and diagnoses.

It's important for every one of these things to have a specific name — just as it's important that you have your own unique name — because otherwise how would medical professionals be able to communicate clearly with one another? You might be able to visit your doctor and say, "I have a pain in my shoulder," and have him solve the mystery of what is causing that pain. But when your doc communicates that information to, say, a surgeon, it's crucial to be more specific.

The beauty of medical terminology is that it makes such vital communication more succinct and to the point. A medical term usually describes in one word a disease or condition that, under normal circumstances, would take several words to describe. *Appendectomy* is a one-word medical term to describe "surgical removal of the appendix." Now that saves you plenty of breath for more important things, like singing an aria or rooting for the your favorite sports team.

The foundation of medical terminology is based in both Greek and Latin origin. The Greeks were the founders of modern medicine, but Latin is the basic source of medical terms. With origins in ancient Rome, Latin quickly made its way through the world, solidifying its rep as the language of choice for medicine and science. Building on guidance from the Greek and Latin origins, medical terms began to be professionalized in the mid-1800s. The first medical dictionary appeared in the 1830s shortly after the first edition of *Webster's American Dictionary of the English Language.*

Making Terminology Work for You

Thankfully, there are ways to wade through the quagmire of medical terms and figure out how to pronounce and use them like a champ. But you have to start at the beginning by breaking down the parts of each word and then deciphering its meaning. Or, to put it in a fancy-schmancy way, you should use etymology. *Etymology* helps you find the origin and historical development of a term. You can use etymology to decipher words with Latin and Greek origins, eponyms (words named after people), and acronyms (modern language terms that stand for longer phrases).

Back to those word parts that you'll break down. There are three you need to know: roots/combining forms, prefixes, and suffixes.

Roots are the glue that holds all medical terms together. They are the basic form around which the final word is formed. A *combining form* is a combining vowel (usually *o* or *i*) plus the root word, usually with a prefix or suffix added. *Prefixes* appear at the beginning of a word and tell the how, why, where, when, how much, how many, position, direction, time, or status. The *suffix*, always at the end of a word, usually indicates a procedure, a condition, or a disease. While the prefix gives you a clue into what to expect in a word's meaning, the suffix tells you what is happening with a specific body part or system. And, usually, it either entails what is wrong with you or the procedure used to diagnose or fix it.

The breaking down of words that you will learn in this book also helps you with pronunciation. With medical terminology, sounds are not always pronounced the same as in English, and there are no steadfast rules that a combination of specific letters will always be pronounced in the same way. One thing that helps in both the standard English and medical worlds, though, is to learn how to pronounce phonetically, by breaking up the word into smaller parts.

Building a Foundation of Vocabulary

Getting the basics of word formation and pronunciation down pat is the hard part. Once you can do that, you can move on to building your word vocabulary. Even though medical professionals like to joke that terminology is like a foreign language (sometimes, yes), don't throw this book out the window just yet. The good news is that you probably already know a lot of medical terms and you can use those to build up the rest of your new-found vocabulary.

Remember your grade school days when you used all kinds of little tricks to remember things like multiplication tables and the state capitals? The same principle applies to new medical terms. You can make lists of word parts, list words by similar sound, map words, or memorize terms by body system. And those are just a few ideas. Do whatever works for you, even if it's singing terms to the tune of "Sunrise, Sunset" in the shower. We promise not to tell.

In Terms of Anatomy

For our purposes in the land of medical terms, we can compare anatomy to the infrastructure of a building. The walls, floors, bricks, plaster, electrical system, plumbing, and so forth all help keep the building working for the people who inhabit it. Your body's anatomy is no different, which is why you are going to read about these particular terms first. Once you get the basics of what holds your body together, you can go on to find out about the physiological systems that make your body react to both internal and external circumstances.

First on our anatomy checklist is the skeletal system. This is your body's frame, much like the frame of a building. This system, along with its joints, works together with the muscles to give you the support and movement you need every day. The bony skeleton provides the jointed framework for the body, giving it shape, protecting vital organs from external injury, and providing attachment points for muscles, ligaments, and tendons.

Working together with the skeleton is the muscular system, in which several different major muscle groups work together. Made up of over 600 muscles and joints, this system is responsible for movement.

Covering all this infrastructure is the integumentary system. Your skin, glands, nails, and hair work like the façade, or outside covering, of a building. They are the things people see when they look at you. The outside of your "building" often shows the world how healthy the rest of your body is. Healthy skin, along with accessory organs glands, hair, and nails, are the hallmarks of healthy insides, so care for them accordingly.

Your sensory system is all the "fun stuff" in your building. The windows, amenities, sound system, and dining facility all bring aesthetic delight to the building's inhabitants, and your senses work in a similar fashion.

It may be hard to imagine that words can describe all the amazing things your anatomy can do, but believe us when we say that it's all possible through terminology. And who knows? Perhaps there's a word out there that hasn't been created yet — until you came along.

All Systems Go

Once you get those basic working parts ingrained in your brain, you will move on to the physiology terminology. Physiology deals with the remaining body systems that help your fabulous body do its day-to-day work.

First up is the thing that keeps your blood pumping and your life moving forward each day: your heart. More specifically, the cardiovascular system. Your heart does not work in a vacuum. It has supporting players, namely your blood cells and vessels. These parts all work together to supply your body with fresh, clean, oxygenated blood.

Then there is the separate but complementary lymphatic system that works to flush your body of impurities. Most directly associated with immunity, the lymphatic system works in the same context as the cardiovascular system due to the similar makeup of the system and the fact that, once cleaned by the lymph nodes, lymphatic fluid is released directly into the bloodstream. Lymph vessels are arranged in a similar pattern as the blood vessels.

Speaking of oxygenating your blood, think about how that oxygen finds its way into your body. You may not consciously think about it every day, but breathing makes it all possible. The body's trillions of cells need oxygen and must get rid of carbon monoxide, and this exchange of gases is accomplished by the respiratory system. External respiration is the repetitive, unconscious exchange of air between the lungs and the external environment.

You have to breathe, but you also have to eat, and eating is way more fun. Your good buddy the gastrointestinal system helps turn those tasty meals and treats into usable energy for your body. Also called the alimentary or digestive tract, this system provides a tubelike passage through a maze of organs and body cavities, beginning at the mouth, the food entrance into the body, and ending at the anus, where solid waste material exits the body and your delicious Chinese takeout magically turns into . . . well, you know.

Moving on, the complicated endocrine system maintains the chemical balance of the body. It does this by sending chemical messengers called hormones throughout the body via the bloodstream. Hormones regulate and control activity of specific cells or organs. Slowly released hormones control organs from a distance. Endocrine glands are located in different parts of the body. They are said to be ductless, because they have no duct system to transport their secretions. Instead, hormones are released directly into the bloodstream to regulate a variety of functions of body organs. One can stimulate growth, another matures sex organs, and yet another controls metabolism. Your body has both central and peripheral glands.

Even more complicated (are we having fun yet?) is the nervous system. Working like the body's built-in computer system, it is far more complex than your laptop. Messages from the brain are relayed via the spinal cord through nerve fibers that provide connections for incoming and outgoing data. The body has more than *ten billion* nerve cells whose function is to coordinate activities of the body. This system controls our voluntary activities as well as involuntary activities. We speak, hear, taste, see, think, move muscles, and have glands that secrete hormones. We respond to pain, danger, temperature, and touch. We have memory, association, and discrimination. These functions are only a small part of what the nervous system controls.

The nervous system is made up of the central nervous system (CNS), which includes the brain and spinal cord. The peripheral nervous system (PNS) is composed of cranial nerves (that extend from the brain) and spinal nerves (that extend from the spinal cord). The autonomic nervous system (ANS) controls and coordinates the functions of the body's vital organs, such as heartbeat and rate of breathing — functions we don't even think about.

Down-Under Details

Speaking of things you don't usually think about, the urinary system is made up of the kidneys (two), ureters (also two), bladder, and urethra. This system's main function is to remove urea (the nitrogenous waste products of metabolism) from the bloodstream, and excrete it in urine from the body.

Urea is formed in the liver from ammonia. The bloodstream carries it (in the same manner as hormones and lymph) to the kidneys, where it passes with water, salts, and acids out of the bloodstream into the kidneys. The kidneys produce the urine that travels through each ureter into the bladder to be excreted via the urethra. Now that's a whole lot of information to impress your friends with at a dinner party. On second thought, maybe not.

When food and oxygen combine in cells to produce energy, the process is known as *catabolism*. In the process, food and oxygen are not destroyed, but small particles making up the food and oxygen are rearranged in a new combination, and the results are waste products. Waste in the form of gas (carbon dioxide) is removed from the body by exhaling through the lungs.

Think about how you were made. No, you weren't discovered under a cabbage leaf. Your mom and dad made you (see *Sex For Dummies* if you don't get our drift here) using their reproductive systems. In the male, it has two main functions: to produce spermatozoa, the male reproductive cell, and to secrete testosterone, the male hormone. The reproductive organs, or gonads, are the testes. They are supported by accessory organs, ducts, glands, and supportive structures. The ducts include the epididymides (epididymis-singular) vas deferens, ejaculatory ducts, and the urethra. Glands include seminal vesicles, prostate, and bulbourethral glands (or Cowper's glands). The supporting structures include the penis, scrotum, and spermatic cords.

The female reproductive system produces the female reproductive cell, or sex cell, secretes the hormones estrogen and progesterone, and provides the conditions to establish a pregnancy, together with providing a safe place for the pregnancy to develop and grow. The gonads (ovaries in the female), together with the internal accessory organs consisting of the fallopian (uterine) tubes, uterus, vagina, external genitalia, and breasts (mammary glands) make up the reproductive system in the female. Reproduction is achieved by the union of the female reproductive cell, an ovum, and the male reproductive cell, a spermatozoon (sperm for short), resulting in fertilization.

This is just a quick glance at the kinds of stuff you're going to learn about your body. Of course, the appropriate terms are discussed in detail along with the simple biology background.

The Ultimate Resource: You

A listing of well-known term references, recall devices, and word-building activities will help you apply terminology to your own personal real-world situation. The references mentioned in this book are some of the most well respected in the field, and ones we highly recommend. Of course, there are thousands of online and print resources, most of which are decent, if not downright reputable. Use your own good judgment when it comes to choosing one as your go-to source.

As you go on this journey, remember that ultimately you are your own best source of tips and tricks. Maybe you're a flash card aficionado. Perhaps you do best when you can visualize the term with the appropriate body system. Does your smartphone rule your world? Then you know there's an app (or two, or ten) for learning medical terms on the fly. Or maybe you like a good old pneumonic device like "*i* before *e* except after *c*." No matter how you choose to learn and recall these terms, do what is most comfortable and useful for you. You're the captain of this boat. Now, hoist the sail!

IN THIS CHAPTER

- Getting an understanding of what medical terminology is
- Finding out how medical terms are used in the real world
- Tracking the evolution of terminology
- Exploring Greek and Latin roots

Chapter 2

Medical Terminology: The How and Why

Repeat after us: Context is a good thing. You love context. Mmmmm, context. It is a good idea to get to know something about your subject matter before you dive head-first into studying it. This is particularly true with medical terminology because so much of the theory and history behind this topic shows up in the actual words and terms you will use every day.

Defining Medical Terminology

First, let's ponder what medical terminology is. It's a whole lot more than just medical words and phrases. Each word and each term is *organic*, meaning you can trace each part of the word back to a specific meaning. Cobbled together, these parts make up the meaning of the word. Medical terminology is made up of terms that describe human anatomy and physiology (body organs, systems, and their functions), body locations, diseases, diagnostic imaging and laboratory testing, together with clinical procedures, surgeries, diagnoses, and pharmacology.

REMEMBER

A medical term usually describes in one word a disease or condition that, under normal circumstances, would take several words to describe.

For example, consider two terms commonly known to most people. *Tonsillitis* is a one-word medical term to describe "inflammation of the tonsils," and *appendectomy* is a one-word medical term to describe "surgical removal of the appendix." It's much easier to use one word than a long, drawn-out phrase to describe these conditions, don't you think?

Medical Terminology in the Real World

The need or desire to learn medical terminology is not limited to the healthcare professionals. For example, a firefighter has to relay information to paramedics, such as the condition of a burn victim being placed in an ambulance. A police officer must complete a written report after delivering a baby in the back seat of a car. Or closer to home, think about trying to understand when a doctor tells you that your child needs surgery, or why an aging parent needs to be placed in a long-term care facility. Medical terminology allows you to convey the greatest quantity of information, with the least confusion and most precision, to anyone in the world. For example, saying someone has a badly broken wrist doesn't convey as much as saying someone has a Salter-Harris II fracture of the right distal radius with moderate lateral displacement and 28 degrees of anterior angulation. Now who's the coolest kid in the clinic?

In theory and practice

You don't need prior knowledge of Greek and Latin or anatomy and physiology to build a medical vocabulary. But you do need to master the fundamentals, or the ABCs, so to speak, to be comfortable and confident with medical terminology. Once you master what makes up a word, it will get easier and easier to swap out those parts to make and understand new terms on the fly.

TIP

You accomplish this by breaking down each word and identifying its parts (prefix, suffix, and root). A basic knowledge of the human anatomy helps, but more important is to know how each body system works independently and together with other systems. Knowing that helps the puzzle pieces fit into place more easily. As you'll read later, the root word is the primary building block for a medical term: It clues you in to the primary body part or system that the word is about. Then the prefix and suffix clue you in to what is happening with that part or system, whether it's a condition, disease, procedure, diagnostic, or pharmacological term.

Mastering medical terms is much easier than you think. It is certainly easier than acquiring a whole new language from scratch. New terms become easier once you know the reasoning behind most medical terms. Many terms are made up of interchangeable parts, used over and over again, in different combinations. Once you understand this, you will be well on your way to translating even the toughest medical terms — including terms you have never heard or seen before.

TIP

As you begin to familiarize yourself with roots, prefixes, and suffixes, make yourself (or purchase) simple flashcards that you can use to drill down the basics. Even running through them once per day will help you get in the habit of speaking with and understanding medical terms.

Writing it down

One thing that gives some people pause with medical terminology is spelling the words correctly. Again, defer to the rule of breaking down the word into parts. If you can spell each small prefix, root, or suffix and put them all together, then you can spell medical terms with ease.

TIP

One of the best ways to practice the spelling is, of course, to write it down.

Whether you are a list maker or prefer to draw maps, there is a way for you to incorporate writing terms as spelling and word-recognition practice. Some useful ideas for writing and recalling terms are

- Make lists of similar prefixes, roots, and suffixes based on what body system they are associated with.
- Make lists of prefixes, suffixes, and roots based on some other memorable moniker, such as sound similarity or similar meaning.
- Draw simple maps of each system and label body part terms.
- Use your body system map to identify diseases affecting each specific part. You can also use this technique to identify locations of specific procedures.
- Create simple worksheets based on root words and/or systems. Remember "minute math" in grade school? Well, you can just as easily crank out some basic fill-in-the-blank worksheets for various systems or root words and time yourself as you memorize terms.
- Got a blank wall? Grab various colors of sticky notes and start making a "word wall." Using a different color for each system (or word part), start creating movable tables with the sticky notes. This way, you can swap out root words, prefixes, and suffixes quickly as you learn words.
- Draw a "mind map" for yourself based on root words and their various prefixes and suffixes. A mind map is the creative version of a flowchart, with a primary concept in the middle and nodes of secondary concepts branching out from it.

REMEMBER

Building a medical vocabulary involves breaking down a word by identifying its prefix, suffix, and root word. The root word is the foundation or basic meaning of the word. It can appear with a prefix and suffix or between a prefix and suffix, as prefixes and suffixes never stand alone. They must be attached to a root word.

TIP

In this book we outline roots, suffixes, and prefixes and include the anatomy for each body system to help you to understand how everything fits together. When in doubt, look at the table of contents and check a specific body system's chapter.

Changes in Medical Terminology

Medical language is an entity unto itself and follows a historical development. Common medical vocabulary used today includes terms built from Greek and Latin word parts, some of which were used by Hippocrates and Aristotle more than 2,000 years ago.

TECHNICAL STUFF

One type of medical term is the *eponym*, a term named after someone. An example would be Parkinson's disease, named after the English physician Dr. James Parkinson.

With the great advancements in medicine throughout the 20th century, medical language changed with the times and continues to do so today. Some words are discarded or considered obsolete, whereas others are changed, and new words are continually added.

Building on guidance from the Greek and Latin origins, medical terms began to be professionalized in the mid-1800s. *Dorland's Illustrated Medical Dictionary* was first published in 1890 as the *American Illustrated Medical Dictionary*, consisting of 770 pages, over 50 years after the first edition of *Webster's American Dictionary of the English Language*. Dr. William Alexander Dorland was the editor, and when he died in 1956 the dictionaries were renamed to include his name, thus they are known today as *Dorland's Illustrated Medical Dictionary*. Electronic medical publishing took off during the 1980s thanks to advancements in database publishing and electronic storage. In the mid-1990s, medical dictionaries — most notably from Dorland's, Stedman's, and Taber's — became available in electronic form with many various editions and publications available on disk, CD-ROM, and via Internet downloading. Check out Chapter 24 for a list of great resources.

It's Greek and Latin to Me

You can thank the two founding fathers of medical terminology for getting the ball rolling: Hippocrates and Aristotle. Hippocrates, considered the father of medicine, was a student, teacher, and great physician. Aristotle was a Greek philosopher and a physical scientist. He stressed observation and induction. His major studies were of comparative anatomy and physiology. The Hippocratic Oath — an oath of professional behavior sworn by physicians beginning a medical career — is attributed to Hippocrates.

The Greeks were the founders of modern medicine, but Latin is the basic source of medical terms. With origins in ancient Rome and thanks to good, old-fashioned conquest, Latin quickly made its way through the world, solidifying its rep as the language of choice for medicine and science. Approximately 75 percent of all medical terms are based on Latin or Greek terms, even though modern-day changes are made to make the terms more comprehensive.

Look no further than the study of etymology to help you crack the code of medical terms. *Etymology* indicates the origin and historical development of a term. Some examples of etymology, or word history, include

- **Words with Latin origins:** *Femur,* for example, is a Latin term referring to a bone in the leg.
- **Words with Greek origins:** *Hemorrhage,* for example, is a word with Greek origin indicating a rapid, uncontrollable loss of blood.
- **Eponyms:** Words named after people, such as Parkinson's disease.
- **Acronyms:** These are modern language terms that stand for longer phrases such as *laser,* which stands for "light amplification by stimulated emission of radiation."

Etymologies were listed in early medical dictionaries, assuming the reader had studied languages and could read Greek or Latin. But gradually the Greek alphabet was cast aside when it was later recognized that few, aside from specialists, were actually studying ancient Greek.

Modernizing Medicine

With the advent of the medical dictionary, terminology came to the masses with full force. Today, medical terminology has evolved into modern applications from basic anatomy to include alternative, holistic, naturopathic, and complementary medicine. Other modern applications of medical terminology include (but are certainly not limited to):

- CAT scans
- DNA advancement
- Hundreds of new drugs on the market
- Investigative and diagnostic medicine
- Joint replacements and other surgical procedures
- Laparoscopic surgeries
- MRIs
- Organ transplants
- Stem-cell research
- Advancements in orthopedic procedures and replacement limbs

Today medical terminology is used and needed in any occupation that is remotely related to medicine and the normal functioning of the body. Here are a few careers involving the need for medical terminology:

- Athletic therapy
- Audiology
- Biomedical engineer
- Cytotechnology
- Dentistry and dental hygiene
- Emergency medical services
- Health records and health information technicians
- Massage therapy
- Medical statistics
- Medical transcription
- Nursing Home administrator
- Nutrition
- Occupational therapy

- Personal training
- Pharmacy
- Physical therapy
- Radiology technicians
- Speech language
- Veterinary medicine

All these applications exist in addition to the obvious groups of healthcare professionals who use terminology in their day-to-day activities, including associates, the medical secretary in a doctor's office, the insurance claims adjuster, even the compensation board adjudicator.

IN THIS CHAPTER

- Finding your roots
- Getting to know prefixes
- Taking a brief look at suffixes

Chapter 3

Introducing the Big Three: Prefixes, Roots, and Suffixes

Introducing the starting lineup for your medical terminology team! Whether you realize it or not, most words are made up of individual parts that contribute their own meaning. The big three — roots, prefixes, and suffixes — of medical terms all work together to clue you in to what that word means. Often, they tell you where it comes from, too.

Starting at center, you have the root. The *root* is the main part of the word, telling you in general the thing you are dealing with. The word root specifies the body part.

Playing forward is the prefix. A *prefix* appears at the beginning of a word and tells you more about the circumstances surrounding the meaning of the word.

The suffix would be the goalkeeper, to really stretch this metaphor. The *suffix* is always at the end of a word and, in the medical world, usually indicates a procedure, a condition, or a disease.

Almost every medical term can be broken down into some combination of prefixes, roots, and suffixes. Because they are the core of a word's meaning, the root words are great in number. There are many more roots than prefixes and suffixes put together.

Rooting Around for Answers

So what makes the root of a word so darned important? Maybe it's because the root lights the way to understanding the body system in question. The combining form, or word root, specifies the body part the word is either describing or associated with. Just by doing that, it helps rule out hundreds of other possibilities, allowing you to think only about a specific set of body parameters. This section shows two big lists of all the important roots that can appear after any prefix or before any suffix. They divide into two categories: exterior root words, which describe the exterior of the body, and interior root words, which deal with — you guessed it — the inside. These are the big daddies, the glue that holds all medical terms together. Think of this section as one-stop shopping. If you can't find your root word here, you won't find it anywhere! We will not be undersold!

Exterior root words

Table 3-1 lists the root words and combining forms that pertain to the exterior of the body.

TABLE 3-1 **Your Fabulous Façade: Exterior Root Words**

Exterior Root	What It Means
Acr/o	Extremities
Amb/i	Both sides/double
Anter/o	Front
Aut/o	Self
Axill/o	Armpit, axilla
Blephar/o	Eyelid or eyelash
Brachi/o	Arm
Bucc/o	Cheek (on the face!)

Exterior Root	What It Means
Canth/o	Angle formed where eyelids meet
Capit/o	Head
Carp/o	Wrist
Caud/o	Tail/downward
Cephal/o	Head
Cervic/o	Neck or cervix (neck of uterus)
Cheil/o, chil/o	Lip
Cheir/o, chir/o	Hand
Cili/o	Eyelash or eyelid, or small hairlike processes
Cor/e, cor/o	Pupil of eye
Crani/o	Skull
Cubit/o	Elbow
Dactyl/o	Fingers or toes
Derm/a, derm/o, dermat/o	Skin
Dors/i, dors/o	Back or posterior
Faci/o	Face
Gingiv/o	Gums in mouth
Gloss/o	Tongue
Gnath/o	Jaws
Inguin/o	Groin
Irid/o	Iris of eye
Labi/o	Lips
Lapar/o	Abdomen, loin, or flank
Later/o	Side
Lingu/o	Tongue
Mamm/a, mamm/o	Breast
Mast/o	Breast

(continued)

TABLE 3-1 *(continued)*

Exterior Root	What It Means
Nas/o	Nose
Occipit/o	Back of the head
Ocul/o	Eye
Odont/o	Teeth
Omphal/o	Umbilicus
Onych/o	Nails
Ophthalm/o, ocul/o	Eyes
Optic/o, opt/o	Seeing, sight
Or/o	Mouth
Ot/o	Ear
Papill/o	Nipple
Pelv/o, pelv/i	Pelvis
Phall/o	Penis
Pil/o	Hair
Pod/o	Foot
Rhin/o	Nose
Somat/o	Body
Steth/o	Chest
Stomat/o	Mouth
Tal/o	Ankle
Tars/o	Foot
Thorac/o	Chest / thorax
Trachel/o	Neck or necklike
Trich/o	Hair or hairlike
Ventr/i, ventr/o	Front of body

COPYCATS AND OPPOSITES

Some prefixes might look very different but have the same meaning. Here are some examples:

- *Anti-* and *contra-* mean against.
- *Dys-* and *mal-* mean bad or painful.
- *Hyper-*, *supra-*, and *epi-* all mean above.
- *Hypo-*, *sub-*, and *infra-* all mean below.
- *Intra-* and *endo-* mean within.

However, other, more troublesome prefixes mean the opposite of each other even though they look or sound similar. These are contentious prefixes:

- *Ab-* means away from (abduct), but *ad-* means toward.
- *Ante-*, *pre-*, and *pro-* mean before, but *post-* means after.
- *Hyper-*, *supra-*, and *epi-* mean above, but *hypo-*, *infra-*, and *sub-* mean below.
- *Macro-* means large, while *micro-* means small.
- *Tachy-* means fast, but *brady-* means slow.
- *Hyper-* also means excessive, yet *hypo-* also means deficient.

Interior root words

Now it's time to meet the movers and shakers that best define your inner self. Table 3-2 lists the root words and combining forms associated with the body's interior workings.

TABLE 3-2

Beautiful on the Inside: Interior Root Words

Interior Root	What It Means
Abdomin/o	Abdomen
Acanth/o	Spiny or thorny
Acetabul/o	Acetabulum
Acromi/o	Acromium
Aden/o	Gland

(continued)

TABLE 3-2 *(continued)*

Interior Root	What It Means
Adip/o	Fat
Adren/o	Adrenal gland
Alveoli/o	Air sac
Angi/o	Vessel
An/o	Anus
Aort/o	Aorta
Arteri/o, arter/o	Artery
Arteriol/o	Arteriole
Aspir/o	To breathe in
Ather/o	Plaque, fat
Athr/o, articul/o	Joint
Atri/o	Atrium
Audi/o, aur/i	Hearing
Balan/o	Glans penis
Bio-	Life
Bronch/i, bronch/o	Bronchus
Bronchiol/o, bronchiol/i	Bronchiole
Carcin/o	Cancer
Cardi/o	Heart
Cellul/o	Cell
Cerebell/o	Cerebellum
Cerebr/i, cerebr/o	Cerebrum
Cholangi/o	Bile duct
Chol/e	Bile
Cholecyst/o	Gallbladder
Choledoch/o	Common bile duct
Chondr/i, chondr/o	Cartilage
Chrom/o, chromat/o	Color

Interior Root	What It Means
Col/o, colon/o	Colon
Colp/o	Vagina
Cost/o	Rib
Cry/o	Cold
Crypt/o	Hidden
Cutane/o	Skin
Cyan/o	Blue
Cysti, cyst/o	Bladder or cyst
Cyt/o	Cell
Dipl/o	Double, twice
Duoden/o	Duodenum
Encephal/o	Brain
Enter/o	Intestine
Episi/o	Vulva
Erythr/o	Red
Esophag/o	Esophagus
Fibr/o	Fibers
Galact/o	Milk
Gastr/o	Stomach
Glyc/o	Sugar
Gynec/o	Female
Hemat/o, hem/o	Blood
Hepat/o, hepatic/o	Liver
Heter/o	Other, different
Hidr/o	Sweat
Hist/o, histi/o	Tissue
Hom/o, home/o	Same, alike
Hydr/o	Water, wet

(continued)

TABLE 3-2 *(continued)*

Interior Root	What It Means
Hyster/o	Uterus
Iatr/o	Treatment
Ile/o	Ileum (intestine)
Ili/o	Ilium (pelvic bone)
Intestin/o	Intestine
Jejun/o	Jejunum
Kerat/o	Cornea of eye, horny tissue
Lacrima	Tears
Laryng/o	Larynx
Leuk/o	White
Lipid/o	Fat
Lith/o	Stone (in gallbladder or kidney)
Lymph/o	Lymph vessels
Melan/o	Black
Men/o	Menses, menstruation
Mening/o	Meninges
Metr/a, metr/o	Uterus
My/o	Muscle
Myel/o	Bone marrow or spinal cord
Myring/o	Eardrum
Nat/o	Birth
Necr/o	Death
Nephr/o	Kidney
Neur/o	Nerve
Oophor/o	Ovary
Orchid/o, orchi/o	Testis
Oss/eo, oss/i, ost/e, ost/eo	Bone
Palat/o	Roof of mouth
Path/o	Disease

Interior Root	What It Means
Peritone/o	Peritoneum
Pharmac/o	Drug
Pharyng/o	Pharynx
Phleb/o	Vein
Phren/o	Diaphragm
Pleur/o	Pleura, rib (side)
Pneum/a, pneum/o	Lungs
Pneum/ato, pneum/ono	Lungs
Poli/o	Gray matter of nervous system
Proct/o	Rectum, anus
Pulmon/o	Lungs
Py/o	Pus
Pyel/o	Pelvis of kidney
Rect/o	Rectum
Ren/i, ren/o	Kidney
Sacr/o	Sacrum
Salping/o	Fallopian tube
Sarc/o	Flesh
Scapul/o	Scapula
Sept/o	Infection
Splen/o	Spleen
Spondyl/o	Vertebra
Stern/o	Sternum
Tend/o, ten/o, tendin/o	Tendon
Testicul/o	Testis
Therm/o	Heat
Thorac/o	Chest
Thym/o	Thymus

(continued)

TABLE 3-2 *(continued)*

Interior Root	What It Means
Thyr/o	Thyroid gland
Thyroid/o	Thyroid gland
Tonsill/o	Tonsils
Trache/o	Trachea
Tympan/o	Eardrum
Ur/e, ur/ea, ur/eo, urin/o, ur/o	Urine
Ureter/o	Ureter
Urethr/o	Urethra
Uter/o	Uterus
Vas/o	Vas deferens
Vas/o, ven/o, ven/i	Vein
Vesic/o	Bladder
Viscer/o	Viscera (internal organs)
Xanth/o	Red, redness
Xer/o	Dry

IT'S JUST SEMANTICS

It is only appropriate, then, that you take a moment to digest what exactly is meant by the word *semantics*. *Semantics* is, quite simply, the study of meaning in communication.

Have you ever heard someone say, "Let's drill down to semantics"? What she probably meant was that she wanted to discuss the actual meaning of whatever it was you were discussing. So, remember that when you are trying to decipher the meaning of a medical term, you do, in fact, want to talk semantics.

The word *semantics* is derived from the Greek *semantikos,* meaning "significant."

This may be a book about medical terms, but we're talking morphemes here, not morphine. A *morpheme* is the smallest linguistic unit that has semantic meaning. For example, *un* means not, or opposite. So the next time you look at a two-letter prefix and think it's just window dressing, think again. Chances are it has plenty of important meaning.

Prefix as Precursor

Think of the prefix as the welcome wagon for a term. It invites you into a whole new world. It tells you something about what you are going to find inside. Prefixes and suffixes are modifiers or adjectives that alter the meaning of the root word, in the same ways as regular English terms. A prefix appears at the beginning of a word and tells the how, why, where, when, how much, how many, position, direction, time, or status.

TIP

An easy word-building activity is to use the prefixes you know and draw connections to medical terms you are familiar with. For example, you probably know that *ultra-* means something is extra, or beyond its normal scope. And you're probably familiar with the word *ultrasound*, a procedure that provides — you guessed it — a look at your insides that is beyond the normal scope of visual exam. See? You're a medical terminology whiz already. Okay, maybe we're exaggerating slightly.

You might recognize many of the prefixes associated with medical terminology, because they have similar meanings in regular, everyday vernacular. For example, the most basic prefix of *a-* means without, or not, in medical terminology, just as it does in any other word. If something is atypical, it is not typical. *Hemi-* means half, as in *hemisphere*. The moral of this story is that prefixes aren't just window dressing. They have a unique and specific goal, which is to tell the reader more about the circumstances surrounding the word's meaning.

Common Prefixes

You can read a lot more about prefixes in Chapter 6, but to whet your appetite Table 3-3 gives you a quick look at some of the most common prefixes that play a huge role in both common, everyday English and medical terminology.

TABLE 3-3 **Preview of Important Prefixes**

Prefix	What It Means
A-, an-	Lack of, without, not
Ante-	Before, in front of, or forward
Anti-	Opposing or against
Bi-	Double, two, twice, both
Co-, con-, com-	Together or with

(continued)

TABLE 3-3 *(continued)*

Prefix	What It Means
De-	Down, or from
Di-	Twice or two
Extra-, extro-	Beyond, outside of, or outward
Hemi-, semi-	Half, half of
Hyper-	Above, excessive, beyond
Hyp-, hypo-	Below, beneath, deficient
Infra-	Below or beneath
Inter-	Between
Intra-	Within, inside
Intro-	Into, or within
Macro-	Large
Micro-, micr-	Tiny, small
Post-	After, or following, behind
Pre-, pro-	In front of, before, preceding
Retro-	Behind, backward
Semi-	Half
Trans-	Through or across
Tri-	Three
Ultra-	Excessive, beyond

Suffixes: Final Thoughts

The suffix, always at the end of a word, usually indicates a procedure, a condition, or a disease. Whereas the prefix gives you a clue into what to expect in a word's meaning, the suffix pulls no punches and tells you what is happening with a specific body part or system. And, usually, it either entails what is wrong medically or indicates the procedure used to diagnose or fix it.

The scope of suffix meanings is extremely wide. Like prefixes, many of these have similar meanings in plain old, everyday English that you hear on the street. For example, the suffix *-meter* simply indicates an instrument used to measure something, just as it does in other fields of study. Geography, a term feared by many fifth graders the world over, ends with *-graphy* and means the process of recording. You'll meet several other forms of *-graphy* in our medical term discussions.

Table 3-4 gives you a preview of the delights that await you in Chapter 7.

TABLE 3-4

Summarizing Important Suffixes

Suffix	What It Means
-ac, -ic, -al, -ous, -tic	Related to, or pertaining to
-ate, -ize	Subject to, use
-ent, -er, -ist	Person, agent
-genic	Produced by
-gram	A written record
-graph	Instrument used to record
-graphy	Process of recording
-ism	Condition or theory
-itis	Inflammation
-ologist	One who studies, specialist
-ology	Study of, process of study
-oma	Tumor
-pathy	Disease, disease process
-phobia	Morbid fear of or intolerance
-scope	Instrument used to visually examine
-scopy	Process of visual examination

IN THIS CHAPTER

- Checking out acronyms, eponyms, and homonyms
- Discovering the common plural forms
- Applying different rules of pluralization to medical terms

Chapter 4

Acronyms, Eponyms, Homonyms, Multiples, and Plurals — Oh My!

After you've got the basics under your belt, it's time to branch out. Really branch out — in multiple directions. You might think that in medical terminology, multiples and plurals work just like they do for regular words in the English language. Psych! Read on to find out about the wily world of medical multiples.

Pluralized medical terms would be pretty easy to comprehend and remember if all examples followed the same rules. The fun (fun?) of the English language is that there are several words that do *not* follow the rules. To see this, all you have to do is look to some basic examples from everyday conversation.

The standard rule is to add an *s* to make a noun plural, so one cat and one dog become two or more *cats* and *dogs*. Simple. But how about one woman, one man, and one child? This pluralization becomes two or more *women*, *men*, and *children*. So much for simply adding the *s*. *Women*, *men*, and *children* are irregular plurals.

For the most part, terms of Latin or Greek origin *do not* follow English rules when it comes to pluralizing. However, luckily for you, it is becoming more and more acceptable for medical terms to be pluralized by the English method. But first, take a quick look at three common kinds of common medical terminology: acronyms, eponyms, and homonyms.

Acronyms

An *acronym* is a word (or abbreviation) formed by the first letters or syllables of other words. Most acronyms are expressed in uppercase letters, but not always. For example, you might be familiar with the words *scuba* and *laser*. These terms are so well known that they have become acceptable as words in their own right. *Scuba* began life as an acronym for *self-contained underwater breathing apparatus*. *Laser* was an acronym for *light amplification by stimulated emission of radiation*. These two humble acronyms went on to greater glory as bona fide words.

There are, to put it mildly, many acronyms in medical terminology, some of which are common, some not so common. It is important to know the context in which they are used, because many are identical or sound similar, but have quite different meanings. Here are some common medical acronyms.

- **AMA:** American Medical Association
- **AMA:** Against medical advice
- **CAT:** Computerized axial tomography (scan)
- **CAT:** Children's apperception test
- **COPD:** Chronic obstructive pulmonary disease
- **COPE:** Chronic obstructive pulmonary emphysema
- **ECT:** Electroconvulsive therapy (shock therapy)
- **ECT:** Enteric-coated tablet
- **ECT:** Euglobulin clot test
- **MRI:** Magnetic resonance imaging
- **MRI:** Medical Research Institute
- **MRI:** Medical records information

WARNING

As you can see, many acronyms look the same, but actually mean something different. Knowing the *context* in which an acronym is being used is very important. Many common acronyms can be misinterpreted.

TECHNICAL STUFF

A favorite acronym of many medical professionals is BM. If you have ever been a patient in hospital, the usual question always asked by the nurse is, "Have you had a BM today?" Of course, most people know the nurse is referring to a bowel movement, but BM also could mean basal metabolism, body mass, bone marrow, basement membrane, blood monocyte, breast milk, or Bachelor of Medicine. Face it — everyone loves a good BM joke.

Next on the tour of plural forms is the antonym, proving once and for all that opposites do attract. An *antonym* is a word that means the opposite of another word. Examples would be right/wrong, right/left, up/down, and front/back. With reference to medical terms, some prefixes can be paired as opposites. Table 4-1 lists some of the most popular.

TABLE 4-1

Medical Antonyms

Prefix	What It Means
Ab-	Moving away from (abduction)
Ad-	Drawing toward (adduction)
Anterior-	Front
Posterior-	Back
Bio-	Life
Necro-	Death
Brady-	Slow
Tachy-	Fast
Cephalo-	Head (upward)
Caudo-	Tail (downward)

(continued)

TABLE 4-1 *(continued)*

Prefix	What It Means
Endo-	Within, inside
Exo-	Outside
Eu-	Normal, well
Dys-	Difficult, unwell
Hyper-	Above or excessive
Hypo-	Below or deficient
Leuko-	White
Melano-	Black
Pre-	Before or in front of
Post-	After or behind
Proximal-	Near (think proximity)
Distal-	Away from (think distance)
Superior-	Above
Inferior-	Below

Eponyms

Eponyms are an unusual and interesting facet of the plural world. An *eponym* is a person, place, or thing from which a person, place, or thing gets (or is reputed to get) its name. For example, Romulus is the eponym of Rome. It can also refer to a person whose name is a synonym for something (from the Greek *eponymos*: *epi* [to] + *onyma* [name]). In the medical field, a disease, sign, operation, surgical instrument, syndrome, or test is often named after a certain physician, surgeon, scientist, or researcher.

TIP

In current usage, it is now acceptable to drop the possessive apostrophe from most eponyms, so either is acceptable. For example, you can use Alzheimer's or Alzheimer.

Here are some of the most popular medical eponyms:

- **Apgar score:** Named after Virginia Apgar, American anesthesiologist (1909–1974). A numbering expressing the condition of a newborn infant at 1 minute of age and again at 5 minutes.
- **Alzheimer's disease:** Named for Alois Alzheimer, a German neurologist (1864–1915). A progressive degenerative disease of the brain.
- **Cushing's syndrome:** Named for Harvey Williams Cushing, American surgeon (1869–1939). A complex of symptoms caused by hyperactivity of the adrenal cortex.
- **Down syndrome:** Named after John Haydon Down, English physician (1828–1896). A chromosomal disorder, also called trisomy 21, formerly called mongolism.
- **Gleason grade:** Named for Donald Gleason, American pathologist (1920–2008). A rating of prostate cancer assigning scores of 1–5 for degrees of primary and secondary growth.
- **Hodgkin's disease:** A form of malignant lymphoma. Named for Thomas Hodgkin, an English physician (1798–1866).
- **Homans' sign:** Named for John Homans, American surgeon (1877–1954). Pain on dorsiflexion of the foot; a sign of thrombosis of deep veins of the calf.
- **Ligament of Treitz:** Located in the intestinal tract. Named after Wenzel Treitz, a Czech physician (1819–1872).
- **Lyme disease:** A multisystemic disorder transmitted by ticks. Named after a place, Old Lyme, Connecticut, where the disease was first reported in 1975.
- **Peyronie's disease:** Named for Francois de la Peyronie, a French surgeon (1678–1747). It means a deformity or curvature of the penis caused by fibrous tissue within the tunica albuginea. When distortion of the penis is severe it causes erectile dysfunction or severe pain during intercourse.
- **Parkinson's disease:** Named for James Parkinson, English physician (1755–1824). A group of neurological disorders including tremors and muscular rigidity.

As you can see, most of those famous people are no longer with us. So you had a much better chance of having something named after you if you were born a hundred years ago.

Homonyms

Similar to the antonyms is the homonym. A *homonym* is a word that has the same pronunciation as another, but a different meaning, and in most cases a different spelling (from the Greek *homonymos: homos* [same] + *onyma* [name]. Some common English language homonyms would be meat and meet, peal and peel, bare and bear, feet and feat, or pain and pane. While the list could go on and on with everyday English words, there are a few true homonyms in medical terminology. Table 4-2 shows the most likely suspects.

TABLE 4-2 **Medical Homonyms**

Word	What It Means
Cholic	An acid, related to bile
Colic	Severe abdominal pain
Humerus	A long bone in the upper arm
Humorous	Funny
Ileum	A portion of the colon
Ilium	A part of the pelvic bone
Jewel	A precious stone
Joule	A unit of energy
Lice	A parasite
Lyse	To break
Loop	An oval or circular ring, by bending
Loupe	Magnifying glass or lens
Mnemonic	To assist in remembering
Pneumonic	Pertaining to the lungs (the "p" is silent)

Word	What It Means
Mucus	Secretion of the mucous membranes
Mucous	Adjective form of mucus (resembling mucus)
Plane	Anatomic (imaginary) level
Plain	Not fancy (plain x-rays)
Plural	More than one
Pleural	Pertaining to the lung
Psychosis	Mental disorder
Sycosis	Inflammation of hair follicles
Radical	Extreme or drastic
Radicle	A vessel's smallest branch
Venus	A planet
Venous	Pertaining to a vein

Deriving a Plural the Medical Way

As you read earlier in this chapter, medical plurals are a bit different from the standard, everyday English variety. Read on to familiarize yourself with the nuances of medical plural building.

Medical rules for forming plurals

Some rules for pluralizing medical terms are as follows, with examples of the rule and exceptions to the rule.

Medical Rule 1: Change the a ending to ae

In other words, *vertebra* becomes *vertebrae*.

By adding the *e* to the plural, the "aah" sound ending pronunciation becomes "eh."

- Axilla, axillae
- Bursa, bursae
- Conjunctiva, conjunctivae
- Scapula, scapulae
- Sclera, sclerae

Medical Rule 2: Change the um ending to a

The *a* at the end is pronounced "aah."

- Acetabulum, acetabula
- Antrum, antra
- Atrium, atria
- Bacterium, bacteria
- Diverticulum, diverticula
- Labium, labia
- Medium, media

Medical Rule 3: Change the us ending to i

The *i* at the end is pronounced "eye."

- Alveolus, alveoli
- Bronchus, bronchi
- Coccus, cocci
- Embolus, emboli
- Fungus, fungi
- Glomerulus, glomeruli

- Meniscus, menisci
- Syllabus, syllabi (but syllabuses is also acceptable)

The exceptions to this rule include the following:

- Corpus, corpora
- Meatus, meatus (stays the same)
- Plexus, plexuses
- Viscus, viscera

Medical Rule 4: Change the is ending to es

The *es* is pronounced "eez."

- Analysis, analyses
- Diagnosis, diagnoses
- Exostosis, exostoses
- Metastasis, metastases
- Prognosis, prognoses
- Testis, testes

The exceptions to this rule are

- Epididymis, epididymides
- Femur, femora
- Iris, irides

Medical Rule 5: Change the ma or oma ending to mata

- Carcinoma, carcinomata
- Condyloma, condylomata
- Fibroma, fibromata
- Leiomyoma, leiomyomata

TIP

In the Rule 5 examples, the English plural is also acceptable: condylomas, carcinomas, leiomyomas, and fibromas.

Medical Rule 6: When a term ends in yx, ax, or ix, change the x to c and add es

- Appendix, appendices
- Calyx, calyces
- Calix, calices (Strange but true, both are correct)
- Thorax, thoraces

Medical Rule 7: When a term ends in nx, change the x to g and add es

- Larynx, larynges
- Phalanx, phalanges

Medical Rule 8: For Latin medical terms that consist of a noun and adjective, pluralize both terms

- Condyloma acuminatum, condylomata acuminata
- Placenta previa, placentae previae
- Verruca vulgaris, verrucae vulgares

There are (of course!) some exceptions to all these rules:

- Cornu, cornua
- Pons, pontes
- Vas, vasa

English rules of forming plurals

Many medical terms apply basic English rules for forming plurals. Thank goodness! You will no doubt recognize many of these common English language plural rules.

English Rule 1: Add an s

- Bronchoscope, bronchoscopes
- Disease, diseases
- Endoscope, endoscopes
- Finger, fingers
- Vein, veins

English Rule 2: When a term ends in s, x, ch, or sh, add es

- Crutch, crutches
- Distress, distresses
- Patch, patches
- Stress, stresses

English Rule 3: When a term ends in y after a consonant, change the y to i and add es

- Artery, arteries
- Bronchoscopy, bronchoscopies
- Endoscopy, endoscopies
- Ovary, ovaries
- Therapy, therapies

English Rule 4: When a term ends in o after a consonant, add nes

- Comedo, comedones

Exceptions:

- Embryo, embryos
- Placebo, placebos

Welcome to the Peanut Gallery: More Exceptions to the Plural Rules

Medical professionals, including physicians, clinicians, and pharmacists, often use measurements and their abbreviations to convey important information. In regard to *multiples*, the plural has no place in measurement abbreviations if coupled with a number value.

For example, the phrase "The incision was several centimeters long" is acceptable because it is a vague, not an exact amount. But if coupled with a number value and a measurement abbreviation, it then becomes, "The incision was 7 cm long." The measurement abbreviation *cm* is always used with a number value and is always singular. It is never pluralized as *cms*, as the number value provides the clue that someone is talking about more than one centimeter.

Another example of common measurement is the tablespoon. When made plural, this word becomes *tablespoons*. Used with a specific number value, it becomes 2 *tablespoons*. When abbreviated, it is always 2 *tbsp.*, not 2 *tbsps*.

REMEMBER

Abbreviation of measurement with numbers is always left singular.

Single-digit numbers are made plural by adding an *s*. For example, "Several 4 × 4s were needed to build the porch" and "The patient was asked to count by 7s." However, no apostrophe is used to form the plural of multiple-digit numbers, including years. "He is in his early 20s" (not his 20's). "She was born in the 1950s" (not the 1950's). Get the picture?

Similarly, to pluralize uppercase abbreviations or acronyms, use a lowercase *s* without an apostrophe. Some medical examples include

- CVA, CVAs
- EEG, EEGs
- WBC, WBCs

But if the abbreviation is expressed in lowercase, then an *'s* (with the apostrophe) is added to pluralize.

- rbc's, not rbcs
- RBCs, not RBC's

The real culprits in medical terminology are what are called the *soundalikes*. These words are pronounced almost the same, but with a different spelling and often a very different meaning. Not knowing the difference can get you into a lot of trouble and can cause a great deal of confusion. Table 4-3 shows several examples.

TABLE 4-3

Troublesome Soundalikes

Word	What It Means
Ablation	Surgical removal
Oblation	A religious offering
Access	A means of approaching
Axis	Center
Afferent	Towards the center
Efferent	Away from the center
Anecdote	A funny story
Antidote	A remedy to treat poisoning
Anuresis	Retention of urine in the bladder
Enuresis	Bed-wetting
Apparent	Clear, obvious
Aberrant	Off course, abnormal
Aural	Pertains to the ear
Oral	Pertains to the mouth
Callous	Hard like a callus, hardened thinking

(continued)

TABLE 4-3 ***(continued)***

Word	What It Means
Callus	Hardened area of skin
Carotid	Artery
Parotid	Gland
Cecal	Pertains to the cecum
Fecal	Pertains to feces
CNS	Central nervous system (abbreviation)
C&S	Culture and sensitivity (lab test)
Discreet	Reserved or private
Discrete	Separate
Dysphagia	Difficulty eating or swallowing
Dysphasia	Difficulty speaking
Effusion	Escape of fluid into tissue
Infusion	To introduce fluid into vein or tissue
Eczema	A type of dermatitis
Exemia	Loss of fluid from blood vessels
Ethanol	Alcohol
Ethenyl	Vinyl
Flanges	Projecting borders or edges
Phalanges	Bones of the fingers or toes

Word	What It Means
Graft	Tissue implant from one area to another
Graph	Diagram
Irradiate	To treat with radiation
Radiate	To spread out from a center
Joule	Energy
Jowl	Flesh on the jaw
Labial	Liplike
Labile	Unstable
Liver	Body organ
Livor	Discoloration of skin after death
Nucleide	A compound of nucleic acid
Nuclide	A species of atom
Osteal	Bony
Ostial	Pertaining to an ostium
Palpation	To feel with the fingers
Palpitation	Rapid heartbeat
Perfusion	Pouring over or through
Profusion	Abundant, much

(continued)

TABLE 4-3 *(continued)*

Word	What It Means
Protrusion	Jutting out
Perineal	Referring to the perineum (genital area)
Peritoneal	Referring to the peritoneum (in abdominal, pelvic cavities)
Peroneal	Vein in the leg
Pleuritis	Inflammation of the pleura of the lung
Pruritus	Itching
Precede	To come before
Proceed	To carry on or continue
Prostatic	Pertaining to the prostate gland
Prosthetic	An artificial device replacing a body part
Radical	Extreme; atoms in uncombined state (free radicals)
Radicle	Small branch of a vessel
Scleroderma	Hardening of the skin
Scleredema	Swelling of the face
Shoddy	Poor quality of work
Shotty	Resembles buckshot

WARNING

Perineal, peritoneal, and *peroneal* are famous screwups among many in the medical field. Don't join the crowd!

IN THIS CHAPTER

- Simplifying your pronunciation methods
- Distinguishing prefix sounds from suffix sounds
- Applying pronunciation tips to everyday usage and word building

Chapter 5

Say What? Pronunciation and Usage

If you read Chapter 4, you now have a better idea of how medical terms are formed. But unless you work on the set of a silent medical movie, you're going to have to learn how to pronounce these words. Even the Hollywood hotshots who rush around the sets of *Grey's Anatomy* and *Chicago Med* have to learn how to say medical terms, and are paid well to do it convincingly. Though you may not net seven figures for shouting, "Get an MRI of this man's duodenum and jejunum, stat!" you will fit right in with your medical counterparts by knowing the correct way to pronounce medical terms.

Hooked on Phonics

With medical terminology, sounds are not always pronounced the same as in your everyday English pronunciation, and there are not even steadfast rules that a combination of specific letters will always be pronounced in the same way. One thing that helps in both the standard English and medical worlds, though, is to learn how to pronounce *phonetically* — by breaking up word sounds into smaller parts.

The variety of possible letters and sound combinations can make — or at least can seem to make — medical terms difficult to pronounce, especially if you've never seen or heard the term before. What may seem familiar to you from everyday English might take on a whole new sound in a medical term.

TIP

We can't repeat this enough: By breaking the word down into basic parts — prefix, root, and suffix — you can simplify the task of pronunciation.

Take a closer look at the prefixes and the combining forms or root words when you start vocalizing the terms you know. You will find that by adding a variety of suffixes, not only does the prefix and suffix change the definition of the term, more importantly, in many instances it changes the way the term is pronounced. What does this mean for you? It means dive into this book and start memorizing! This in itself is a difficult task, but thankfully, there are some basic rules and tips that you can apply to help you along the way.

Pronouncing Common Prefixes and Beginning Sounds

You have to start somewhere, so why not at the beginning? Because many medical terms start with an odd (to the English speaker's eye) combination of letters, the pronunciation isn't always obvious. Some letters are silent that aren't normally in the English language, whereas some letters take on a whole new sound. Clear as mud, right? Let's take a look at some common rules to help clarify things a bit.

The sound of silence

Terms beginning with the letters *ps* are pronounced with an "s" sound. The *p* is silent, as it usually is when it appears at the beginning of a medical word.

TIP

Remember that the "pee" is silent — like it is in a swimming pool.

Examples:

Psychiatry: (sigh-KIYA-tree)

Psychology: (sigh-CALL-ogy)

Terms beginning with *pn* are pronounced only with the "n" sound. Again, the *p* is silent.

Example:

Pneumonia: (new-MOAN-ia)

Terms beginning with *pt* work exactly the same. Once again, the *p* is silent.

Example:

Ptosis: (TOE-sis)

Terms beginning with *ch* often take on the hard consonant sound like a "k."

Examples:

Chronic: (KRON-ic)

Chromatin: (KROME-a-tin)

Terms beginning with *c* or *g* can take on sound of "s" or "j" if they come before *e*, *i*, or *y*.

Examples:

Cycle: (SIGH-cull)

Cytoplasm: (SIGH-toe-plazm)

Genetic: (je-NET-ic)

Giant: (J-EYE-unt)

But *c* and *g* have a hard sound before other letters.

Examples:

Cast: (CAst)

Cardiac: (CARD-iak)

Gastric: (GAS-trick)

Gonads: (GO-nadz)

From your ear to the dictionary

That's a pretty good start, but now it's time to throw a wild card into the mix. What if you cannot see the term, but only hear it? Could you find it in a medical dictionary? Some good, old-fashioned memorization rules will help you recall those hard-to-pronounce beginnings.

If it begins with an "s" sound, it could begin with *c*, *ps*, or *s*:

Cytology: (sigh-TOL-oh-jee)

Psychiatrist: (sigh-KIY-a-trist)

Serology: (sir-ROL-oh-jee)

If it begins with a "z" sound, it could begin with *x* or *z*:

Xeroderma: (zero-DER-mah)

Zygote: (zEYE-goat)

If it begins with an "f" sound, it could begin with *f* or *p*:

Flatus: (FLAY-tus)

Phlegm: (FLEM — also note the silent *g* before *m*)

If it begins with a "j" sound, it could be *g* or *j*:

Gingivitis: (JIN-jih-VIT-is)

Jaundice: (JOHN-dis)

If it begins with a "k" sound, it could be *c*, *ch*, or *k*:

Crepitus: (KREP-i-tus)

Cholera: (CALL-er-ah)

Kyphosis: (kie-FOE-sis)

Pronouncing Common Suffixes and Endings

You're not out of the woods yet. One might think that pronouncing the endings of words is fairly self-explanatory. But again, medical terminology is kind of like the curve ball of modern language. As such, letters don't always sound like what they look like. This section lists some things to remember about saying word endings.

For terms ending in *i* (usually to form a plural), the *i* is always pronounced "eye."

Examples:

Calculus, calculi: (KAL-kyul-eye)

Glomerulus, glomeruli: (glom-MERUL-eye)

Radius, radii: (RAID-ee-eye)

Terms ending in *ae* (again often plurals) are pronounced "ay" (or sometimes "eh")

Example:

Vertebra, vertebrae: (VERT-e-bray)

In terms ending in *es* (you guessed it — often plurals), the *es* is pronounced as if it were a separate syllable.

Examples:

Naris, nares: (nar-EEZ)

Testis, testes: (test-EEZ)

Pronouncing Common Combinations

Now that you have established a few pronunciation rules, consider what happens to the pronunciation of a term when you combine a prefix with a root word or combining form, together with a suffix, and often a combining vowel. The combinations are endless.

TIP

Keep a few simple explanations in mind before you start combining word parts. To review:

- **Prefix:** Always at the beginning of a term. Modifies the word root that it precedes. It almost always indicates a location, number, time or period of time, or status.
- **Word root/combining form:** Usually indicates a body part, such as *cardi/o* for heart, *gastr/o* for stomach, and *neur/o* for nerve.
- **Suffix:** Appears at the end of a medical term. Usually, though not always, indicates a condition, procedure, disorder, or disease.

TECHNICAL STUFF

A *combining vowel* can be used to change the spelling of a term, making the pronunciation easier. A combining vowel is *not* used when the suffix begins with a vowel because this would make pronunciation difficult. A combining vowel is only used when the suffix begins with a consonant. For example, *gastr/o* pertains to the stomach. Adding the suffix *-itis*, meaning inflammation, results in the term *gastritis* (GAS-TRY-tis). If the combining vowel *o* were not removed, the result would be *gastroitis* creating a double vowel and a word more difficult to pronounce (GAS-TRO-it-is).

Putting It All Together

You've got all the tools, now you just need to use them to build your pronunciation skills. To do that, you have to get brave and start adding all the word parts together. A long medical term must be broken up into the word parts in order to arrive at a definition and a pronunciation. You can do this in two ways.

Some people like to look at the suffix first to determine if the term is a condition, a procedure, disorder, or disease. Once the suffix is defined, you can then move to the beginning of the word to define the prefix, if there is one, and the word root. This method is preferred by many people just getting their feet wet in the world of medical terms.

Others prefer to tackle the term from the beginning, establishing a meaning for the prefix first, then moving to the word root, and to the suffix last of all.

The pronunciation of a word can sometimes change when you take some prefixes, couple them with root words, and add vowels and suffixes. Following are some examples:

- **Euthyroid (YOU-thyroid):** The prefix *eu* means normal. Before thyroid, it means that the thyroid is normal.
- **Febrile (FEB-ril):** Means to have a fever. Add the prefix *a*, which means being away from or without, and the word becomes *afebrile* (ay-FEB-ril), meaning without a fever.
- **Hypertension (high-per-TEN-shun):** High blood pressure.
- **Hypotension (high-poh-TEN-shun):** Low blood pressure. Though there is not much difference in the pronunciation of hypertension and hypotension, and one means the opposite of the other, it is important to hear — and see — the different spelling of the prefix application.

- **Oliguria (ol-ig-YOUR-ee-ah):** Scanty or infrequent urination.
- **Polyuria (pol-ee-YOUR-ee-ah):** Excessive or frequent urination.

Suffixes can also affect the pronunciation of a word. Different suffixes can mean different pronunciations, particularly in respect to colors. Check out these two combinations and how the pronunciation and meaning change with altered suffixes:

- **Erythrocytes (eh-RITH-roh-sites):** Red blood cells
- **Erythrocytosis (eh-RITH-ROH-sigh-TOE-sis):** Having increased erythrocytes
- **Melanosis (mel-ah-NO-sis):** Unusual black pigmentation
- **Melanocytes (mel-ah-no-SITES):** Pigmentation cell in the skin layer

Even the more grounded basis of a word, the root or combining form, can change the way you say and see words. The combining vowel, in particular, can change the meaning and pronunciation:

- **Arthritis (ar-THRI-tis):** Inflammation of a joint (arthr/o)
- **Arthropathy (ar-THROP-a-thee):** A condition of a joint
- **Arthroplasty (AR-thro-plas-tee):** Surgical repair of a joint
- **Neuritis (noo-RYE-tis):** Inflammation of a nerve (neur/o)
- **Neuropathy (noo-ROP-a-thee):** A condition of a nerve
- **Neuroplasty (NOOR-o-plas-tee):** Surgical repair of a nerve

TERMINOLOGY TREASURE HUNTING IN THE DICTIONARY

It is important to remember that not every medical term you see or hear may appear in a medical dictionary as it is commonly spelled or pronounced. With so many root words, prefixes, and suffixes, the possible combinations would be endless, and the medical dictionary would become a set of encyclopedias. So when trying to find a term in a medical dictionary, you might have to look under the root word first and the prefix and suffix separately. Most commonly used terms are now listed alphabetically, but just because you can't find a term in the dictionary right away doesn't mean it doesn't exist. It just means you might have to piece together your own definition.

What Condition Your Condition Is In

Pronouncing terms for conditions can be easy if you familiarize yourself first with the root word of the condition, and then with the suffix. Let's use the simple, everyday stomach ailment as an example. By first pronouncing the root word, then adding different suffixes, you can up your vocabulary by a few points:

- **Gastro (GAS-troh):** Stomach
- **Gastritis (gas-TRY-tis):** Inflammation of the stomach (-itis)
- **Gastrodynia (gas-troh-DYNE-ee-ah):** A pain in the stomach (-dynia)
- **Gastropathy (gas-TROP-a-thee):** A stomach condition (-pathy)

On the other hand, you can grow your condition vocabulary and usage skills by applying the suffix to a variety of roots:

- **-megaly (MEG-ah-lee):** Enlargement of
- **Cardiomegaly (kar-dee-oh-MEG-ah-lee):** Enlargement of the heart
- **Hepatosplenomegaly (he-PA-TO-splen-oh-MEG-ah-lee):** Enlargement of the liver and the spleen (*splen/o* for spleen) and *hepat/o* for liver
- **Splenomegaly (splen-oh-MEG-ah-lee):** Enlargement of the spleen

Suffering Suffixes

Suffixes play the most major role in the different ways procedural terms are spelled and pronounced. Lucky for you, there is a short list of very common suffixes that pertain to procedures. So, again, make the acquaintance of a short list of word parts and you get a world of words in return.

Here are some of the suffixes pertaining to procedures that create changes in pronunciation:

- **-centesis:** A surgical puncture to withdraw or aspirate fluid
- **-ectomy:** Surgical removal of
- **-otomy:** Surgical incision or cutting into
- **-ostomy:** Surgical creation of an artificial opening

- **-plasty:** Surgical repair
- **-scope:** An instrument used for visual examination
- **-scopy:** To see, or a visual examination
- **-gram:** Resulting record or picture
- **-graphy:** The process of recording a record or picture

Using those suffixes, watch the change in pronunciation depending on the suffix used:

- **Appendicitis (a-pen-di-SITE-is):** Inflammation of the appendix
- **Appendectomy (ap-pen-DEK-toe-me):** Surgical removal of the appendix
- **Abdominocentesis (ab-DOM-in-o-sen-TEE-sis):** Surgical puncture of the abdominal cavity
- **Abdominoplasty (ab-DOM-in-o-plasty):** Surgical repair of the abdomen
- **Bronchoscope (BRONK-o-scope):** Instrument used to examine bronchus
- **Bronchoscopy (bronk-OSK-oh-pee):** Visual examination of bronchus using a bronchoscope
- **Cardiogram (CARD-ee-oh-gram):** Film produced by a cardiography
- **Cardiography (car-dee-OG-rah-fee):** Process of recording heart activity
- **Colostomy (koh-LOST-oh-me):** Surgical creation of an opening in the colon
- **Colotomy (koh-LOT-oh-me):** Surgical cutting into the colon
- **Endoscope (EN-DO-scope):** Instrument used for internal visual examination
- **Endoscopy (en-DOS-koh-pee):** Visual examination using an endoscope
- **Hypertropic (hi-per-TROF-ic):** Pertaining to hypertrophy
- **Hypertrophy (hi-PER-tro-fee):** Increase in size of an organ or body part
- **Mammogram (MAMM-oh-gram):** Resulting record of a mammography
- **Mammography (mamm-OG-rah-fee):** Process of examining breasts
- **Mammoplasty (mamm-oh-PLAS-tee):** Surgical repair to the breast
- **Oophoritis (ou-for-EYE-tis):** Inflammation of an ovary
- **Oophorectomy (ou-for-ECT-om-ee):** Surgical removal of an ovary
- **Prostatectomy (pros-ta-TEK-toe-mee):** Surgical removal of the prostate
- **Prostatomegaly (PROS-ta-toe-MEG-a-lee):** Enlargement of the prostate

- **Salpingectomy (sal-pin-JECT-oh-me):** Surgical removal of a fallopian tube
- **Salpingogram (sal-PING-oh-gram):** Resulting record from salpingography
- **Salpingography (sal-pinj-OG-rah-fee):** Procedure to examine fallopian tube

Some of the examples here demonstrate how the pronunciation of a medical word can change just by adding *gram* versus *graphy* or *ectomy* versus *otomy*. Something as small as a one-letter change can change the sound and meaning entirely. Take *scope* versus *scopy*. One letter difference changes an instrument into an examination, and more importantly, changes the pronunciation even more.

TIP

So practice your pronunciation. Say the terms out loud and get the emphasis on the right syllable! (SILL-ab-el!)

AND NOW FOR THE GRAND FINALE

So what, you ask, is the craziest medical term to pronounce? What can you wow your friends with at cocktail parties and class reunions? What would make even the technical advisors of *Grey's Anatomy* shudder in delight?

Try these two 25-cent words on for size:

- **Salpingo-oophorectomy (sal-PING-oh/ou-for-ECT-om-ee):** Surgical removal of an ovary and tube
- **Oophorosalpingectomy (OU-for-oh-sal-pin-JECT-om-ee):** Also meaning surgical removal of an ovary and tube

And, just so you're clear, here is the inside information on *oophorectomy*. This crazy word is only pronounced "ou-ou-for-oh" by the surgeon when he or she is dictating notes to be sure the transcriptionist spells it correctly with the double-O. Otherwise, the double O at the beginning of oophorectomy — or in the middle, as in *salpingo-oophorectomy*, is always "ooo." If it sounds like people are mooing, then you know they're saying it correctly.

2 Mapping Words and Bodies

IN THIS PART . . .

The possibilities of prefixes and suffixes

Recognizing words on your own terms

Breaking words down to make better sense of them

A more in-depth picture of the body and its systems, organs, and cavities

IN THIS CHAPTER

- Defining common prefixes
- Categorizing prefixes by meaning
- Getting to know most likely prefix uses
- Reviewing some root words

Chapter 6

As It Was in the Beginning: Prefixes

You first met your new friends, the prefixes, in Chapter 3. To recap: *Prefixes* show up at the beginning of a word and tell the how, why, where, when, how much, how many, position, direction, time, or status.

Prefixes have a very important job: They act as modifiers or adjectives, altering the meaning of the root word of the medical term. Though you see in this chapter some new and unfamiliar prefixes that only exist in the medical world, for the most part medical prefixes work just like any other prefix in the English language.

Common Prefixes

TIP

Keep the other word part functions in mind when dealing with prefixes. The *combining form* or *root*, as explained in Chapter 3, specifies the body part. The *suffix*, always at the end of a word, usually indicates a procedure, condition, or disease. When all three work together, they make one powerful word.

First things first: Let's take a look at the most common prefixes in simple, easy-to-memorize alphabetical order. Later in the chapter, we go over how these prefixes fit into everyday medical life and language.

A–E prefixes

- **A-, an-:** Lack of, without, not
- **Ab-:** Away from, take away
- **Ad-:** Towards or to, near
- **Ambi-, ambo-:** Both
- **Amphi-:** Double, both sides
- **Ana-:** Up, apart
- **Ante-:** Before, in front of, or forward
- **Anti-:** Opposing or against
- **Ap-, apo-:** Separated or derived from
- **Aut-, auto-:** Self, by yourself
- **Bi-:** Double, two, twice, both
- **Brady-:** Slow; most often refers to heart rhythm/rate
- **Brachy-:** Short
- **Cata-:** Lower, down, against
- **Circum-:** Around
- **Co-, con-, com-:** Together or with
- **Contra-:** Against or opposed to
- **De-:** Down or from
- **Di-:** Twice or two
- **Dia-:** Through, apart, across, between
- **Dis-:** Apart from or free from
- **Dys-:** Bad, painful, difficult
- **E-, ec-, ex-:** From, away from, out of
- **Ect-, exo-, ecto-:** Outside, outer, on
- **Em-, en-:** In
- **End-, endo-, ent-, ento-:** Within or inner
- **Epi-, ep-:** Upon, over, or on
- **Eu-:** Normal
- **Extra-, extro-:** Beyond, outside of, or outward

KISSING COUSINS: DIFFERENT NAMES, SAME MEANINGS

Some prefixes look totally different, but have the exact same meaning. Check out these proxy prefixes:

Hyper-, supra- and *epi-* all mean "above."

Anti- and *contra-* mean "against."

Dys- and *mal-* both mean "bad" or "painful."

Hypo-, sub-, and *infra-* all mean "below."

Intra- and *endo-* mean "within."

WARNING

Be on the lookout for prefixes that sound similar but mean slightly different things, such as *ab-* and *ad-*, *ambi-* and *amphi-*, and *dis-* and *dys-*.

F–J prefixes

- **Hemi-, semi-:** Half, half of
- **Hyper-:** Above, excessive, beyond
- **Hyp-, hypo-:** Below, beneath, deficient
- **Im-, in-:** Into, in, within
- **Infra-:** Below or beneath
- **Inter-:** Between
- **Intra-:** Within, inside
- **Intro-:** Into or within
- **Iso-:** Same or equal

WARNING

Infra-, *inter-*, and *intra-* are always mixed up and used inappropriately.

K–O prefixes

- **Macro-:** Large
- **Mal-:** Bad
- **Mes-, meso-:** Middle
- **Meta-:** Beyond or changing
- **Micro-, micr-:** Tiny, small
- **Mono-, uni-:** One
- **Mult-, multi-:** Many, multiple
- **Neo-:** New or recent
- **Oligo-:** Scanty
- **Ortho-:** Straight, normal

TIP

If you can't recall the meaning of a prefix, try putting into everyday English context. For example, you might remember the meaning of *macro-* by thinking about the word *macroeconomics*, which is about economics on a large scale.

NOT EVEN CLOSE: OPPOSITE PREFIXES

Some prefixes mean the opposite of each other:

Ab- means "away from" (*abduct*), but *ad-* means "toward."

Ante-, pre-, and *pro-* all mean "before," but *post-* means "after."

Hyper-, supra-, and *epi-* mean "above," but *hypo-, infra-,* and *sub-* mean "below."

Tachy- means "fast," whereas *brady-* means "slow."

Macro- means "large," whereas *micro-* means "small."

Hyper- means "excessive," but *hypo-* means "deficient."

P–Z prefixes

- **Pan-:** All
- **Para-:** Beyond, beside, or after
- **Per-:** Through
- **Peri-:** Around
- **Poly-:** Many, excessive
- **Post-:** After or following, behind
- **Pre-, pro-:** In front of, before, preceding
- **Presby-:** Old age
- **Pseudo-:** False
- **Quadri-:** Four
- **Re-:** Backward or again
- **Retro-:** Behind, backward
- **Semi-:** Half
- **Sub-:** Under or beneath
- **Super-, supra-:** Above, excessive, superior
- **Sym-, syn-:** With or together
- **Tachy-:** Rapid or fast
- **Trans-:** Through or across
- **Tri-:** Three
- **Ultra-:** Excessive, beyond

Matching Prefixes to Situations

The next step in prefixes is applying them to the words used every day in medical terminology. Keep in mind that the following is not by any stretch the end-all, be-all, conclusive list of medical words, but it's a nice sampling of prefixes at work.

In your body

Here are some common examples of prefixes in body-related words. You can see a nice mix of amounts, directions, and changes in these prefixes:

- **A**menorrhea: Without period or menses, as in pregnancy
- **An**ovulatory: Ovaries not releasing eggs, can be hormonally induced
- **Bi**lateral: Lateral meaning side; both sides
- **Brady**cardia: Slow heart rate
- **Brady**arrhythmia: Slow, irregular heartbeat
- **Circum**ferential: Around the outside
- **Dys**functional: Difficult or painful; dysfunctional uterine bleeding
- **Exo**cervix: Part of the cervix away from the uterus
- **Endo**cervix: Inner part of cervix, within the uterus
- **Hyper**tension: Excessive or high blood pressure
- **Hyper**emesis: Excessive vomiting
- **Hypo**tensive: Low or below normal blood pressure
- **Infra**umbilical: Below or beneath the umbilicus
- **Multi**loculated: A tumor or cyst having many or multiple locules, small spaces or cavities often filled with fluid
- **Oli**guria: Scanty, inadequate amount of urine production
- **Oligo**menorrhea: Scanty menstrual flow
- **Para**ovarian: Beside an ovary
- **Peri**cardial: Around the heart
- **Peri**urethral: Around the opening of the urethra
- **Poly**dipsia: Excessive thirst (symptom of diabetes)
- **Poly**uria: Excessive urination (also symptom of diabetes)
- **Pseudo**cyst: A structure resembling a cyst; but not an actual cyst
- **Sub**costal: Beneath or under the ribs
- **Sub**umbilical: Area beneath or under the umbilicus

In the doctor's office and hospital

Check out this sampling of words you might hear around the physician's office or in the hospital ER:

- **Ab**duction: Moving a body part away from the point of origin

  This term is used in orthopedics to test range of motion of an arm or leg. In medical transcription, it is often dictated as "A-B-duction" to distinguish from "A-D-duction," meaning the opposite.
- **Ad**duction: Moving towards the point of origin; opposite of abduction; usually dictated or pronounced "A-D-duction"
- **Auto**logous bone graft: Bone taken from donor site on body to use as a graft on another part of the body
- **Di**ssection: To cut or slice into two parts
- **Intra**uterine device: Contraceptive device inside or within uterus
- **Intra**venous: Within a vein; injection within a vein (not between)
- **Intra**muscular: Injection into a muscle, not between
- **Macro**scopic: Large enough to be seen with the naked eye
- **Multi**parous: Condition of having had many children
- **Peri**operative: Period of time around or during an operative procedure
- **Post**natal: After or following giving birth
- **Post**operative: Period of time following an operative procedure
- **Pre**operative: Period of time before an operative procedure
- **Pre**natal: Period of time before giving birth (a.k.a. "the pregnancy")
- **Pre**menstrual: Period of time before a menstrual period begins
- **Pseudo**pregnancy: A false pregnancy
- **Tachy**cardia: Rapid or fast heart rate
- **Tachy**arrhythmia: Rapid or fast heart arrhythmia

In the pharmacy and research lab

Heaven knows there are tons of long, hard-to-spell, 25-cent words used in the pharmacy and the lab. Here's a quick taste:

- **Anti**-inflammatory: Agent opposing or fighting against inflammation
- **Contra**indication: Inadvisable, to be avoided

  In drug therapy, certain drugs are contraindicated in the presence of other drugs with which they interact.
- **Micro**scopic: Very small; only seen using a microscope
- **Neo**plasia: Condition of new or recent (cell) growth
- **Neo**plasm: New or recent growth; could be a tumor or cyst

Retro Root Rewind A–M

So you know the prefixes. Great! Now, can you remember the wide range of root words they match up with to create medical terms? Table 6-1 gives you a quick refresher course on roots from A–M. For the N–Z root words, see the table at the end of this chapter.

TABLE 6-1 Recapping Root Words (A–M)

Root Word	What It Means
Abdomin/o	Abdomen
Acetabul/o	Acetabulum
Acro	Extremity
Aden/o	Gland
Adren/o	Adrenal gland
Alveoli/o	Air sac
Andr/o	Male
Angi/o	Vessel
An/o	Anus
Arteri/o	Artery

Root Word	What It Means
Arteriol/o	Arteriole
Arthr/o, articul/o	Joint
Ather/o	Fatty degeneration
Atri/o	Atrium
Audi/o	Hearing
Bacteri/o	Bacteria
Balan/o	Glans penis
Bio-	Life
Blephar/o	Eyelid
Brachi/o	Arm
Bronch/i, bronch/o	Bronchus
Bronchiol/o	Bronchiole
Carcin/o	Cancer
Cardi/o	Heart
Carp/o	Wrist
Cellul/o	Cell
Cephal/o	Head
Cerebell/o	Cerebellum
Cerebr/i, cerebr/o	Cerebrum
Cervic/o	Neck or uterine cervix
Chol/e	Bile
Cholecyst/o	Gallbladder
Choledoch/o	Common bile duct
Chondr/i, chondr/o	Cartilage
Chrom/o	Color
Clavic/o	Clavicle
Col/o	Colon
Colp/o	Vagina

(continued)

TABLE 6-1 *(continued)*

Root Word	What It Means
Cost/o	Rib
Crani/o	Cranium - (skull)
Cry/o	Cold
Crypt/o	Hidden
Cutane/o	Skin
Cyan/o	Blue
Cysti, cyst/o	Bladder or cyst
Cyt/o	Cell
Dactyl	Fingers, toes, or digits
Dermat/o, derm/o	Skin
Dipl/o	Double, twice
Duoden/o	Duodenum
Encephal/o	Brain
Enter/o	Intestine
Episi/o	Vulva
Esophag/o	Esophagus
Erythr/o	Red
Fibr/o	Fibers
Galact/o	Milk
Gastr/o	Stomach
Gingiv	Gums
Gloss/	Tongue
Glyc/o	Sugar
Gynec/o	Female
Hemat/o, hem/o	Blood
Hepat/o, hepatic/o	Liver
Heter/o	Other, different
Hidr/o	Sweat

Root Word	What It Means
Hist/o, histi/o	Tissue
Hom/o, home/o	Same, alike
Hydr/o	Water, wet
Hyster/o	Uterus
Iatr/o	Treatment
Ile/o	Ileum (intestine)
Ili/o	Ilium (pelvic bone)
Intestin/o	Intestine
Ischi/o	Ischium
Jejun/o	Jejunum
Kerat/o	Cornea of eye, horny tissue
Lacrim/o	Tears
Lact/o, lact/i	Milk
Lapar/o	Abdomen
Laryng/o	Larynx
Leuk/o	White
Lingul/o	Tongue
Lipid/o, lip/o	Fat
Lith/o	Stone or calculus
Lymph/o	Lymph vessels
Mamm/o	Breast
Mast/o	Breast
Melan/o	Black
Mening/o	Meninges
Men/o	Menses, menstruation
Metr/a, metr/o	Uterus
Myel/o	Bone marrow or spinal cord
My/o	Muscle
Myring/o	Eardrum

Retro Root Rewind N–Z

Break time. That was a lot of roots. Like, more roots than *The Tonight Show* band The Roots. This might be a good time for a breather. Once you've wrapped your mind around A–M, get ready to cover the rest of the alphabet in Table 6-2.

TABLE 6-2

Recapping Root Words (N–Z)

Root Word	What It Means
Nas/o	Nose
Nat/o	Birth
Necr/o	Death
Neo	New
Nephr/o	Kidney
Neur/o, neur/i	Nerve
Ocul/o	Eye
Odont/o	Tooth
Onych/o	Nail
Oophor/o	Ovary
Ophthalm/o	Eye
Orchid/o, orchi/o	Testis
Oss/eo, oss/i, ost/e, ost/eo	Bone
Oto	Ear
Palat/o	Roof of mouth
Pancreatic/o	Pancreas
Path/o	Disease
Ped	Children
Perine/o	Perineum
Peritone/o	Peritoneum (membrane lining abdominal and pelvic cavities)
Phac/o, phak/o	Lens (eye)

Root Word	What It Means
Pharmac/o	Drug
Pharyng/o	Pharynx (throat)
Phleb/o	Vein
Phren/o	Diaphragm
Physio	Nature or function of
Pleur/o, pleur/a	Pleura, rib (side)
Pneum/a/o, pneum/ono, pneum/ato	Lungs
Pod	Foot
Poli/o	Gray matter of nervous system
Proct/o	Rectum, anus
Psych	Mind
Pulmon/o	Lungs
Pyel/o	Pelvis of kidney
Pylor/o	Pylorus
Py/o	Pus
Rect/o	Rectum
Ren/i, ren/o	Kidney
Rhino	Nose
Sacr/o	Sacrum
Salping/o	Fallopian tube
Sarc/o	Flesh
Scapul/o	Scapula
Sept/o	Infection or septum
Sigmoid/o	Sigmoid
Spermat/o, spermat/a	Sperm
Splen/o	Spleen
Spondyl/o	Vertebra
Stern/o	Sternum

(continued)

TABLE 6-2 *(continued)*

Root Word	What It Means
Stomat/o, stom/a	Mouth or orifice
Tend/o, ten/o, tendin/o	Tendon
Testicul/o	Testis
Therm/o	Heat
Thorac/o	Chest
Thym/o	Thymus
Thyr/o, thyroid/o	Thyroid gland
Tonsill/o	Tonsils
Trache/o	Trachea
Tympan/o	Eardrum
Ung/o	Nail
Ur/e, ur/ea, ur/eo, urin/o, ur/o	Urine
Ureter/o	Ureter
Urethr/o	Urethra
Uter/o	Uterus
Vas/o	Vas deferens
Vas/o, ven/o	Vein
Vesic/o	Bladder
Viscer/o	Viscera
Xanth/o	Yellow
Xer/o	Dry

IN THIS CHAPTER

- Defining common suffixes
- Categorizing suffixes by meaning
- Getting to know the most likely suffix uses
- Reviewing some root words

Chapter 7

So It Shall Be in the End: Suffixes

The suffix has a job that's as important as the prefix's and the root word's. It is a third clue to the mystery of each medical term. The suffix is always at the end of a word and usually indicates a procedure, a condition, or a disease. All medical terms have suffixes. The suffix is all business and tells us what is happening with a specific body part or system — usually what is wrong with the body or which procedure is being used to diagnose or fix it.

Common Suffixes

The scope of suffix meanings is extremely wide. Like prefixes, many suffixes have similar meanings to those used in plain old, everyday English, whereas some are wildly different. You will get to know the usual suspects of suffixes fairly quickly — the following three in particular.

-itis

The suffix *-itis* simply indicates an inflammation of some kind. The *-itis* is quite popular in medical terminology because it can be applied to just about any body part within any body system. Here's a quick sample:

- **Tonsillitis:** Inflammation of the tonsils
- **Bronchitis:** Inflammation of the bronchi
- **Arthritis:** Inflammation of a joint

-oma

Remember the goofy yet memorable David Letterman joke, "Oprah, Uma. Uma, Oprah."? Well, meet *-oma*. The *-oma* suffix can often stand for something certainly not as pretty as Uma Thurman: a tumor. It can also pertain to a neoplasm, or new growth. Again, *-oma* is one of the most versatile suffixes because a tumor or neoplasm can happen on or near any body part, in any body system. Some *-oma*s you might have heard of:

- **Carcinoma:** Malignant (cancerous) tumor or growth.
- **Leiomyoma:** Benign (non-cancerous) tumor derived from smooth muscle. Commonly called a fibroid or fibroid tumor.
- **Melanoma:** Tumor of the *melanocytic* (melanocytes in the skin) system of the skin, a highly malignant and quickly metastasizing (spreading) tumor.

TECHNICAL STUFF

A tumor can be benign or malignant depending on the type and composition, and amount of cell division and growth.

-pathy

The last of the big three is the *-pathy* suffix, which indicates a disease process. Once again, the wide-ranging use of this suffix is made possible by the large number of body systems it can help describe.

- **Cardiomyopathy:** Disease process involving the muscles of the heart
- **Cardiopathy:** Disease process involving the heart
- **Neuropathy:** Disease process involving the nervous system
- **Osteopathy:** Disease process involving bone

And lots more suffixes

There are, of course, many, many more suffixes that are just as important as the big three, though they may not be quite as recognizable to you (yet). As with English terms, many of the suffixes make their terms into adjectives. Table 7-1 lists several you should get to know.

TABLE 7-1 Suffixes: Wrapping It Up

Suffix	What It Means
-ac, -ic, -al, -ous, -tic	Related to or pertaining to
-algia, -dynia	Pain, discomfort
-arche	Beginning
-ate, -ize	Subject to, use
-cele	Protrusion (hernia)
-centesis	Surgical puncture to withdraw or aspirate fluid
-cidal, cide	Kill or destroy
-cle, -cule, -ule, -ulus	Small
-cyte	Cell
-desis	Surgical fusion or binding
-dynia	Pain
-ectasis, ectasia	Stretching, dilatation
-ectomy	Cutting out, surgical removal
-emesis	Vomit
-emia	Pertaining to blood, a blood condition
-ent, -er, -ist	Person, agent
-esis, -ia, -iasis, -ity, -osis, -sis, -tion, -y	State of or condition of
-esis, iasis	Condition
-form, -oid	Looking like, resembling, or shaped like
-genesis	A beginning process, origin of
-genic	Produced by

(continued)

TABLE 7-1 *(continued)*

Suffix	What It Means
-gram	A written record
-graph	Instrument used to record
-graphy	Process of recording
-ism, -ia, -ac	Condition or theory
-itis	Inflammation
-lysis	Destruction, breakdown, or separation
-malacia	Softening
-megaly	Enlargement
-meter	Instrument used to measure
-metry	Process of measuring
-ologist	One who studies, a specialist
-ology	Study of, process of study
-oma	Tumor, neoplasm, swelling
-opia	Vision condition
-opsy	To view
-osis	Process, condition
-ostomy, -stomy	Artificial surgical opening
-otomy	Process of incision or cutting into
-pathy	Disease, abnormality
-penia	Lack of or deficiency
-pexy, -pexis	Surgical fixation
-phagia, -phagy	Eating
-phobia	Morbid fear of or intolerance
-plasia	Formation, development
-plasty	Surgical reconstruction, or shaping of
-plegia	Paralysis
-pnea	Breathing
-poiesis, poietic	Production or manufacture of

Suffix	What It Means
-ptosis	Downward displacement, or drooping
-rrhage, -rrhagia	Excessive flow or discharge
-rrhaphy	Suturing in place, fixation
-rrhea	Flow or discharge
-rrhexis	Rupture or breaking away
-sclerosis	Hardening
-scope	Instrument used to visually examine
-scopy	Process of visual examination
-spasm	Sudden or involuntary
-stasis	To stop, stopping
-tome	Instrument
-tripsy	Crushing
-trophic, -trophy	Growth or development

TECHNICAL STUFF

The suffixes, *-rrhagia* or *rrhage,-rrhaphy,-rrhea,* and *-rrhexis* are known as The Four R's. All four are difficult to pronounce and are almost always misspelled — usually with one *r* being left out.

Matching Suffixes to Situations

Tired yet? Hang in there just a bit longer, because now it's time to take a look at some examples of suffixes in the real medical world. Let's start with the place closest to you: your own body.

In your body

- Acro**phobia:** Fear of heights
- Ane**mia:** Low hemoglobin in blood
- A**pnea:** Condition of not breathing
- Cardio**megaly:** Enlargement of the heart

- Claustro**phobia:** Fear of enclosed or small area
- Col**ostomy:** Artificial opening into the colon
- Dia**rrhea:** Frequent flow of watery or loose stools
- Dys**phagia:** Painful or difficult eating (or swallowing)
- Dys**pnea:** Difficult or painful breathing
- Erythr**ocytes:** Red blood cells
- Gastro**dynia:** Stomach pain or discomfort
- Hemi**plegia:** Paralysis of one side of body
- Hemo**rrhage:** Excessive flow of blood
- Hepato**megaly:** Enlargement of the liver
- Hepatosplen**omegaly:** Enlargement of the liver and spleen
- Hyper**emesis:** Excessive vomiting
- Ile**ostomy:** Artificial opening into the ileum
- Leuk**emia:** Blood condition of white blood cells
- Leuko**cytes:** White blood cells
- Meno**rrhea:** Heavy menstrual period
- My**algia:** Muscle pain
- Nephr**osis:** Kidney condition
- Ortho**pnea:** Inability to breathe properly except in an upright position
- Osteo**penia:** Deficiency in bone mass
- Photo**phobia:** Visual intolerance of light
- Quadri**plegia:** Paralysis of all four quadrants of the body
- Splen**omegaly:** Enlargement of the spleen
- Trache**ostomy:** Artificial opening into the trachea; follows a tracheotomy

In the doctor's office and hospital

- Abdomino**plasty:** Plastic surgery on the abdomen
- Amnio**centesis:** Procedure to withdraw fluid from amniotic sac during pregnancy

- Appendec**tomy:** Surgical removal of appendix
- Broncho**scope:** Instrument used to perform a bronchoscopy
- Cardio**gram:** Hard copy record of cardiography
- Cardio**graph:** Machine used to perform a cardiography
- Cardio**graphy:** Process of recording activity of the heart
- Hernio**rrhaphy:** Surgical fixation or repair of a hernia
- Hysterec**tomy:** Surgical removal of uterus
- Laparo**scope:** Instrument used to perform a laparoscopy
- Lapar**otomy:** Cutting into the abdomen
- Mammo**graphy:** Process of examination of breast tissue
- Myo**rrhaphy:** Suture or fixation of a muscle
- Myo**rrhexis:** Suturing of a ruptured muscle
- Naso**plasty:** Repair of deviated nasal septum
- Oste**otomy:** Cutting into bone
- Psych**ologist:** Person who studies psychology
- Rhino**plasty:** Nose job
- Trache**otomy:** Cutting into the trachea
- Urethro**pexy:** Surgical fixation of the urethra

In the pharmacy and research lab

- Latro**genic**: Produced by doctor and/or treatment. (For example, an iatrogenic effect of chemotherapy can be hair loss.)
- Latro**phobia**: Morbid fear of doctors and/or treatment.
- Path**ologist**: Doctor who studies causes and effects of diseases.
- Pharmac**ology**: The study of drugs.
- Ultrasono**gram**: A written record of a diagnostic imaging technique using sound waves.

IN THIS CHAPTER

- Appreciating Greek and Latin origins
- Surveying terms describing the body's interior
- Checking out terms covering the body's exterior
- Looking at pathological terms

Chapter 8

Hey, I Know You: Word Recognition

Getting the hang of medical prefixes, roots, and suffixes is just the beginning of reaching your goal of becoming a terminology expert. Once you do that, you can move on to general word recognition.

Root words remain the basic component of word building, and you can look directly to them to recognize all sorts of words that associate with specific body parts and regions. Because you have spent so much time going over these individual building blocks, you can now begin to use what you know to piece together the larger puzzle of knowing whole words.

Blame it on Aristotle and Hippocrates. Approximately 75 percent of all medical terms are based on Latin or Greek terms.

The Inside Story: Terms for Your Interior

Inside all these cavities, of course, lies a bounty of body part-related medical terms. All the root words and combining forms from Chapter 3 (and Chapters 6 and 7) can morph into all kinds of different words that explain everything from everyday common conditions and procedures to pathology and pharmacology.

TIP

Remember that you can take any root word or combining form and create several different medical terms.

Table 8-1 lists many examples of where these root words can take you on your medical terminology journey.

TABLE 8-1 **Interior Affairs**

Root Word	What It Means	Example(s)
Abdomin/o	Abdomen	Abdominoplasty: Surgical repair or reconstruction of the abdomen
Angi/o	Vessel	Angioplasty: Surgical repair or reconstruction of a vessel
Arteri/o	Artery	Arterioplasty: Surgical repair or reconstruction of an artery
Arthr/o	Joint	Arthritis: Inflammation of a joint Arthroplasty: Surgical repair or reconstruction of a joint
Audi/o	Hearing	Audiometry: Measurement of hearing using an audiometer
Bio	Life	Biology: The study of life and living organisms
Bronch/i, bronch/o	Bronchus/lung	Bronchitis: Inflammation of the bronchi Bronchoscopy: Visual examination of the bronchi
Cardi/o	Heart	Cardiomegaly: Enlargement of the heart Cardiac: Pertaining to the heart Carditis: Inflammation of the heart
Cholecyst/o	Gallbladder	Cholecystectomy: Removal of the gallbladder Cholecystitis: Inflammation of the gallbladder
Chondr/i, chondr/o	Cartilage	Chondromalacia: Softening of cartilage
Col/o	Colon	Colonoscopy: Visual examination of the colon Colonoscope: Instrument used in colonoscopy
Cry/o	Cold	Cryobiology: Branch of biology dealing with effects of low temperatures
Cysti, cyst/o	Bladder, or cyst	Cystectomy: Surgical removal of a simple cyst or of the urinary bladder Cystitis: Inflammation of the bladder Cystogram: Radiograph of the bladder Cystopexy: Surgical fixation of the bladder to abdominal wall

Root Word	What It Means	Example(s)
Cyt/o	Cell	Cytology: Study of cells
Duoden/o	Duodenum	Duodenotomy: Surgical cutting into the duodenum Duodenectomy: Surgical removal of the duodenum Duodenitis: Inflammation of the duodenum
Encephal/o	Brain	Encephalitis: Inflammation of the brain
Episi/o	Vulva	Episiotomy: Surgical cutting of the vulva
Erythr/o	Red	Erythrocytes: Red blood cells Erythema: Reddening of the skin
Esophag/o	Esophagus	Esophagitis: Inflammation of the esophagus Esophagogastroduodenoscopy (EGD): Visual examination of the esophagus, stomach, and duodenum by scope
Galact/o	Milk	Galactorrhea: Spontaneous flow of milk when nursing
Gastr/o	Stomach	Gastritis: Inflammation of the stomach Gastrectomy: Surgical removal of the stomach Gastrodynia: Stomach ache
Glyc/o	Sugar	Glycosuria: Sugar in the urine
Gynec/o	Female	Gynecologist: Physician who studies and treats diseases of female reproductive organs
Hemat/o, hem/o	Blood	Hematocyte: Blood cell
Hepat/o, hepatic/o	Liver	Hepatitis: Inflammation of the liver
Heter/o	Other, different	Heterosexual: Sexually attracted to the opposite sex
Hist/o, histi/o	Tissue	Histology: Study and function of tissue
Hom/o, home/o	Same, alike	Homosexual: Sexually attracted to the same sex
Hydr/o	Water, wet	Hydromassage: Massage by means of moving water
Hyster/o	Uterus	Hysterectomy: Surgical removal of the uterus
Ile/o	Ileum (intestine)	Ileostomy: Artificial opening into the ileum Ileitis: Inflammation of the ileum
Ili/o	Ilium (pelvic bone)	Ilioinguinal: Pertaining to the ilium and inguinal regions

(continued)

TABLE 8-1 *(continued)*

Root Word	What It Means	Example(s)
Jejun/o	Jejunum	Jejunitis: Inflammation of the jejunum Jejunostomy: Artificial opening into the jejunum
Lacrima	Tears	Lacrimatory: Causing a flow of tears
Laryng/o	Larynx	Laryngitis: Inflammation of the larynx Laryngectomy: Surgical removal of the larynx
Leuk/o	White	Leukocyte: White blood cell
Lith/o	Stone or calculus	Lithotripsy: Crushing of a stone or calculus
Men/o	Menstruation	Menorrhea: Menstrual flow Menorrhagia: Excessive or heavy menstrual flow
Myel/o	Bone marrow/spinal cord	Myelogram: Recording of the spinal cord
My/o	Muscle	Myositis: Inflammation of a muscle Myalgia: Pain in a muscle or painful muscle
Nat/o	Birth	Prenatal: Before birth Postnatal: After birth
Necr/o	Death	Necrosis: Death of a cell Necrophobia: Morbid fear of death or dead bodies
Nephr/o	Kidney	Nephrectomy: Surgical removal of a kidney
Neur/o, neur/i	Nerve	Neurologist: Physician who studies and treats conditions of the nervous system
Oophor/o	Ovary	Oophorectomy: Surgical removal of an ovary Oophoritis: Inflammation of an ovary
Orchid/o, orchi/o	Testis	Orchialgia: A pain in the testicle Orchiectomy: Surgical removal of a testicle
Peritone/o	Peritoneum	Peritoneal: Pertaining to the peritoneum Peritonitis: Inflammation of the peritoneum
Pharyng/o	Pharynx	Pharyngitis: Inflammation of the pharynx (sore throat)
Pleur/o, pleur/a	Pleura, rib (side)	Pleurisy: Inflammation of the lining of the chest cavity Pleurolysis: Surgical separation of pleural adhesions

Root Word	What It Means	Example(s)
Pneum/a/o/ato/ono	Lungs	Pneumonitis: Inflammation of the lung
Proct/o	Rectum, anus	Proctologist: Physician who studies and treats diseases of rectum and anus
Pulmon/o	Lungs	Pulmonary: Pertaining to the lungs
Pyel/o	Renal pelvis	Pyelography: Radiograph (x-ray) of the pelvis of the kidneyPyelolithotomy: Removal of a stone from the kidney pelvis
Rect/o	Rectum	Rectosigmoid: Pertaining to the rectum and sigmoid
Salping/o	Fallopian tube	Salpingectomy: Surgical removal of a fallopian tube
Sarc/o	Flesh	Sarcoid: Resembling flesh
Splen/o	Spleen	Splenomegaly: Enlargement of the spleen Splenectomy: Surgical removal of the spleen
Tend/o, ten/o, tendin/o	Tendon	Tendinitis (or tendonitis): Inflammation of a tendon
Testicul/o	Testis	Testicular: Pertaining to a testis or testicle Testitis: Inflammation of a testis
Thorac/o	Chest	Thoracotomy: Incision into the chest cavity Thoracentesis: Surgical puncture into chest cavity
Tonsill/o	Tonsils	Tonsillectomy: Surgical removal of tonsils Tonsillitis: Inflammation of the tonsils
Ureter/o	Ureter	Ureterolithotomy: Removal of a calculus (stone) from a ureter by means of incision Ureteropelvic: Pertaining to the ureter and pelvis of the kidney
Urethr/o	Urethra	Urethritis: Inflammation of the urethra Urethropexy: Surgical fixation of the urethra
Vas/o	Vas deferens	Vasectomy: Surgical removal of portion of vas deferens for male sterilization
Viscer/o	Viscera (organs)	Viscerography: Radiography of the viscera

Terms for the Outside of Your Body

Whew! Now let's take a look at some of the words you can conjure for the exterior of your body. Table 8-2 is your ticket.

TABLE 8-2 **Out of Bounds: External Terminology**

Root Word	What It Means	Example(s)
Blephar/o	Eyelid or eyelash	Blepharoplasty: Surgical repair of the eyelids
Cephal/o	Head	Cephalocentesis: Surgical puncture of the head (skull) Cephalomegaly: Enlargement of the head (skull)
Cervic/o	Neck or cervix	Cervicodynia: Pain in the neck Cervicitis: Inflammation of the cervix
Cheil/o, chil/o	Lip	Cheilophagia: Biting of the lips
Derm/a/o, dermat/o	Skin	Dermatitis: Inflammation of the skin Dermatologist: Physician who studies and treats diseases of the skin Dermatome: Instrument used for cutting thin skin slices for skin grafting
Dors/i, dors/o	Back or posterior	Dorsalgia: Pain in the back
Gingiv/o	Gums in mouth	Gingivitis: Inflammation of the gums
Inguin/o	Groin	Inguinodynia: Pain in the groin
Irid/o	Iris of eye	Iridectomy: Surgical removal of the iris
Lapar/o	Abdomen, loin, flank	Laparotomy: Cutting into the abdomen Laparoscopy: Visual examination into the abdomen
Lingu/o	Tongue	Sublingual: Under the tongue
Mamm/a, mamm/o	Breast	Mammoplasty: Surgical repair or reconstruction of the breast
Mast/o	Breast	Mastectomy: Surgical removal of the breast
Odont/o	Teeth	Odontalgia: Toothache
Onych/o	Nails	Onychophagia: Habit of biting the nails Onychomalacia: Softening of the nails
Ophthalm/o, ocul/o	Eyes	Ophthalmologist: Physician studying eyes and treatment of eye disease

Root Word	What It Means	Example(s)
Optic/o, opt/o	Seeing, sight	Optician: One who fills the ophthalmologist's prescription for corrective eye glasses
Or/o	Mouth	Orolingual: Pertaining to the mouth and tongue
Ot/o	Ear	Otitis media: Inflammation of the middle ear Otodynia: Earache
Pelv/o	Pelvis	Pelvimetry: Measurement of dimensions and capacity of the pelvis
Pod/o	Foot	Podarthritis: Inflammation of the joints of the foot
Rhin/o	Nose	Rhinoplasty: Nose job Rhinorrhea: Discharge of mucus from the nose (runny nose)
Stomat/o	Mouth	Stomatitis: Inflammation of the oral mucosa or lining of the mouth
Thorac/o	Chest	Thoracentesis: Surgical puncture into the chest cavity Thoracotomy: Surgical incision into the chest cavity

Pathological Conditions

Any medical term can be used in everyday settings like the doctor's office or hospital. Some, such as those in Table 8-3, specifically detail the different kinds of pathological conditions associated with root words.

TABLE 8-3 **Quick Glance: Pathology**

Root Word	What It Means	Example(s)
Aden/o	Gland	Adenomegaly: Enlargement of a gland Adenitis: Inflammation of a gland
Atri/o	Atrium	Atriomegaly: Abnormal enlargement of an atrium of the heart
Carcin/o	Cancer	Carcinogen: A cancer-producing substance
Cheir/o, chir/o	Hand	Cheiromegaly: Abnormal enlargement (megaly) of the hand
Cholecyst/o	Gallbladder	Cholelithiasis: Stones in the gallbladder
Choledoch/o	Common bile duct	Choledocholithiasis: Stones in the common bile duct of the gallbladder

(continued)

TABLE 8-3 *(continued)*

Root Word	What It Means	Example(s)
Cyan/o	Blue	Cyanosis: Bluish discoloration of the skin Cyanotic: Pertaining to or characterized by cyanosis
Cysti, cyst/o	Bladder or cyst	Cystocele: Hernial protrusion of urinary bladder through vaginal wall
Dipl/o	Double, twice	Diplopia: The condition of double vision
Encephal/o	Brain	Encephalopathy: A disorder or disease of the brain
Hemat/o	Blood	Hematemesis: Vomiting of blood
Hepat/o, hepatic/o	Liver	Hepatomegaly: Enlargement of the liver
Hydr/o	Water, wet	Hydropenia: Deficiency of water in the body (dehydration)
Melan/o	Black	Melanoma: Black-colored tumor or growth
Necr/o	Death	Necrosis: Condition of death of a cell
Nephr/o	Kidney	Nephrolithiasis: Condition of kidney stones
Path/o	Disease	Pathology: Branch of medicine that deals with the study of disease and its effects Forensic pathology: Pathology dealing with personal injury, murder, and legal issues Pathologist: Physician who diagnoses diseases by examining tissues and cells under a microscope. Also performs autopsies.
Pneum/ato, pneum/ono	Lungs	Pneumoconiosis: Condition of abnormal deposits of dusts or other matter in the lungs
Salping/o	Fallopian tube	Hydrosalpinx: Accumulation of fluid in a fallopian tube
Sept/o	Infection	Septicemia: Toxins or pathogenic organisms in the blood (blood poisoning)
Ureter/o	Ureter	Ureterolith: Calculus or stone lodged in the ureter
Urethr/o	Urethra	Urethrorrhea: Abnormal discharge from the urethra
Viscer/o	Viscera (organs)	Visceromegaly: Enlargement of internal organs, also called organomegaly

TECHNICAL STUFF

There are well over 100 types of cancers and over 100 causes for the common cold. Knowing the correct terminology is vital to your understanding (and communicating) of all of them.

IN THIS CHAPTER

- Identifying word parts
- Defining meanings of prefixes, suffixes, and root words
- Adding up individual word meanings

Chapter 9

Deconstruction Junction: Breaking Down Words

A necessary and important component to learning medical terminology is being able to break down or dissect a word to establish its meaning. Knowing your word parts and how to break down a medical term by its word parts is a vital method you can use to understand its definition. This means hard-to-pronounce or long medical terms used by physicians and healthcare workers are *not* as difficult as they seem.

When you understand a word part and understand the word part's meaning, it is easy to analyze the definition of a medical term. Many medical words are very close in spelling but have different meanings. When you know the correct meaning of a word, there is less chance of using a sound-alike word inappropriately.

TIP

When in doubt, look it up in a medical dictionary.

Now, let's take on some larger words and try to break them down using the rules.

Finding Parts of Words

Don't worry — you're not backtracking, you're just reminding yourself about the three major parts of every medical term so that you can more easily discover its meaning.

Identifying word elements

At the beginning of a medical term, you often (but not always) find the prefix, which can indicate the direction, the where, the when, and the amount.

Next comes the root word, indicating the body part involved. Some root word meanings are obvious and easy to understand, like *arteri/o* for artery, *abdomin/o* for abdomen, *testicul/o* for testicle, and *tonsill/o* for tonsil. Many are not so easy: What about *blephar/o* for eyelids, *aden/o* for gland, *nephr/o* for kidney, *hepat/o* for liver, or *oophor/o* for ovary? Obviously, you're going to have to break out your best memorization skills for words like these.

The suffix at the end of a term is often your first clue to the definition of the term. It can indicate a procedure, a condition, or a disease.

REMEMBER

There is *always* a suffix at the end of a medical term.

The meaning of a suffix, just as with some root words, may not be obvious. It's important to remember that the suffix always has the same meaning, no matter what root word it's tacked on to.

TIP

The suffix, then, is the first place to look when trying to analyze or break down a medical term. From the suffix, back up to the prefix, if there is one, and finally, look at the root word.

Defining the prefix

The prefix and suffix are "adjectives," in a way, telling you something about the root word in the middle. Changing the prefix or the suffix changes the meaning of the term.

Let's look at some commonly used prefixes, *pre-* (before), *peri-* (during), and *post-* (after or following), all coupled with the same term. Watch how the prefix changes the time frame. We can use the word *operative* for example, beginning with *preoperative*, referring to the time period or events before an operative procedure. Changing the prefix to *peri-* would be *perioperative*, indicating the time or the events around or during an operation. Then changing the prefix to *post-* would result in *postoperative*, meaning the time or events after the surgery is completed. By using the three different prefixes, these words sound somewhat alike but are quite different in their meanings.

Some prefixes often mistaken one for another are the prefixes *ab-*, meaning "away from," and *ad-*, meaning "towards" or "in the direction of."

REMEMBER

Remember *abduction*, a kidnapping, or being taken away, as a memory key to tell the two apart.

Another example is the prefix *dys-*, often used in medical terms. Think of *dysfunctional* (not the *dis* in *discomfort*). *Dys-* used as a prefix in front of a medical term means "difficult," "bad," or "painful."

The prefix *inter-*, meaning "between or among," is often mistaken for *intra-*, which means "within or inside." Think of an *interstate* highway, winding between and among states. For *intra-*, think of an *intrauterine contraceptive device*, used within or inside the uterus.

TECHNICAL STUFF

The definition of a prefix is always the same, no matter what it's paired with.

Each time you see *intra-* before a root word, it always means "within or inside of." *Inter-* always means "between or among."

TIP

Prefixes are joined to a root word without the use of a hyphen, even when a double vowel results as in *perioperative, intrauterine*. The only exception to this rule is that a hyphen is used when the prefix joins up with a proper name: *non-Hodgkin's lymphoma*.

Defining the root word

The root word describes the body parts involved in the medical term. So, if you are having a hard time remembering the meaning of a word, you can parse it out by identifying the root word. At the very least, you'll know what body part it refers to, which can help you narrow down the possible prefix and suffix suspects. Take a look at some common examples:

- **Arthro:** Joint
- **Colo:** Colon
- **Laryngo:** Larynx
- **Myelo:** Bone marrow

- **Myo:** Muscle
- **Neuro:** Nerve
- **Osteo:** Bone

As always, a little memory work is needed here.

WARNING

Medical terms always have a suffix *but not always a prefix.* Some medical terms have a combination of two or more root words, coupling multiple body parts together: for example, *hepatospleno* comes from *hepato* (liver) and *spleno* (spleen).

Identifying the combining vowel

The *combining vowel,* usually an *o,* joins the root word to a suffix. If a suffix begins with a vowel, the combining vowel *o* is not used, because it would create a double vowel.

Take the root word *neuro* (for "nerve," right?) as an example. Let's join it to the suffix *-itis,* which means "inflammation." Using the combining vowel *o* to join these together, we would have *neuroitis,* which is not only difficult to pronounce but also contains a double vowel. Therefore, the *o* is dropped, and inflammation of a nerve becomes *neuritis.*

TECHNICAL STUFF

O is the most commonly used combining vowel. Whether using it to combine word parts to make a medical term about disease like osteoporosis (bone disease common in women) or a phobia like parthenophobia (the fear of virgins), O is your go-to guy for combining.

Defining the suffix

As you know, the suffix indicates a procedure, disease, disorder, or condition, and you look at it first. For example, the suffix *-itis* is common. It means "inflammation," so every time you see *-itis,* you know it means something is inflamed. Taking a word that you know — tonsil — you know that *tonsillitis* means "inflammation of the tonsil." *Gastr/o* is the root word for "stomach," so *gastritis* is "inflammation of the stomach."

The commonly used suffix *-ectomy* means "surgical removal or excision of." When you put *-ectomy* with *tonsil,* you have *tonsillectomy,* removal of the tonsils. *Gastrectomy* would therefore be what? Right: Surgical removal of the stomach (yikes).

TIP

The word tonsil (or tonsils) has only one *l*, but when it's made into a combining form such as *tonsillitis* or *tonsillectomy*, the *l* is doubled. *Tonsillitis* is a commonly misspelled medical word. More memory work!

Suffixes as "adjectives" help describe the root word. For instance, the suffixes *-al*, *-ic*, *-ous*, and *-eal* are all suffixes that mean "pertaining to." The suffix *-ologist* refers to "one who studies or practices a specialized medical field." The suffix *-ology* is "the study of." The common suffix *-pathy* means "disease."

Take an easily identifiable root word, *cardio* or *cardiac*, meaning "heart," and apply different suffixes. *Cardiology* is the study of heart diseases. The *cardiologist* is the physician who practices cardiology, and *cardiopathy* means some form of heart disease. *Neurology*, then, is the study of nerves or the nervous system, and the *neurologist* is the physician who specializes in neurology. Any disease of the nervous system or the nerves is *neuropathy*.

Going Deeper into Suffixes

Check out some more suffix examples. Suffixes related to procedures include *-centesis*, referring to surgical puncture to remove fluid for diagnostic purposes or to remove excess fluid. That means *abdominocentesis* is surgical puncture of the abdominal cavity.

Want to talk about removing something? The suffix *-ectomy* means "surgical removal of." When you see *-ectomy* at the end of any term, no matter how long or how difficult or confusing the first part of the word is, it means surgical removal of something. Another term we all know that ends in *-ectomy* is *appendectomy*, surgical removal of the appendix.

But, sadly, it's not always that easy. Take a look at a more complicated word and then break it down. How about the word *salpingo-oophorectomy*? The *-ectomy* we know indicates the surgical removal of something. But what? *Salpingo* is the root word referring to the fallopian tube; *oophoro* is the root word for ovary. Therefore, *salpingo-oophorectomy* is surgical removal of a fallopian tube and ovary. Surgical removal of an ovary only would be *oophorectomy*. Surgical removal of a fallopian tube only would be *salpingectomy*.

TIP

The eagle eyes among you may have noticed this: There is a hyphen in salpingo-oophorectomy. This is there mainly to aid with pronunciation and to avoid a triple "o" vowel with the combining of the two roots. The word can also be expressed as *oophorosalpingectomy*, which means the same thing.

Another suffix related to procedures is *-graphy*, meaning the process of recording a picture or a record. *Radiography* is the process of recording a picture by radiograph or an x-ray. Suffixes *-gram* and *-graph* are used to describe the finished product, the recording or picture. An *arteriography* is the process of recording the picture of arteries. The *arteriogram* or *arteriograph* is the film that is produced by the arteriography. The suffix *-ostomy* means to surgically create an artificial opening or *stoma*. A *colostomy* is a surgical creation of an opening between the colon and the body surface. The root word *colo* means colon. The suffix *-otomy* means "surgical cutting into," or a surgical incision. In order, then, to perform a *tracheostomy* (the surgical creation of an opening in the trachea), a *tracheotomy* (the surgical incision into the trachea) must be performed.

TIP

It is important to know the difference between "ostomy" and "otomy" — there is only one letter difference, but a big difference in the meaning.

A similar suffix in meaning is *-plasty*. The suffix *-plasty* means "surgical repair." The rule of thumb to remember here is when you hear or see *-plasty* think of the plastic surgeon, because, in most cases, *-plasty* surgical procedures *are* performed by the plastic surgeon. A term associated with this suffix is *mammoplasty*. The root word *mammo* refers to the breast. A *reduction mammoplasty* would be surgical reduction in the size of the breast.

Another commonly used suffix with regards to procedures is *-scopy*. This involves the visual examination of the interior of a body cavity or organ using an endoscope. The *endoscope* is the instrument, and *endoscopy* is the actual visual examination being performed with the endoscope.

TECHNICAL STUFF

In medicine today, more and more diagnostic procedures are being performed using the endoscopic method. Endoscopic surgery is less invasive. Small incisions (also known as *portals*) are made into skin, and the laparoscope is inserted through the portals. This provides visualization for excisions to be made through these very small incisions — as opposed to a full thickness, muscle-splitting incision to fully open up (in most cases) the abdominal wall.

TECHNICAL STUFF

Female sterilizations, hysterectomies, gallbladder removal, and appendectomies, just to name a few, are now being done laparoscopically. Less time is spent in the hospital, and the recovery period is reduced by as much as a month. For example, a gallbladder removed by routine upper abdominal incision requires a recovery period of four to six weeks; performed laparoscopically, with only portals to heal, the time is cut to two weeks.

Suffixes related to conditions are used over and over again. You have already covered a few, but let's look at some. We have *-algia*, meaning "pain and suffering." *Arthralgia* would refer to the pain and suffering of joints. *Myalgia* means "pain or suffering in the muscle." The suffix *-dynia* also means "pain." The word *gastrodynia* (*gastro* is a root word for "stomach") means "pain in the stomach."

We already know *-itis* means "inflammation." You can have *gastritis, tonsillitis, laryngitis, thyroiditis, neuritis, cellulitis, dermatitis, colitis, enteritis,* and *arthritis* (though you certainly wouldn't want to). You could have an *-itis* of almost any part of your body.

REMEMBER

Inflammation has two *m*'s, but inflamed has only one.

The suffix *-malacia* means "abnormal softening," most often used referring to bone disorders, but it does mean abnormal softening, and *arteriomalacia* refers to abnormal softening of the walls of an artery or arteries.

The suffix *-megaly* means "large" or "enlarged." It can be coupled with many body parts or organs. *Cardiomegaly* means enlargement of the heart, *splenomegaly* enlargement of a spleen. *Hepatomegaly* is enlargement of the liver. *Thyromegaly* would be enlargement of the thyroid gland. And *hepatosplenomegaly* would be enlargement of the liver *and* spleen, a double-barreled root word.

The suffix *-osis* means "a disease or abnormal condition," a general suffix associated with many of the root words. *Gastrosis* means a disease (any disease) of the stomach. *Scoliosis* is a curvature of the spine. *Diverticulosis* means outpouchings of the intestinal wall. *Psychosis* (*psyche* is the root word for "mind") covers many varieties of mental disorders.

Adding Up Individual Word Meanings

Just as in a math problem, you can add up the parts of a word and get one coherent answer, one complete meaning. Here's one example to get you started: Break the word *gastroenterologist* into root words and suffixes:

gastroenterologist = gastro + entero + logist

Look at the suffix first: *-logist* says this is a person, the physician. Now go back to the beginning. *Gastro* is the root word for stomach, and *entero* is the root word for intestines. Broken down, then, a gastroenterologist is a physician who studies and treats diseases of the stomach and intestines, performing a medical service known as *gastroenterology.*

TIP

With two root words, the meaning of both root words must be researched to know the true meaning of the term.

Let's take a trip through the body to find some not so easy terms. Using the rules of dissection, you should be able decipher some brainteasers.

- **Ana/tomy:** -tomy ("process of cutting") + ana ("apart") = study of body structure (to study, one must cut up or dissect)
- **Arthro/-ophthalmo/pathy:** -pathy ("condition or disease") + arthro ("joint") + ophthalmo ("eye") = disease affecting joints and eyes
- **Auto/psy:** -opsy ("to view") + auto ("self") = examination of body after death (yes, it's a stretch)
- **Bio/logy:** -logy ("the study of") + bio ("life") = study of living things
- **Cerebro/malacia:** -malacia ("softening") + cerebro ("brain") = softening of the brain
- **Cerebro/vascul/ar:** -ar ("pertaining to") + cerebro ("brain") + vasculo ("vessel") = pertaining to the brain and blood vessels
- **Choledocho/litho/tripsy:** -tripsy ("crushing") + choledocho ("common bile duct of the gallbladder") + litho ("stone") = crushing of stones in the common bile duct of the gallbladder
- **Chondro/malacia:** -malacia ("softening") + chondro ("cartilage") = softening of cartilage
- **Chondr/oma: -oma** ("mass or tumor") + chondro ("cartilage") = tumor of cartilage
- **Costo/chondr/al:** -al ("pertaining to") + costo ("rib") + chondro ("cartilage") = pertaining to the ribs and cartilage
- **Crani/otomy:** -otomy ("cutting into") + cranio ("skull") = cutting into the skull
- **Dermat/itis:** -itis ("inflammation") + dermato ("skin") = inflammation of the skin
- **Dermato/plasty:** -plasty ("surgical reconstruction") + dermato ("skin") = surgical reconstruction of the skin
- **Encephalo/megaly: -**megaly ("enlargement") + encephalo ("brain") = enlargement of the brain
- **Encephalo/pathy:** -pathy ("disease") + encephalo ("brain") = brain disease
- **Esophago/gastro/duodeno/scopy:** -scopy ("visual examination") + esphago ("esophagus") + gastro ("stomach") + duodeno ("duodenum") = visual examination of the esophagus, stomach, and duodenum
- **Glyc/emia:** -emia ("blood condition") + glyco ("sugar") = sugar in the blood

  Then, by adding prefixes to glycemia, we get

  Hyper/glyc/emia: -hyper ("excessive") = excessive sugar in blood

Hypo/glyc/emia: -hypo ("insufficient") = insufficient or low amount of sugar in the blood

- **Gyneco/mastia:** -mastia ("breast") + gyneco ("woman/female") = excessive development of male breast tissue
- **Hemat/emesis:** -emesis ("vomiting") + hemato ("blood") = vomiting of blood
- **Hemi/gastr/ectomy:** -ectomy ("surgical removal of") + hemi ("half") + gastro ("stomach") = surgical removal of half the stomach
- **Hemo/lysis:** -lysis ("breakdown or destruction") + hemo ("blood") = breakdown of blood
- **Hyper/cholesterol/emia:** -emia ("blood condition") + hyper ("excessive or above normal") + cholesterol = excessive amount of cholesterol in blood
- **Hyper/emesis:** -emesis ("vomiting") + hyper ("excessive") = excessive vomiting
- **Hyper/hidr/osis:** -osis ("abnormal condition") + hyper ("excessive or above normal") + hidro ("sweat") = excessive secretion of sweat or excessive sweating
- **Hystero/salpingo/gram:** -gram ("a record") + hystero ("uterus") + salpingo ("fallopian tube") = x-ray record of the uterus and fallopian tubes
- **Inter/vertebral:** -vertebral ("pertaining to vertebrae or a vertebra") + inter ("between") = between vertebrae or a vertebra
- **Intra/cranial:** -cranial ("pertaining to the skull") + intra ("within") = pertaining to within the skull
- **Jejuno/ile/ostomy:** -ostomy ("artificial surgical opening") + jejuno ("jejunum") + ileo ("ileum") = surgical opening or new connection between the jejunum and ileum
- **Labio/glosso/pharyng/eal:** - eal ("pertaining to") + labio ("lips") + glosso ("tongue") + pharyngo ("pharynx") = pertaining to the lips, tongue, and throat
- **Laryngo/tracheo/bronch/itis:** -itis ("inflammation") + laryngo ("larynx") + trachea ("trachea") + broncho ("bronchus") = inflammation of the larynx, trachea, and bronchus *(croup)*
- **Leio/myo/sarcoma:** -sarcoma ("malignant tumor") + leio ("smooth") + myo ("muscle") = tumor of smooth muscle
- **Leuko/penia:** -penia ("lack of or deficiency") + leuko ("white/white blood cells") = deficient amount of white blood cells
- **Micro/dactyly:** micro ("small") + dactyly ("fingers or toes") = pertaining to small fingers and/or toes
- **Nephro/pexy:** -pexy ("surgical fixation") + nephro ("kidney") = surgical fixation of a kidney

- **Neur/itis:** -itis ("inflammation") + neuro ("nerve") = inflammation of a nerve
- **Oligo/sperm/ia:** -ia "(condition") + sperm ("spermatozoa") + olio ("too little, too few") = a subnormal concentration or number of spermatozoa in seminal fluid
- **Osteo/arthro/pathy:** -pathy (condition or disease) + osteo ("bone") + arthro ("joint") = condition or disease affecting bones and joints
- **Oto/rhino/laryngo/logist:** -logist ("person who studies") + oto ("ear") + rhino ("nose") + laryngo ("larynx/throat") = doctor specialized in otorhinolaryngology = ear, nose, and throat
- **Para/nasal:** -nasal ("pertaining to nose") + para ("beside or near") = beside or near the nose
- **Peri/neur/itis:** -itis ("inflammation") + peri ("around") + neuro ("nerve") = inflammation around a nerve
- **Pneumo/conio/sis:** -sis ("condition") + conio ("dust") + pneumo ("lung") = lung condition caused by inhalation of dust particles
- **Post/mortem:** -mortem ("death") + post ("following or after") = after death
- **Presby/cusis:** -cusis ("hearing") + presby ("old age") = diminished hearing due to aging
- **Presby/opia:** -opia ("vision") + presby ("old age") = vision impaired due to aging
- **Respiro/meter:** -meter ("to measure") + respiro ("to breathe") = instrument to measure extent of respiratory movements
- **Rhabdo/myo/sarcoma:** -oma ("tumor") + rhabdo ("rod shaped") + myo ("muscle") + sarc ("flesh/tissue") = malignant tumor of muscle tissue made up of rod-shaped cells
- **Rhino/kyphosis:** -kyphosis ("humped condition" + rhino ("nose") = a hump-back condition of the nose
- **Sialo/lith/otomy:** - otomy ("surgical incision into") + sialo ("salivary gland") + lith ("stone or calculus") = incision into a salivary gland or duct to remove a stone
- **Somn/ambul/ism:** -ism ("condition") + somn ("sleep") + ambulo ("to walk") = condition of sleep walking
- **Thoraco/myo/dynia:** -dynia ("pain") + thoraco ("chest/thorax") + myo ("muscle") = pain in the muscles of the chest wall
- **Thrombo/phleb/itis:** -itis ("inflammation") + thrombo ("clot") + phlebo ("vein") = inflammation of a vein with clot formation
- **Torti/collis:** -is ("condition") + torti ("twisted") + collum ("neck") = condition in which the neck is twisted to one side

IN THIS CHAPTER

- Distinguishing the different branches of science that help you study the body
- Discovering the building blocks of the body
- Getting to know anatomical regions, planes, and cavities

Chapter 10

An Org Chart to Live By: Organization of the Body

Before we get into the real nitty-gritty of the source of all these magnificent medical terms — your body, that is — you may want to first get to know the big picture of your body. In this chapter, we review the structure and organization of the body. The body appears to be a solid structure from the outside. Inside, body regions, organs, and cavities fit nicely together to provide that solid structure. Your body really *is* a wonderland — made up of complementary systems and parts. Let's explore!

Looking at the Big Picture

There are all sorts of ways to look at the human body. You can study it from different angles, both literally and figuratively. Let's start with the figurative, as in the different kinds of science used to analyze the body. Then later, you can move on to the more concrete ways of looking at your beautiful bod.

The branches of science that cover the study of the body are as follows:

- **Anatomy** means "cutting apart." This is the science that studies the structure of the body and the relationships of its parts to each other. The "cutting apart" is the method used *(dissection)* to study the structure of the human body.
- **Biology** is the study of all forms of life and living things.
- **Embryology** studies the origin (beginnings) and the development of an organism. This covers from the 2nd to the 8th week after conception, which is referred to as the *embryonic stage.* After eight weeks, the developing organism is known as a *fetus.*
- **Histology** studies the body microscopically — the minute structures and their composition, plus the functions of normal cells, tissue, and organs.
- **Pathology** studies the changes caused by disease to the structures of the body or changes due to disease that alter the functions of the body.
- **Physiology** studies the normal activity and functions of the body.

Cells

The *cell* is the basic, smallest unit of life. Cells that perform similar functions join together, or group together, to form *tissue.* Groups of different types of tissue join together to form an *organ.* Groups of organs that work together to perform a complex function, form a *body system.*

TECHNICAL STUFF

The body is maintained by metabolism (*meta* means "change," *bolus* refers to "mass," and *ism* is "a condition"). *Metabolism* consists of the total processes of *anabolism* (*ana* means to build up) and *catabolism* (*cata* means to break down). When metabolism stops, an organism dies.

Each of us has trillions of cells that vary in size and shape according to their purpose or function. Specialized cells are responsible for the functions of growth, secretions, excretions, nutrition, and reproduction. Mechanical, chemical, and nervous stimulation activate the cells. The shapes of most typical cells are as follows:

- **Epithelial or skin cell:** May be square and flat
- **Adipocyte or fat cell:** Contains large vacant spaces for fat storage
- **Muscle cell:** Long and slender

- **Nerve cell:** May be long and have fingerlike extensions, which carry impulses
- **Gamete (sex) cell:** Two types only: sperm and egg

Each cell has a *membrane*, forming the exterior boundary; *cytoplasm* that makes up the body of the cell; and a *nucleus*, the small control center of the cell that contains the *chromosomes*. There are 46 chromosomes (23 pairs) in a human cell. *Genes* are regions within the chromosomes. Each chromosome has thousands of genes that all determine hereditary characteristics. Each gene is composed of *DNA(deoxyribonucleic acid)*, the chemical that regulates the activities of the cell. The mature *reproductive* (sex) cell has only 23 chromosomes, and at conception, the male and female sex cells join together to contribute to innumerable possible combinations. That's why no two individuals are alike, except for identical twins.

TECHNICAL STUFF

The body's largest single cell is the female sex cell, an ovum, while the smallest single cell is the male sex cell, a sperm.

Tissues

In the building blocks of body structures, cells of similar characteristics and specific tasks join together to form tissue. The body is made up of four different types of tissue:

- **Connective tissue** supports and encases body structures. It is the most widespread kind of tissue throughout the body. It holds organs in place and connects body parts to each other. The main types of connective tissue include *bone* that supports the body; *cartilage*, firm but bendable; *dense fibrous* that makes up the tendons and ligaments; *loose* that connects adjoining structures; and *apidose* tissue that pads and protects, stores fat, and insulates the body against heat loss.
- **Epithelial tissue:** Found in the skin and in the lining of blood vessels, this makes up the outer covering of external and internal body surfaces (such as skin and mucous membranes) and the lining of the digestive, respiratory, and urinary tracts.
- **Muscle tissue** provides movement. The main function of muscle tissue is to contract.
- **Nerve tissue** conducts impulses to and from the brain and is composed of nerve cells called neurons. Nervous tissue needs more oxygen and more nutrients than any other body tissue.

TECHNICAL STUFF

The skin contains about 45 miles of nerves, and one square inch of skin tissue has 3 million cells and 4 yards of nerve tissue. You will shed 40 pounds of skin in your lifetime. That's a lot of tissue!

Organs and Systems

When two or more kinds of tissue work together to perform a specific function, you have an organ. For example, the skin is an organ made up of connective, nerve, and epithelial tissue.

Although organs act as units, they do not function alone. Several organs join together to form a system and perform a body function. Each system has a special function.

Some of the major body systems include the following:

- **The cardiovascular system** includes the heart and blood vessels and carries the blood throughout the body.
- **The digestive or gastrointestinal system** includes the mouth, esophagus, stomach, and small and large intestines. This system digests and absorbs food and excretes waste.
- **The endocrine system** is made up of a variety of glands and manufactures and distributes hormones.
- **The integumentary system** includes the hair, skin, nails, and sweat and oil glands and provides an outer protective covering.
- **The lymphatic system** works with the cardiovascular system to protect the body against disease-causing organisms.
- **The musculoskeletal system,** composed of bones, muscles, tendons, and ligaments, provides the framework for the body, supports organs, and permits movement in the body.
- **The reproductive systems,** the uterus, ovaries, testes, and prostate, provide for reproduction.
- **The respiratory system** includes the trachea, lungs, and bronchi and provides the exchange of gases, absorbs oxygen, and expels carbon dioxide.
- **The sensory or special senses system,** made up of the eyes, ears, nose, and mouth, along with the nervous system composed of the brain and spinal cord, processes stimuli and allows the body to act and respond.
- **The urinary system** manufactures and excretes urine.

TECHNICAL STUFF

For every organ that you have two of (kidneys, lungs, for example) you just need one to survive. Talk about having an heir and a spare!

Cavities of the Body

The body is not as solid a structure as it appears on the outside. It has five body cavities. Each *cavity* contains organs that are organized (no pun intended) in a neat and orderly fashion.

The five body cavities include the following:

- **The abdominal cavity** contains the stomach, intestines, liver, spleen, gallbladder, pancreas, ureters, and kidneys.
- **The cranial cavity,** the cavity inside the skull, or the *cranium,* contains the brain.
- **The pelvic cavity** contains the urinary bladder, urethra, part of the large intestine, and the rectum, uterus, and vagina in the female, and prostate in the male.
- **The spinal cavity** consists of the spinal column connecting to the cranial cavity.
- **The thoracic or chest cavity** contains the esophagus, trachea, lungs, heart, and aorta. This cavity can be divided into two smaller areas. The *pleural cavity* surrounds the lungs. (Each pleural cavity is lined with a membrane called *pleura. Visceral pleura* is closest to the lungs. *Parietal pleura* is closest to the outer wall of the cavity.) The *mediastinum* is the area between the lungs. It contains the heart, aorta, trachea, esophagus, and thymus gland.

REMEMBER

The cranial and spinal cavities are *dorsal* body cavities, because they are located on the back part of the body. The thoracic, abdominal, and pelvic cavities are *ventral* body cavities, as they are on the front or belly-side of the body.

The thoracic and abdominal cavities are separated by a muscular partition called the diaphragm. The abdominal and pelvic cavities are not separated and, to really confuse you, together they are frequently referred to as the *abdominopelvic cavity.*

Table 10-1 lists some root words related to body structure and organization.

TABLE 10-1 **Roots of Structures**

Root	What It Means	Example Term	What It Means
Cyt/o	Cell	Cytology	Study of cells
Epitheli/o	Epithelium	Epithelioma	Tumor of the skin
Fibr/o	Fibrous	Fibrosis	Condition of the fibrous tissue
Hist/o	Tissue	Histologist	Physician who studies tissue
Lip/o	Fat	Liposuction	Removal of fat cells by suction
Myo	Muscle	Myositis	Inflammation of a muscle
Neur/o	Nerve	Neuropathy	Condition of the nerve
Organ/o	Organ	Organomegaly	Enlargement of an organ
Viscer/o	Internal organs	Viscera	Internal organs

Table 10-2 lists some suffixes pertaining to body structure and organization.

TABLE 10-2 **Structural Suffixes**

Suffix	What It Means	Example Term	What It Means
-cyte	Cell	Erythrocyte	Red blood cell
-gen	Agent that causes	Carcinogen	Agent causing cancer
-genic	Producing	Carcinogenic	Has cancer-causing properties
-ologist	One who studies/practices	Cytologist	Physician who studies cells
-oma	Tumor or swelling	Myoma	Tumor in the muscle
-osis	Abnormal condition	Cytosis	Abnormal condition of cells
-pathy	Disease	Neuropathy	A disease of the nerves
-plasm	Growth or formation	Neoplasm	A new growth
-sarcoma	Malignant tumor	Myosarcoma	Malignant muscle tumor

Directional Terms and Anatomical Planes

An *anatomical plane* is an imaginary flat plate or field. Imagine a slice view through the body and you're on the right track. Anatomic planes provide further division of the body, again to identify a specific location or area. Visualize dividing the body in half, top from bottom, and then right from left, and finally front from back.

- **The frontal or coronal plane** is a vertical plane dividing the body into *anterior* (front) and *posterior* (back) portions.
- **The midsagittal plane** is a horizontal plane that divides the body into right and left halves at the body's midpoint.
- **The sagittal plane** is a vertical plane that passes from front to back, dividing the body into right and left sides.
- **The transverse plane** is a horizontal (cross-section) plane, parallel to the ground and through the waistline, dividing the body into upper and lower halves.

The anatomical planes of the body are used in radiology when specific body location or direction is necessary.

TIP

When thinking about all these terms, planes, and regions, think of the body as if it is standing, arms at each side, with palms facing forward and the feet side by side. Whether a patient is standing, or lying down face up, the directional terms are always applied in the same manner. Directional terms are used to pinpoint or specifically locate an area on the body.

When referring to the front of the body, the terms *anterior* and *ventral* are used. When referring to the back of the body, it's *posterior* and *dorsal.* With the waistline of the anatomical position as a guideline, above the waistline is referred to as *cephalad* ("head" or "upward") or *superior* ("above"). Below the waistline is referred to as *caudal* ("tail" or "downward") or *inferior* ("below"). Superior and inferior are also used to describe body parts in relation to one another in general.

The sides of the body are referred to as *lateral,* and the middle referred to as *medial.* The term *distal* refers to "away from the point of origin" (think of distance). *Proximal* refers to "nearest the point of origin" (close proximity). Distal and proximal are two directional terms that seem to pose problems. View the torso of the body as the point of origin. Using the arm as an example, the proximal portion of the arm is where the arm joins to the shoulder. The distal, or away-from, portion of the arm, would be the hand. In the leg, the upper thigh would be the proximal portion of the leg, and the foot would be the distal portion of the leg.

Directional terms can be joined together to provide a combined form. *Ipsilateral* pertains to one side, whereas *mediolateral* is a directional term meaning pertaining to the middle and one side (such as right mediolateral pain). It is often used in medical exams and surgical procedures. Here's one use of mediolateral: A right mediolateral abdominal incision would be an incision beginning at the middle of the abdomen and going toward the right side. A similar term is *lateromedial.* A lateromedial incision would be the same as a mediolateral one, but beginning from the side and going toward the middle.

Table 10-3 lists some root words that pertain to directional terms.

TABLE 10-3 **Directional Roots**

Root Word	What It Means
Anter/o	Front
Caud/o	Tail or downward
Cephal/o	Head or upward
Dist/o	Away from (distant) the point of origin
Dors/o	Back
Infer/o	Below
Later/o	Side
Medi/o	Middle
Poster/o	Back or behind
Proxim/o	Near to (proximity) the point of origin
Super/o	Above
Ventr/o	Front or belly

GET IN POSITION

Some frequently used anatomic positions describing body positions are

- **Anatomical position** is when the body is standing, arms at each side, with palms facing forward and the feet side by side. (Whether a patient is standing or lying face up, the directional terms are always applied in the same manner.)
- **Erect** is standing position.
- **Genupectoral** is kneeling with chest resting on examining table.
- **Lateral recumbent** means lying on left side with right thigh and knee drawn up to chest.
- **Prone** means lying face down.
- **Supine (dorsal)** is lying flat on your back.

Regions of the Body

All these body parts don't make a whole lot of sense until you can put them in the context of their general location within the body. Your body can be defined in several different ways, from groups and regions to cavities and planes.

Body *regions*, like the directional terms and anatomical planes we cover later, are used to specifically identify a body area. To illustrate all that's involved with a body region, take a closer look at two major regions: the abdominal and spinal.

The *abdominal area* is divided further into anatomic regions to diagnose abdominal problems with greater accuracy.

Starting with the diaphragm, which is the muscle separating the thoracic cavity from the abdominal cavity, down to the level of the pelvis or groin, the abdominal area is divided into nine equal regions.

Visualize the abdomen divided into nine squares: three across the top, three across the middle, and three across the bottom, like a tic-tac-toe board. The center portion is the *umbilical* region, the region of the navel or the umbilicus. Directly above this is the *epigastric* region, or the region of the stomach. Directly below the umbilical region is the *hypogastric* region.

On either side of the epigastric region are the *right* and *left hypochondriac* regions. To the right and left of the umbilical region are the *right* and *left lumbar regions.* To the right and left of the hypogastric region are the *right* and *left iliac regions.*

TIP

The anatomical divisions of the abdomen are referenced in anatomy textbooks to specify where certain organs are found.

The clinical regions of the abdomen are used to describe the abdomen when a patient is being examined. The clinical regions of the abdomen divide the abdominal area, as above, into four equal quadrants:

- **The right upper quadrant (RUQ)** contains the right lobe of the liver, gallbladder, and parts of the small and large intestines.
- **The left upper quadrant (LUQ)** contains the left lobe of the liver, stomach, pancreas, spleen, and parts of the small and large intestines.
- **The right lower quadrant (RLQ)** contains parts of the small and large intestines, appendix, right ureter, right ovary, and fallopian tube.
- **The left lower quadrant (LLQ)** contains parts of the small and large intestines, left ureter, left ovary, and fallopian tube.

Table 10-4 provides a quick look at some of the smaller body regions, beginning at the head and moving downward.

TABLE 10-4

Small But Mighty Body Regions

Region	Where It Is
Auricular region	Around the ears
Axillary	Axillae (armpits)
Buccal	Cheeks of the face
Carpal	Wrist
Cervical	Neck
Clavicular	On each side of the suprastemal notch (small dip at top of the sternum)
Infraorbital	Below the eyes
Infrascapular	On each side of the chest, down to the last rib
Interscapular	On the back, between *scapulae* (shoulder blades)
Lumbar	Below the infrascapular area
Mammary	Breast area
Mental	Region of the chin
Nasal	Nose
Occipital	Lower posterior head
Orbital	Around the eyes
Pectoral	Chest
Popliteal	Behind the knee
Pubic	Below the *hypogastric region* (above the pubis)
Sacral	Area over the sacrum
Sternal	Over the sternum
Submental	Below the chin
Supraclavicular	Above the clavicles

More body divisions are the regions of the spinal column, also known as the back. Note the difference between the spinal column (the *vertebrae*) and the spinal cord (the nerves running through the column). The *spinal column* is made of bone tissue, and the *spinal cord* is composed of nerve tissue.

The spinal column is divided into five regions. Begin at the top and work downward:

- **The cervical region (abbreviation C)** is located in the neck region. There are seven cervical vertebrae, C1 to C7.
- **The thoracic or dorsal region (abbreviation T or D)** is located in the chest region. There are 12 thoracic or dorsal vertebrae, T1 to T12, or D1 to D12. Each bone in this segment is joined to a rib.
- **The lumbar region (abbreviation L)** is located at the loin or the flank area between the ribs and the hip bone. There are five lumbar vertebrae, L1 to L5.
- **The sacral region (abbreviation S)** has five bones, S1 to S5, that are fused to form one bone, the *sacrum.*
- **The coccygeal region** includes the coccyx, or tailbone, a small bone composed of four fused pieces.

Figures 10-1 through 10-3 illustrate the body's anatomical positions and regions, planes, and cavities.

REMEMBER

It is important to remember that all these terms are for directional purposes only. They provide a road map to the body. In a medical examination, directional planes, regions of the abdomen, and divisions of the spinal column are used often by the examiner.

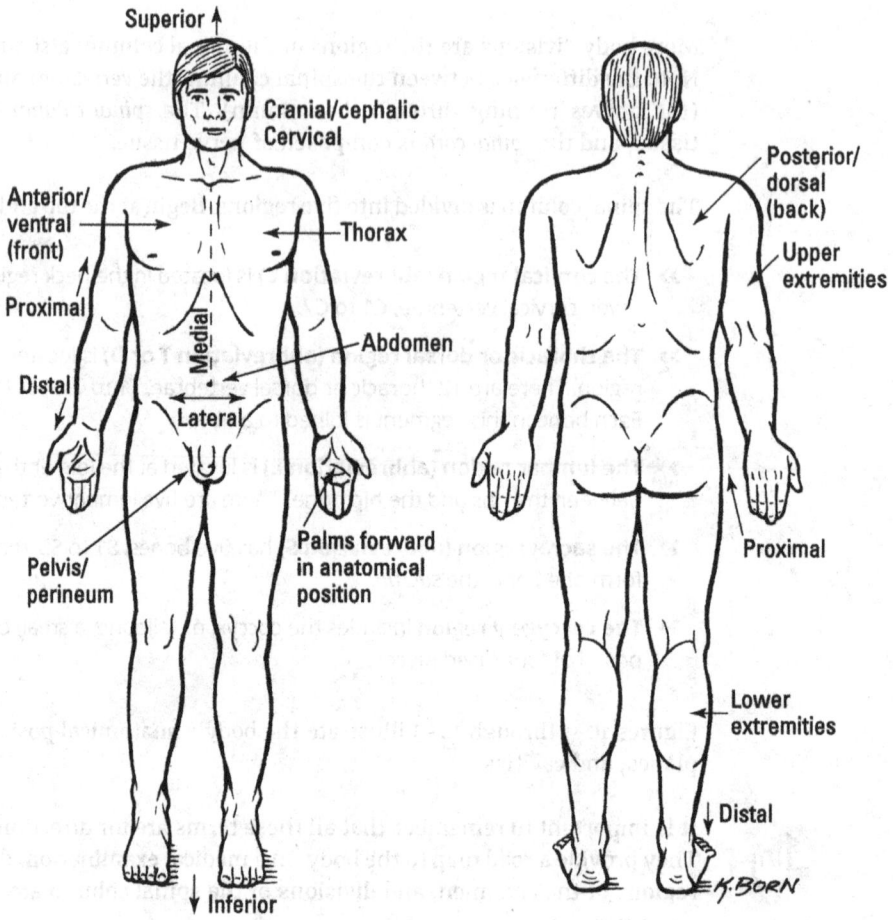

FIGURE 10-1: Anatomical positions and regions of the body.

Illustration by Kathryn Born

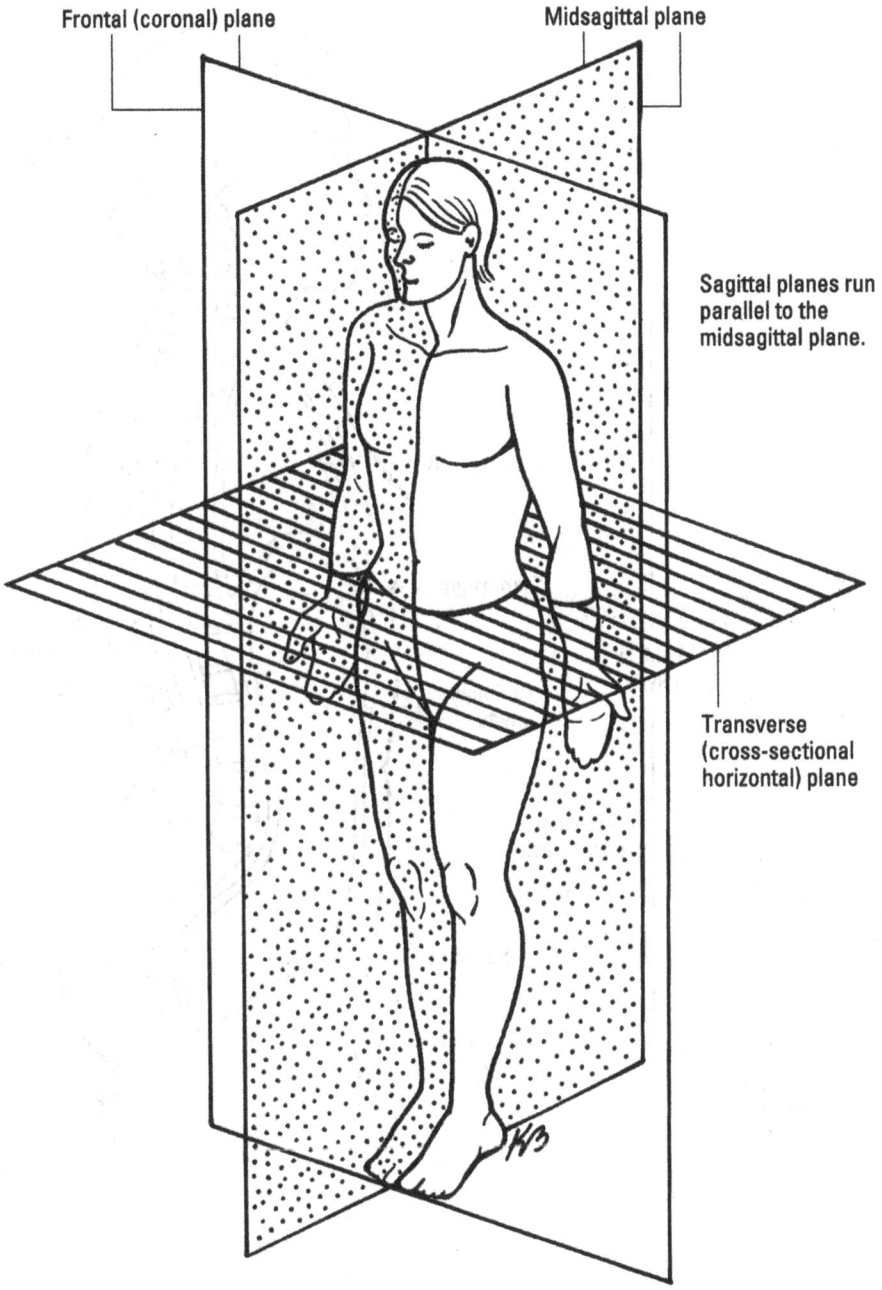

FIGURE 10-2: Planes of the body.

Illustration by Kathryn Born

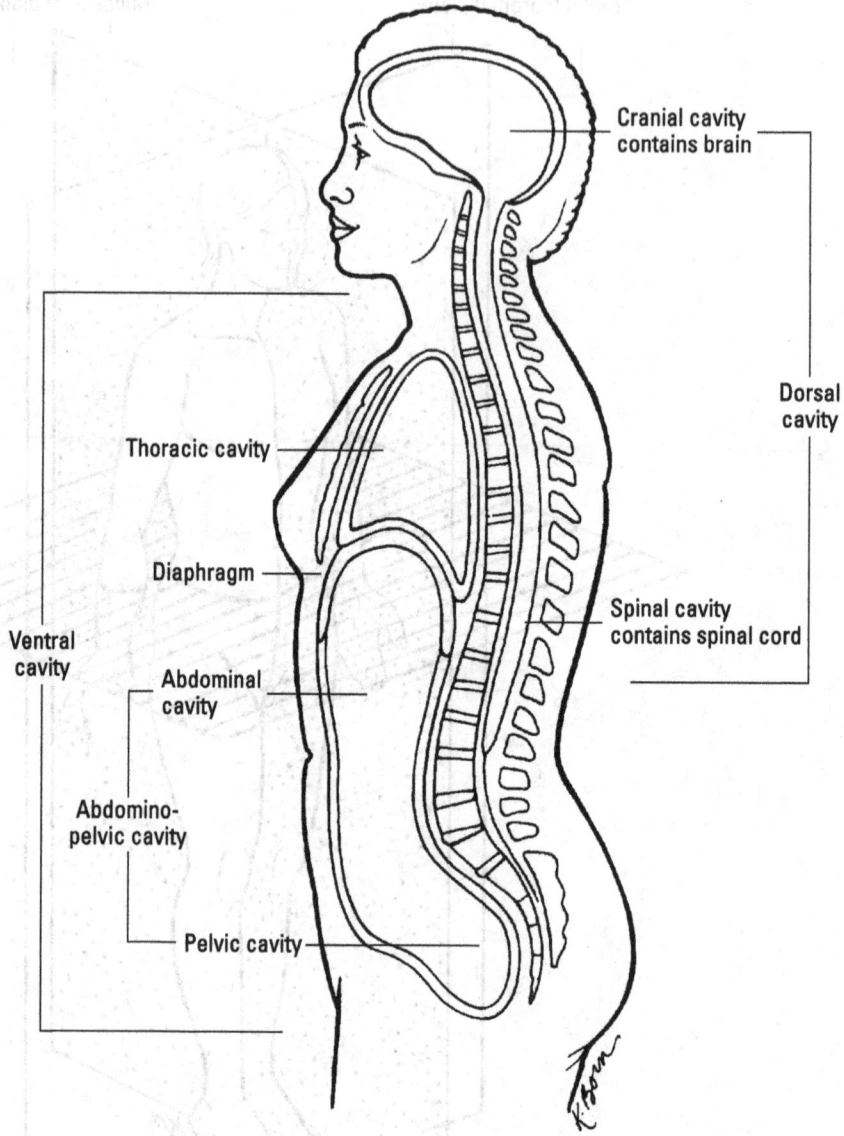

FIGURE 10-3: The body's cavities.

Illustration by Kathryn Born

IN THIS CHAPTER

- Discovering the systems associated with basic anatomy
- Taking a tour of the physiological systems
- Finding out how systems work together

Chapter 11

All Systems Go: When Systems Combine

Teamwork is the key for your body systems. When they all do their own individual jobs, they have a better chance of working together in harmony. Not every single system works with every other system, but many do work together to keep you running at your top performance.

Anatomical Systems Working Together

Everything starts with anatomy. *Anatomy* is the study of the parts of the body, from what you can see on the outside, like the skin covering muscles and bones, to the brain in the skull, or the variety of organs neatly arranged inside the trunk or torso of the body like a well-packed suitcase. Coupled with physiology (which we cover later), a bit of studying your basic anatomical building blocks will help you identify and create tons of medical terms.

A good start to learning about anatomy and physiology is to observe the body as a whole. Parts III and IV of this book cover these systems in detail, but to whet your appetite let's do a quick preview of the systems of the body.

The musculoskeletal system

The *musculoskeletal system* is made up of 206 bones and more than 600 muscles. The bones of the skeleton have tons of jobs. They provide support for the body's framework and protect vital internal organs, brain, and spinal column. Bones store minerals necessary for growth, and red bone marrow makes blood cells. Most importantly, bones make movement possible, providing attachments for muscles.

REMEMBER

Bones are attached to other bones by *ligaments*, whereas *tendons* connect bones to muscles. A *joint* is where two bones meet.

Muscles attach to bone, not only making movement possible but holding the bones of the skeleton together. Muscles allow flexibility of the body and help maintain body temperature. But think about some other functions of muscles. There are all kinds of muscles you probably don't think too much about. Cardiac muscle keeps your heart beating, but the cardiac muscle is *involuntary*. That means you don't have to think about keeping your heart beating. Muscle contraction throughout the body keeps the blood flow moving. The digestive system is lined by smooth muscle that keeps the food moving. And don't forget the muscles that keep the bladder and colon closed up — until you voluntarily relax these muscles when you want.

The integumentary system

The *integumentary* system is a really fancy way of referring to the skin, hair, nails, and glands. The skin is actually the body's largest organ (yes, it is an organ!). It covers about 20 square feet and accounts for nearly 15 percent of your body weight. Skin (obviously) provides an external covering for the body. As a protective membrane, it prevents loss of water, salt, and heat.

The skin provides a protective barrier against bacteria, pathogens, and toxins that want to invade your body. Plus, it's full of glands that do many smaller, but equally important jobs. *Sebaceous* glands secrete oil to lubricate, whereas *sudoriferous* glands secrete sweat, acting as a cooling system. Nerves are involved as well and carry impulses that act as receptors for pain, temperature, and touch. The blood vessels in the skin aid in regulating body temperature.

TECHNICAL STUFF

Dead cells of the epidermis are always being worn and washed away. We get a new outer layer of skin every 27 days.

The sensory system

The eyes and the ears, like the skin, are sense organs. They act as the body's external perception/alarm system by letting in light and sound. Impulses from the eyes are sent to the *occipital lobe* in the brain for processing, and impulses from the ears go to the brain's *temporal lobe*. In these lobes of the brain, nerve impulses are translated into sound sensations and visual images that we experience as vision and hearing.

WARNING

Age sure takes its toll on the eyes and ears. *Presbyopia* is impaired vision due to aging. *Presbycusis* is hearing loss occurring in old age.

TECHNICAL STUFF

The eye is the fastest moving body part. Every hour, the eye can process 36,000 bits of information.

Physiology Systems Working Together

Physiology is the study of the function or day-to-day operation of the parts of the body. This includes the functions of everything from the smallest cell, seen only under a microscope, to a large organ like the heart. You might think that each body part has one function to carry out and works independently on its own to accomplish this function, but in fact, most body parts are team players that work together to accomplish a task. Brisk walking, for example, not only requires the use of leg muscles, but also good lung capacity to keep up the pace. You know that the heart pumps blood through the body via arteries and veins, which are part of the cardiovascular system. Without the lungs performing their function to re-oxygenate the blood as it passes through the lungs, the exchange of gases (the function of the respiratory system) would not happen, and body cells and organs would die.

TECHNICAL STUFF

Pathology (sometimes *pathophysiology*) is the study of the effects of disease on body parts and the ways disease can interfere with an organ or system's functioning ability.

The cardiovascular and lymphatic systems

The *cardiovascular system* (sometimes called the *circulatory system*) has many functions. Blood carries oxygen, nutrients, hormones, and lymph fluid to cells and transports waste products, carbon dioxide, and urea away to be excreted. The heart is the body's pumping station that pumps out freshly oxygenated blood through a vast network of vessels. The heart is divided into four chambers: two upper chambers (the *right atrium* and *left atrium* (plural: *atria*) and two lower chambers, the *right* and *left ventricles.*

TIP

The cardiovascular system could not survive without the assistance of the muscular system — the *myocardium* is the heart muscle — which in turn is kept functional by the *autonomic* section of the nervous system.

Not to be forgotten as a team player with the cardiovascular system is the *lymphatic system.* This system works together with the blood to fight disease. It looks after the body's immune system. This system produces *lymph,* a fluid released into the body through lymphatic vessels, which are linked up with blood vessels to carry lymph throughout the body. This system produces *lymphocytes,* the disease-fighting cells that circulate the body through blood. *Lymph nodes* located throughout the body act as the filtrating centers. Lymph nodes can trap and filter toxic and malignant substances. Special cells can digest foreign substances as well as manufacture antibodies to fight off infection.

TECHNICAL STUFF

The heart pumps more than five quarts of blood a minute. That's 2,000 gallons per day!

A FANTASTIC VOYAGE

Freshly oxygenated blood is pumped from the left ventricle through the *aorta* (the largest artery) into arteries that decrease in size to *arterioles* and to *capillaries,* the smallest branches of the venous system, where the exchange of gases takes place. Oxygen is absorbed into tissue cells, while carbon dioxide is expelled by the cells. The oxygen-depleted blood is carried via *venules* (small veins) through *veins,* to the *superior and inferior venae cavae,* the body's largest veins, back to the heart, where it is received in the right atrium.

But this blood has to be oxygenated before it begins the trip again, so the right atrium sends the stale blood to the right ventricle, where it then gets sidetracked to the lungs to be topped up with oxygen. The blood travels through a vast network of vessels once again, this time through capillaries that wind around the *alveoli* (the air sacs of the lung), where the lungs perform the function of re-oxygenating the blood, getting it ready for its next trip around the body. Through the processes of *inspiration* and *expiration* in the lungs, fresh oxygen enters the bloodstream, and the not-needed carbon dioxide is eliminated by the lungs. This freshly oxygenated blood then comes back to the heart and is received in the left atrium, then on to the left ventricle, where it is pumped through the aorta to begin the trip all over again. Imagine this happening with every heart beat 100,000 times a day, resulting in 1,800 gallons of blood being circulated on a daily basis!

The spleen, tonsils, and thymus are accessory organs of this system, all playing special roles. The *spleen* stores red blood cells, which can be released into the body as needed. The *thymus* gland produces lymphocytes, the disease fighters. The *tonsils* are also made up of lymphatic tissue and act as a filter system for bacteria.

The respiratory system

The *respiratory system* provides the mechanisms that allow you to breathe. You can't live without it, and, as with the other systems, improper functioning would render you dead! Now that would really ruin your day.

TECHNICAL STUFF

The surface area of a lung is equal to a tennis court, and the lung contains 700 million alveoli inside.

The respiratory system works in conjunction with the cardiovascular system to provide the exchange of oxygen and carbon dioxide between the air in the lungs and the blood. Inhaling and exhaling, the movement of air in and out of the lungs *(ventilation)* allows the body to maintain its oxygen requirements for body cells and tissue to survive. The lungs facilitate the exchange of oxygen and carbon dioxide between the blood and the body cells. This system also metabolizes oxygen, resulting in carbon dioxide production in body cells. Air, which is about 15 percent oxygen, enters the nose (sometimes the mouth, as in chronic mouth breathers when sleeping) — where it is moistened and warmed — through to the *pharynx* (throat), consisting of the *nasopharynx*, *oropharynx*, and *hypopharynx*.

Ventilation (breathing) is a process that again is looked after automatically by the nervous system. You don't have to consciously think about breathing. When you breathe in *(inspiration)*, all passageways are opened to allow the air entry. The *diaphragm*, a large muscle separating the chest cavity from the abdominal cavity, pushes down and the ribs move up to give the lungs lots of room to expand. Air pressure within the lungs decreases and air comes in. When you breathe out *(expiration)*, the diaphragm moves up, the rib cage comes down, lung pressure increases, and air is pushed out.

The lungs are contained in the *thoracic cavity* that divides into the pleural and mediastinum cavities. The *pleural cavity* surrounds the lungs, and the *mediastinal cavity* between the lungs holds the heart, trachea, and esophagus. The right lung consists of three *lobes*, and the left lung two lobes. The cavities are the *pleural* and *mediastinum*, but when referring to the area in general you should say *mediastinal cavity*, even though the area is referred to as the mediastinum.

YOU'VE GOT CONNECTIONS

The *hypopharynx* is a common passageway for both food and air to travel to their final destinations. Air taken through the nose to the larynx produces the voice. The *trachea* (windpipe) connects the larynx to a right and left *bronchus,* just above the lungs. The bronchi break down into smaller branches called *bronchioles* that lead into small clusters resembling grapes. These grapelike sacs are called *alveoli,* of which there are approximately 300 million in healthy lungs, surrounded in *capillaries.* Oxygen moves from alveoli into the lung capillaries surrounding them to be exchanged via the bloodstream throughout the body. Carbon dioxide moves from the capillaries into the alveoli to be expelled by the lungs.

The gastrointestinal system

The *gastrointestinal system* (also called the *digestive system* or *alimentary tract*) has three functions: to digest food, absorb nutrients, and carry waste materials to be eliminated. Except for the processes of swallowing food and having a bowel movement, this system pretty much looks after itself for everything that happens in between.

TECHNICAL STUFF

The liver produces over 1,000 enzymes to handle the body's chemical conversion necessary for you to live every day.

We chew food, which we swallow, that goes into the esophagus and then into the stomach. The stomach partially digests the food before it moves on to the *small intestine* (also called small bowel) for further digestion and absorption. The residual food moves into the *large intestine* (large bowel) where it is doomed to be eliminated as solid waste. Except for the pharynx (throat) and esophagus, all gastrointestinal organs are in the abdominal cavity, often referred to as the *gut* or *belly.*

The accessory organs of this system — teeth, salivary glands, liver, gallbladder, and pancreas — all do their special part to add in the process of digestion, absorption, and elimination. The pancreas (also part of the endocrine system) secretes *enzymes* necessary for digestion. The liver (the body's largest gland) secretes *bile* needed for digestion. It metabolizes proteins, fats, and carbohydrates. The liver also acts as a filter system that neutralizes toxins. The gallbladder stores bile that also aids the digestive process.

TECHNICAL STUFF

The liver joins a group of mixed-function organs (working as both organ and gland) that includes the stomach, intestines, kidney, ovaries, and testes. In addition to their regular system functions, they also produce hormones.

Digested food and nutrients are absorbed into the bloodstream through the walls of the small intestine, so blood and the cardiovascular systems again assist another system. All the while, the muscular system provides the *peristalsis*, wave-like contractions of muscle throughout this long tract of passageways, that propel the food onward and outward.

WARNING

This system is very prone to inflammation because of the invasion of foreign material (food). Food poisoning is a perfect example, but let's not forget *gastroenteritis* (inflammation of stomach and intestines), vomiting, and everyone's favorite, *diarrhea*.

The endocrine system

The *endocrine system* maintains the chemical balance in the body. It works in conjunction with the nervous system to regulate body systems. This is accomplished by sending messengers called *hormones* through the body via the bloodstream. The nervous system controls the endocrine system's release of hormones, and hormones control the *metabolic* function in the body. The *pituitary gland*, known as the "master gland," is located in the brain. It works together with the *hypothalamus gland* to aid homeostasis and body functions such as growth, salt and water balance, reproduction, and metabolism.

TECHNICAL STUFF

Homeostasis is an automatic process that maintains stability and balance of the body's internal environment in order to stay healthy.

Glands that make up this system include the thyroid, parathyroids, adrenals, and pineal. All these glands produce hormones. The *pancreas* (also a part of the digestive system) also produces hormones. The pancreas joins a group of mixed-function organs including the stomach, intestines, kidney, ovaries, and testes. In addition to their regular system functions, they also produce hormones.

The *thyroid gland* secretes two hormones that are necessary for the body to maintain a normal rate of metabolism. The *parathyroid glands* secrete a hormone that moves the storage of calcium from bone into the blood (to maintain adequate levels of calcium in the bloodstream).

The *adrenal glands* are made up of the cortex and medulla. The *cortex* secretes *steroids* and mineral *corticoids*, which are essential to life because they regulate the levels of mineral salts, or *electrolytes*. In fact, all adrenal hormones secreted by the cortex are steroids. These include mineralocorticoids, which regulate potassium, sodium and chloride (electrolytes) and glucocorticoids (which includes cortisol) that aids in metabolism of carbohydrates, fat and proteins (tissues release glucose to raise blood sugar levels when needed).

THE THREE LITTLE SYSTEMS

The *central nervous system* includes the brain and spinal cord. The *peripheral nervous system* consists of *cranial* and *spinal nerves,* or all the nerves that branch out from the brain and spinal cord. Impulses are sent to and from the brain via a vast network of nerves. The peripheral system consists of nerves that operate automatically, sending impulses from the central nervous system to glands, the heart, and blood vessels as well as the involuntary muscles in the digestive and urinary systems. This autonomic system also contains sympathetic nerves that stimulate the body when under stress or in a crisis, to increase blood pressure and heart rate.

The *adrenal medulla* secretes catecholamines only, such as epinephrine (adrenaline) and norepinephrine (noradrenaline), which aid the body in stressful situations.

The pancreas has specialized cells called the *islets of Langerhans.* They produce insulin and *glucagon,* which stimulates *gluconeogenesis,* or sugar production, in the liver. *Insulin* is necessary in the blood so sugar can pass from the blood into cells. The *pineal gland* secretes melatonin, thought to affect the brain, help regulate sleep patterns, and influence the rate of gonad maturation.

The endocrine glands all play a part in this large orchestra to maintain the harmonious music of the body. The hypothalamus and pituitary are the orchestra leaders of this complex system, which needs to function properly to maintain good health.

The nervous system

The *nervous system* is one of the most complicated systems in the body. More than 10 *billion* nerve cells function constantly to organize and coordinate the activities of the body. This system controls voluntary as well as involuntary functions. We speak, move muscles, hear, taste, see, and think. We have memory, a word bank, association, and discrimination. These enormous tasks represent just a small number of functions controlled by the nervous system.

TECHNICAL STUFF

The brain is a three-pound organ that uses 17 percent of the body's cardiac output and 20 percent of all available oxygen.

The brain controls *homeostasis,* an automatic checklist your body goes through, to keep all systems running normally. When the body is stressed due to infection, pain, or not enough oxygen, body cells are not at their best and don't function as well as they should. So the brain monitors blood pressure, body temperature, and sugar in the blood. The *hypothalamus*, located in the brain, maintains homeostasis by initiating the release of hormones when needed.

Most major regions of your body host some sort of nervous system worker bee, from your head to your toes.

- The brain's largest part is the *cerebrum*. The lobes of the cerebrum control functions such as speech, recognizing objects, concentration, vision, problem solving, hearing, learning, and almost all functions of consciousness.
- The *cerebellum*, or "hind brain," assists in coordinating voluntary body movement and helps maintain body balance. The hypothalamus controls body temperature, sleep, and appetite.
- The *medulla oblongata* regulates the centers that control respiration, heart rate, and the respiratory system.
- The *spinal cord* passes through the *vertebral canal* from the *medulla* down to the *lumbar vertebrae*. The cord conducts nerve impulses to and from the brain.

You can see why the nervous system is so complex. It is the body's control center, and the spinal cord with its nerve network is the body's communication system.

The urinary and reproductive systems

Think you're running out of systems? Not a chance! Next, consider your urinary system, whose responsibility it is to remove the liquid waste from the body. *Urine* is liquid waste filtered from the blood, collected in the *tubules* of the kidneys, and passed along to the *renal pelvis*, the central collecting portion of each of two kidneys, down each *ureter* (we each have two) to the *urinary bladder*, which is, of course, the holding tank. When urination occurs, urine is released from the bladder, travels down the urethra, and exits the body.

Much of this system also looks after itself automatically. It works in conjunction with the bloodstream to begin the filtration process with the autonomic nervous system, so we don't have to *think* about producing urine, we only have to release it when the bladder is full. The muscular system involves the *sphincter* that we control to open to release urine from the body.

The kidneys play an important role in the process of homeostasis — to keep everything in sync and in order. Kidneys help maintain the proper balance of salt and water content in the blood as well as maintain the proper acid-base balance in the blood. The kidneys work together with the liver and adrenal glands to maintain balance of sodium and potassium in the blood, which affects blood volume and, in turn, affects blood pressure. Once again, this is an example of multiple systems working together to accomplish an important task.

In the male, the *prostate* surrounds the urethra. The urethra passes through the prostate as its connection to the male reproductive system. During urination, urine passes through the male urethra.

TECHNICAL STUFF

During ejaculation, *seminal fluid* passes through the urethra, so the urethra serves two purposes in the male. The *prostate gland* secretes juices that help make up the seminal fluid.

The reproductive systems have one purpose: to secrete hormones (accomplished through the endocrine system) in order to have the ability to reproduce. To accomplish this, a male must fertilize a female, either in person or via one of the many modern fertility clinical procedures.

The female system consists of the *ovaries* (the *gonads*) that produce the hormones *estrogen* and *progesterone*. The *fallopian tube* is the passageway that a mature *ovum* (egg) takes from the ovary to the uterus. The *uterus* is a muscular, very expandable organ that provides a safe place for a pregnancy to grow to maturity (40 weeks). The *vagina* is the birth canal, the route taken by the infant at delivery and also the route taken by the sperm to achieve the pregnancy. Actually, fertilization of a sperm and an ovum takes place in the fallopian tube and then travels to the uterus to grow. Each month the uterus prepares for a possible pregnancy. When conception does not occur, the lining of the uterus is expelled as a *menstrual period*. Then the whole monthly process begins all over again.

TECHNICAL STUFF

The breasts are considered part of the reproductive system because they are the glands that begin producing milk following delivery.

In the male, the *testes* are the gonads. It is in the testes or *testicles*, which are held in the *scrotum*, that the hormone *testosterone* is produced, as well as *spermatozoa*, which are stored in the *epididymis*. At the time of ejaculation, the spermatozoa together with seminal fluid gathered along the route, travels through a duct system that includes the *vas deferens*, *seminal vesicles*, prostate, and urethra, via the penis, to exit the body. During intercourse, it is all deposited into the vagina.

TECHNICAL STUFF

The body has 50,000–100,000 genes in only 46 chromosomes. All of that genetic information gets passed down from parent to child.

We're sure you'll agree that, when all is said and done, the human body is a pretty amazing machine!

3 In Terms of Anatomy

IN THIS PART . . .

Boning up on the skeletal system

Getting pumped about the muscular system

Disentangling terms for hair, skin, and nails

Perceiving the terminology of the sensory systems

IN THIS CHAPTER

- Finding out how your skeletal system works
- Determining root words, prefixes, and suffixes appropriate to this system
- Using terminology of the skeletal system to discuss common conditions and diseases
- Finding the right terms to use when diagnosing problems

Chapter 12

Boning Up on the Skeletal System

Consider the skeletal system to be your body's infrastructure. This system, along with its joints, works together with the muscles to give your body the support it needs to function. The bony skeleton, composed of 206 bones, provides the jointed framework for the body, giving it shape. This framework protects vital organs from external injury and provides attachment points for muscles, ligaments, and tendons to make body movement possible.

Bones are connected to other bones by ligaments. Muscles are connected to bones by tendons, which are located at each end of a muscle because a muscle needs to be attached to two bones to make movement possible. A joint, then, is any place in the body where two or more bones meet.

How the Skeletal System Works

Although bones, muscles, joints, ligaments, and tendons all work together, they each have a special job. Bones provide the framework for your body but ligaments and tendons provide the attachments for muscles to contract and relax.

Bones store mineral salts, and the inner core of a bone is composed of *hematopoietic* (blood cell–forming) red bone marrow. Other areas of the bone are used as storage areas for minerals necessary for growth, such as calcium and phosphorus. And you thought bones just gave your body its shape. In fact, they operate as your body's Fort Knox of vital minerals. Talk about double duty!

Figure 12-1 shows the human skeleton.

Red bone marrow is red because red blood cells form in it. In adults red marrow is eventually replaced by yellow marrow, which stores fat. Bones are complete organs, chiefly made up of connective tissue called *osseous* or *bony* tissue plus a rich supply of blood vessels and nerves.

TECHNICAL STUFF

Colles' fracture was first described by Dr. Andrew Colles, an Irish surgeon in 1814. It is a fracture of the distal end of the radius (*distal* meaning the portion of a body part farthest from the point of origin). But you don't have to be Irish to sustain one. In this case, the point of origin is the shoulder, looking at the limb separately, and not the body as a whole.

Bones and osteology

Now it's time to get down with osteology. No, it's not a slick new dance move. *Osteology* is the study of bones. Notice the root word *osteo?* You might know it as part of the word *osteoporosis* — a common condition typical in women involving the loss of bone density (in fact, four out of five Americans with osteoporosis are women). So *osteo* is the focus in this chapter. The first step into the world of osteology is looking at the actual makeup of our bones.

TECHNICAL STUFF

Bones of the hands and feet make up over half of our 206 total bones, while the skull is composed of 22 bones.

Bones are classified by their shape — long, short, flat, irregular, and sesamoid. Like this:

» **Long bones,** found in arms (the *humerus* is the upper arm) and legs (the *femur* is your thigh) are strong, broad at the ends where they join with other bones, and have large surface areas for muscle attachment.

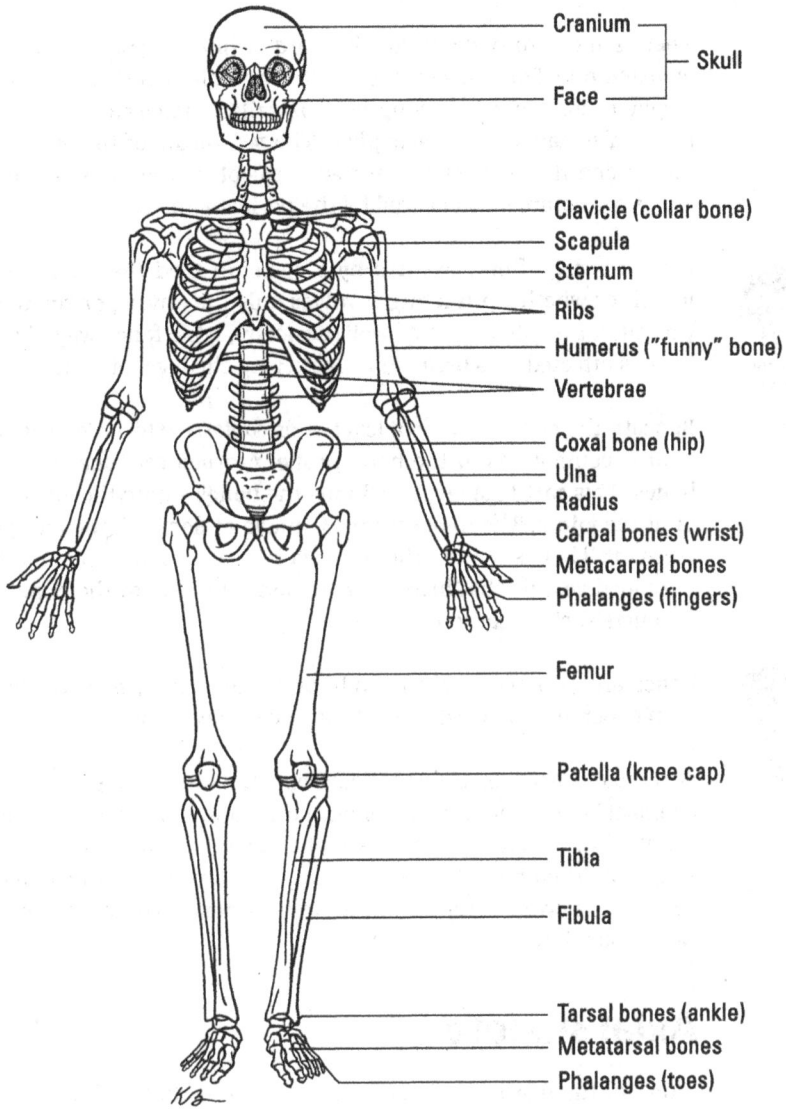

Illustration by Kathryn Born

FIGURE 12-1: Front view of the skeleton showing rib cage, clavicles, upper and lower limbs, and pelvis.

- **Short bones** are found in the wrists and ankles and have small, irregular shapes.
- **Flat bones** are found covering soft body parts. The shoulder blades, ribs, and pelvic bones are examples of flat bones.
- Vertebrae are examples of **irregular bones.**
- **Sesamoid bones** are small, rounded bones found near joints. The kneecap is an example of a sesamoid bone.

There's more to bones than the hard, white substance you think of when you envision one. For starters, the shaft or middle region of a long bone is called the *diaphysis*. Each end of a long bone is called the *epiphysis*. Both are joined by the *physis*, also called the *growth plate*. The *periosteum* of the bone is a strong, fibrous membrane that covers the surface, except at the ends. Bones other than long bones are completely covered by the periosteum.

TECHNICAL STUFF

Fractures are often classified by a system called the *Salter-Harris system*, which identifies whether a fracture involves only the physis, or could involve the epiphysis and/or the diaphysis as well. Basically, it's a fancy way of saying what area of bone is affected by a break and classifying the level of seriousness of that break.

Beneath the periosteum is a level of *osteoblasts*, which deposit calcium and phosphorus compounds in the bony tissue. *Articular cartilage* covers the ends of long bones. This cartilage layer cushions the bones where they meet with other bones, or at the joints. The *compact bone* is made of dense tissue lying under the periosteum in all bones. Within the compact bone is a system of small channels containing blood vessels that bring oxygen and nutrients to the bone and remove waste products such as carbon dioxide.

TECHNICAL STUFF

Bones are 31 percent water, and pound for pound, they are four times stronger than concrete. The hardest of these is your jaw bone.

Cancellous bone, sometimes called *spongy bone*, is more porous and less dense than compact bone. Spaces in cancellous bone contain red bone marrow, which is richly supplied with blood and consists of immature and mature blood cells in various stages of development. The ribs, the pelvic bones, the sternum or breastbone and vertebrae, as well as the epiphyses of long bones, contain red bone marrow within cancellous tissue.

Axial skeleton

Think of the word *axis* when you think about the axial skeleton. The bones that make up this particular part of the skeleton tend to encircle important organs or rotate in an axial motion. The axial skeleton includes the heavy hitters in this section.

Cranium

The bones of the cranium (skull) protect the brain. The bones of the skull include the *frontal bone*, which forms the forehead and bony sockets that contain the eyes. The *parietal bone* forms the roof and upper sides of the skull. Two *temporal* bones form the lower sides and base. The *mastoid process* is a small round part of the temporal bone behind the ear.

The *occipital bone* forms the back and base of the skull and joins the parietal and temporal bones, forming a *suture* (a joining line) of cranial bones. The occipital bone has an opening called the *foramen magnum* through which the spinal cord passes. The *sphenoid bone* extends behind the eyes and forms part of the base of the skull. It joins the frontal, occipital, and ethmoid bones and serves as an anchor to hold these bones together. The *ethmoid bone* is a thin delicate bone, supporting the nasal cavity and forms part of the orbits of the eyes.

WARNING

Be careful when working with a newborn cranium, as the cranial bones of a newborn are not completely joined. There are gaps of *unossified* tissue (tissue that is still in the fibrous membrane stage) in the skull, called the soft spot or *fontanelle.* The lines where the bones of the skull join are called *cranial sutures.* The pulse of blood vessels can be felt under the skin in these areas.

Facial bones

All the facial bones except one are joined together. Only the *mandible,* or lower jaw bone, is capable of moving, which is necessary for chewing and speaking. Other facial bones include the *nasal* bones, and the *maxillary* bones. Two large bones compose the upper jaw. Both the mandible and maxilla contain sockets called *alveoli,* in which the teeth are embedded. The mandible joins the skull at the temporal bone, forming the lengthily named *temporomandibular joint.* The *zygoma* or *zygomatic bones* form the cheek. Together, these bones create a sort of mega-bone that makes up the upper portion of your face.

Vertebral column

The *vertebral column,* or spinal column, is composed of 26 bone segments called *vertebrae* (singular *vertebra*), which are arranged in five *divisions:* cervical, thoracic, lumbar, sacrum, and coccyx (tailbone).

The first seven vertebrae are called the *cervical vertebrae* (C1-C7). These vertebrae do not join with the ribs. The first cervical vertebra, C1 (also known as the *atlas*), articulates with the occipital bone of the skull at the back of neck. It supports the head and allows it to move forward and back. The second cervical vertebra, C2 (the *axis*), acts as a pivot, about which the atlas rotates, allowing head to turn from side to side, extend, and flex.

The second division consists of 12 *thoracic vertebrae* (T1-T12). These vertebrae join with the 12 pairs of ribs. The third division consists of five *lumbar vertebrae* (L1-L5). They are the strongest and largest of the back bones. The *sacrum* is a slightly curved triangular bone, composed of five separate segments, or sacral bones, that gradually become fused. The *coccyx* is the tailbone. It is also a fused bone, formed from four small *coccygeal bones.*

The Greek *diskos* means "flat plate." An example is the lumbar disk. And coccyx comes from the Greek word for cuckoo; it resembles a cuckoo's beak.

A vertebra is composed of a disk-shaped portion called the *vertebral body*, which is the solid anterior portion (closest to body front, farthest from the body back). A *lamina* is a part of the posterior (back) portion of a vertebra. *Spinous processes, thoracic processes,* and *transverse processes* are little wing-like projections that project or extend from each vertebra. The *foramen* is the opening in the middle of each vertebra that the spinal cord passes through.

Between the body of one vertebra and the bodies of vertebrae lying beneath are *vertebral disks,* which help to provide flexibility and cushion shock to the vertebral column.

Thorax

The thorax (not to be confused with a character invented by Dr. Seuss) starts with the *clavicle,* or the collarbone, connecting the sternum (breastbone) to each shoulder. The *scapula* is the shoulder blade, consisting of two flat triangular bones, one on each back side of the thorax. The scapulae extend to join with the clavicle at the *acromion.*

TECHNICAL STUFF

The shoulder blade connects to the body by 15 different muscles but not by a single bone connection.

The *sternum* is the breastbone, the flat bone extending down the midline of the chest. The uppermost part of the sternum joins to the sides of the clavicle and ribs, whereas the other, narrowed portion is attached to the diaphragm. The lower portion of the sternum is the *xiphoid process,* the small, mobile bone tag on the very end of the sternum. This is the thing you would feel for when placing your hands on a chest to perform CPR. The 12 pairs of ribs are close neighbors with the sternum. The first seven pairs join the sternum anteriorly (at the chest) by attachments of *costal cartilage.* Ribs 1–7 are called true ribs. Ribs 8–12 are called false ribs. The false ribs join with the vertebral column in the back, but join the 7th rib anteriorly and do not attach to the sternum. Ribs 11 and 12 are called floating ribs because they are completely free at their anterior end.

TECHNICAL STUFF

The ribs move five million times a year — every time you breathe.

Pelvis

The *pelvic girdle* or hip bone is a large bone that supports the trunk of the body and joins with the femur (thigh bone) and *sacrum.* The adult pelvic bone is composed of three pairs of fused bone: the *ilium,* the *ischium,* and the *pubis.*

The ilium is the uppermost and largest portion. The connection between the iliac bones and the sacrum is so firm that they are often referred to as one bone, the *sacroiliac.* The *iliac crests* are found on both the anterior and posterior portions of the pelvis. They are filled with red bone marrow and serve as an attachment for abdominal wall muscles.

The ischium is the posterior portion of the pelvis. The ischium and the muscles attached to it are what we sit on.

The pubis is the anterior portion containing two parts that are joined by way of a disk. This area of fusion is called the *pubic symphysis.* The region within the bone formed by the pelvic girdle is called the *pelvic cavity.* The rectum, sigmoid colon, bladder, and female reproductive organs are contained in this cavity.

Appendicular skeleton

Think of the word *appendage* when your thoughts turn to the appendicular skeleton. Your reachers, grabbers, and hoofers are all covered in this section. Appendages fall into two major categories of bones.

Upper extremities

Arms and hands are part of this category. The bones of the arm and hand include the *humerus,* the upper arm bone. The large head of the humerus is round and joins the scapula and clavicle. The *ulna* and *radius* are the bones of the lower arm or forearm. The bony prominence of the ulna at the elbow is called the *olecranon. Carpals* are wrist bones. Finally, there are two rows of four bones. The *metacarpals* are five bones radiating to the fingers. *Phalanges* (the singular is *phalanx*) are the finger bones.

Each finger has three phalanges: the proximal, middle, and distal. The *proximal* is the phalange closest to the point of origin, whereas the *distal* is farthest from the point of origin. So, the proximal would be the first after the knuckle, the middle would be in the middle, and the distal at the fingertip. The thumb has only two phalanges: medial and distal at tip of the thumb, which is why it is categorized differently than the rest of your fingers.

Diaphysis comes from Greek *diaphusis,* meaning "state of growing between." Diaphysis is the shaft of long bones that grows as children grow.

Leg and foot

The *femur* is the thigh bone. At the top end of it, a rounded head fits into a socket in the hip bone called the *acetabulum.* The *patella,* or kneecap, is a small flat bone that lies in front of the joint between the femur and one of the lower leg bones called the *tibia*. The tibia is the larger of the two lower bones of the leg, often referred to as the shin bone. The *fibula* is the smaller of the two bones.

The *tarsals*, or ankle bones, are short bones that are much like the carpal bones of the wrist, but larger. The *calcaneus*, the largest of these bones, is also called the heel bone. *Metatarsals* compose the forefoot or bones leading to the phalanges in the toes. There are two phalanges in the big or great toe and three in each of the other four toes. Just like the fingers, all the bones in the toes are phalanges, from proximal to distal. In the big or great toe they are called the proximal and distal, differing slightly from the thumb.

TECHNICAL STUFF

The femur is the longest bone in the body and accounts for one quarter of your total height.

Joints

Now think about the "glue" that holds all these bones together. Okay, joints aren't really made of glue, but they sure do a good job of keeping everything connected. Let us articulate that concept a bit better: Joints, also called *articulations*, are the coming together of two or more bones. Some are not movable, such as the *suture joints* between the cranial bones. Some joints only partially move, such as joints between the vertebrae.

Most joints do allow movement. These freely movable joints are called *synovial joints*. An example is the ball and socket type — the hip joint, for example, in which the head of the femur fits into the acetabulum. Another synovial joint is the hinged type as seen at the elbow, knee, or ankle joints.

The bones of a synovial joint are separated by a *capsule*, composed of fibrous cartilage. Ligaments of connective tissue hold the bones together around the capsule to strengthen it. The bone surfaces at a joint are covered with a smooth surface called the *articular cartilage*. The *synovial membrane* is the inner layer of the capsule, the layer beneath the capsular surface.

The *synovial cavity* is filled with a lubricating fluid produced by synovial membranes. This fluid contains water and nutrients that help to lubricate the joints so that friction on the articular cartilage is minimal.

Bursae (singular *bursa*) are closed sacs of synovial fluid lined with synovial membrane. They lie in the spaces between tendons, ligaments, and bones and lubricate areas where friction would normally develop close to the joint capsule. The *olecranon bursa* at the elbow joint and the *patellar bursa* at the knee are examples of bursae.

Skeletal Root Words

Now that you've gotten to know the specific parts of the skeletal system a bit better, it's time to put your expertise into practice by breaking down the root words into meanings and useful applications. The roots, as always, are essential medical terminology knowledge because once you master these roots (those good ol' Greek and Latin ones, that is), you can break down any skeletal-related word and discover its meaning.

Table 12-1 lists important skeletal system root words and combining forms.

TABLE 12-1 **Digging Up Your Skeletal Roots**

Root Word	What It Means
Kyph/o	Humpback (posterior curvature of thoracic spine)
Lamin/o	Lamina (part of the vertebral arch)
Lord/o	Curve or swayback (*lordosis:* anterior curvature in lumbar spine)
Lumb/o	Lower back, lumbar region
Myel/o	Bone marrow
Oste/o	Bone
Orth/o	Straight
Scoli/o	Crooked, bent (*scoliosis:* lateral curvature of spine)
Spondyl/o	Vertebra (referring to conditions of the structure)
Vertebr/o	Vertebra (referring to or describing the structure)

Table 12-2 lists the combining forms used with bones.

TABLE 12-2 **Bone-Related Combining Forms**

Combining Form	Example	What It Means
Acetabul/o	Acetabulum	Hip joint
Brachi/o	Brachiocephalic	Pertaining to the arms and head
Calcane/o	calcaneus	Heel
Carp/o	Carpals	Wrist bones

(continued)

TABLE 12-2 *(continued)*

Combining Form	Example	What It Means
Clavic/o, clavicul/o	Clavicle	Collar bone
Coccyg/o	Coccygodynia	Pain in and around the coccyx
Cost/o	Costal	Ribs
Crani/o	Cranium	Skull
Femor/o	Femur	Upper leg bone
Fibul/o	Fibula	Lower leg bone
Humer/o	Humerus	Upper arm bone
Ili/o	Ilium	Pelvic bone
Ischi/o	Ischium	Pelvic bone
Lumb/o	Spine	Lumbar region
Malleol/o	Malleolus	Ankle
Mandibul/o	Mandible	Lower jaw
Maxill/o	Maxilla	Upper jaw
Metacarp/o	Metacarpals	Bones of hand
Metatars/o	Metatarsals	Bones of foot
Olecran/o	Olecranon	Elbow
Patell/o	Patella	Knee cap
Phalang/o	Phalanges	Bones of fingers and toes
Pub/o	Pubis	Portion of pelvic bone
Radi/o	Radius	Lower arm bone
Sacr/o	Sacrum	Sacral area of spine
Scapul/o	Scapula	Shoulder blade
Stern/o	Sternum	Breastbone
Tars/o	Tarsals	Ankle bones
Tibi/o	Tibia	Lower leg bone
Uln/o	Ulna	Lower arm bone

Table 12-3 lists the combining forms used with joints.

TABLE 12-3 **Joint-Related Combining Forms**

Combining Form	What It Means
Arthr/o	Joint
Articul/o	Joint
Burs/o	Bursa
Chondr/o	Cartilage
Disk/o	Intervertebral disk
Fibros/o	Fibrous
Menisc/o	Meniscus
Synovi/o	Synovium
Ten/o, tend/o, tendin/o	Tendon

More Anatomical Terms

Although the makeup of the skeletal system is pretty straightforward, there are still more useful terms you need to know in order to communicate about 'dem bones. Try a few of the words in Table 12-4 on for size.

TABLE 12-4 **More Common Skeletal Vocabulary**

Word	What It Means
Ankylosis	Stiffness of a joint
Arthralgia	Pain in the joint
Articulation	Joint
Bradykinesia	Slow movement
Bursa	Sac of fluid at or around a joint
Calcium	One of the mineral constituents of bone
Cancellous bone	Spongy porous bone tissue
Chiropodist	Specialist in diagnosing and treating foot disorders

(continued)

TABLE 12-4 *(continued)*

Word	What It Means
Chiropractics	System of therapy that consists of manipulation of the bones and joints of the entire body
Chiropractor	Specialist in chiropractics
Chondromalacia	Softening of cartilage
Compact bone	Hard, dense bone tissuelation
Condyle	Knucklelike process at the end of a bone — near a joint
Diaphysis	Shaft or midportion of a long bone
Dyskinesia	Difficult movement
Dystrophy	Abnormal development
Epiphysis	End of a long bone
Fissure	Narrow slitlike opening between bones
Fontanelle	Soft spot, incomplete closure of infant's skull sutures
Fossa	Depression or cavity in a bone
Hematopoiesis	Development of blood cells in bone marrow
Hyperkinesia	Excessive movement or overactivity
Intercostal	Between the ribs
Intracranial	Within the cranium
Kyphosis	Abnormal hump of thoracic spine, "hunchback"
Ligament	Connective tissue binding bones to other bones
Mastoid process	Round projection on the temporal bone behind the ear
Orthopedics	Branch of medicine dealing with the study and treatment of diseases and abnormalities of the skeletal system
Orthopedist	Physician specializing in orthopedics
Orthotics	Making and fitting of orthopedic appliances such as arch supports, used to support, align, or correct deformities
Osseous tissue	Bone tissue
Ossification	Process of bone formation
Osteoblast	A bone cell that helps form bone tissue
Osteoclast	A bone cell that absorbs and removes unwanted bone tissue
Osteopath	Physician who specializes in osteopathy

Word	What It Means
Osteopathy	Branch of medicine using the usual forms of diagnosis of treatment but with emphasis on the role of the relationship between the body organs and the skeletal system, and performing manipulations in order to decrease pain and help body function
Osteosarcoma	Malignant tumor of bone
Podiatrist	Specialist in diagnosing and treating foot disorders such as corns and ingrown toenails; some also perform foot surgery
Prosthesis	Artificial substitute or replacement for a missing body part such as an artificial leg, eye, joint, or heart valve
Red bone marrow	Found in cancellous bone, the site of hematopoiesis
Scoliosis	Abnormal lateral curvature of the spine
Subcostal	Below the ribs
Tendinitis or tendonitis	Inflammation of a tendon
Tendon	Connective tissue binding muscles to bones
Tenodynia	Pain in a tendon
Tenosynovitis	Inflammation of the tendon and synovial membrane
Trabeculae	Supporting bundles of bony fibers in cancellous or sponge bone
Trochanter	Large process behind the neck of the femur
Tubercle	Small rounded process on a bone
Tuberosity	Large rounded process on a bone
Yellow bone marrow	The fatty tissue found in the diaphyses of long bones

Common Skeletal Conditions

Breaks, sprains, and bunions are no fun. Many of the most common maladies associated with the skeletal system involve the application of casts or other corrective devices. Good, old-fashioned *fractures* (a sudden break of the bone) top the list of skeletal conditions. Whether a result of an auto accident or just plain clumsiness (come on, like you didn't see that curb jump out at you!), any bone in your body is a potential break waiting to happen.

You are probably familiar with many common bone conditions because you've likely experienced one of them.

- **Bunion** is an abnormal prominence with bursal swelling at the metatarsophalangeal joint near the base of the big toe.
- **Bursitis** is an inflammation of a bursa. Tennis elbow is an example of bursitis of the olecranon bursa.
- **Dislocation** is a displacement of a bone from its joint. Dislocations may be reduced or restored to their normal condition and the joint immobilized with sling or strapping for healing of torn ligaments and tendons.
- **Sprain,** everyone's favorite, is trauma or injury to a joint with pain, swelling, and injury to ligaments.

Possibly the most painful is the *protrusion of an intervertebral disk,* an abnormal extension of the intervertebral pad into the neural canal. This is commonly referred to as a *herniated disk* or *slipped disk.*

The bones can also experience conditions due to deformity and growths. *Talipes,* also known as clubfoot, is a congenital deformity of the bones of the foot. The bones are twisted out of shape or position. *Exostoses* are bony growths (benign tumors) on the surface of a bone.

Let's not forget our old friend, *arthritis,* the inflammation of a joint. Speaking of old, this condition is not limited to seniors. Arthritis knows no age, and it has several permutations:

- **Ankylosing spondylitis** is a chronic arthritis with stiffening of joints, particularly the spine. This condition responds to corticosteroids and anti-inflammatory therapy.
- **Gouty arthritis (gout)** is inflammation of joints caused by excessive uric acid in the body. An inherited defect in metabolism causes excessive uric acid to accumulate in the blood, joints, and soft tissues near the joints. Gout commonly occurs in the big (great) toe.
- **Osteoarthritis,** also called degenerative joint disease or degenerative arthritis, is chronic inflammation of bones and joints due to degenerative changes in the cartilage related to overuse This occurs mainly in the hips and legs. Drug therapy reduces the inflammation and pain, and physical therapy loosens impaired joints.
- **Psoriatic arthritis** is a chronic disease characterized by inflammation of the skin (psoriasis) and joints (arthritis). Patchy red and white areas affect the elbows, knees, and scalp.
- **Rheumatoid arthritis** is a chronic autoimmune disease where joints become inflamed and painful. In rheumatoid arthritis, the small joints of the hands and feet are usually affected first, and the larger joints later.

BREAK IT TO ME GENTLY, DOC

Don't think every fracture is a run-of-the-mill break. You'd be surprised at how complicated a fracture can be. Here's a sampling from the fracture menu:

- **Closed fracture:** Bone is broken with no open wound in the skin.
- **Comminuted fracture:** Bone is splintered, crushed, or has completely detached segments.
- **Compression fracture:** Bone is pushed in on itself; commonly occurs in the vertebrae.
- **Greenstick fracture:** Bone is partially bent and partially broken, like when a green stick breaks. Often occurs in children.
- **Impacted fracture:** Bone is broken with one end wedged into the other.
- **Open (compound) fracture:** Broken bone with an open skin wound.

Treatment of fractures includes *reduction,* restoring the fracture to its normal position. There are two types of reduction:

- **Closed reduction** involves a manipulated reduction without an incision.
- **Open reduction** features making an incision into the skin to gain access to the fracture site and then restoring normal position.

Once the fractured bone is set, a fiberglass or plaster of Paris cast, which is a solid mold of the body part, is applied to the injured area while healing takes place.

Finding the Culprit: Skeletal Diseases and Pathology

Some conditions affecting the skeletal system are more complicated and are considered *pathological,* meaning the result of, or marker for, systemwide disease. Some may sound familiar to you, including *osteoporosis,* a decrease in bone density due to loss of calcium. Osteoporosis may occur as part of the aging process or due to corticosteroid therapy, but can be diagnosed and treated.

Two other diseases with the *osteo-* root are *osteomyelitis* and *osteogenic sarcoma.* The former is an inflammation of the bone and bone marrow due to infection. Bacteria enters the body through a wound, spreads from an infection near the bone, or originates in a skin or throat infection. Infection occurs in the long bones of the arm and leg, which can lead to an abscess and, if the bone dies, a *sequestrum* (a segment of dead bone) may develop. *Osteogenic sarcoma* is a malignant tumor of bone. Similarly, *Ewing's tumor* is a highly malignant metastasizing tumor (Ewing's sarcoma) involving the entire shaft of a long bone. It occurs in children and adolescents.

Paget's disease is a skeletal disease often hereditary in older persons — bone resorption and formation are increased, leading to thickening and softening of bones, causing bending of weight-bearing bones.

TECHNICAL STUFF

Most lesions associated with osteogenic sarcoma occur just above or below the knee.

Inflammation is not just for muscles and soft tissues. Bones can become inflamed as well. *Rickets* is characterized by *osteomalacia*, or softening of bone. It is a disease of infancy and childhood when bones that are forming fail to receive the calcium and phosphorus they need. Bones become soft and bend easily.

Testing, Testing: Skeletal Radiology and Diagnostic Tests

X-rays of bones and joints are common procedures to identify fractures or tumors, to monitor healing of a fracture, and to identify abnormal structures. The major methods to the skeletal madness are as follows:

- **Arthrocentesis:** Surgical puncture of a joint to aspirate fluid for diagnostic purposes
- **Arthrogram:** X-ray film of a joint
- **Arthroscopy:** Visual examination of the interior of a joint using an arthroscope
- **Bone densitometry (DEXA or DXA) (bone density):** Determines the density of bone, performed to diagnose osteoporosis
- **Bone scan (scintigraphy) (nuclear medicine test):** Detects presence of metastatic disease of the bone and monitors degenerative bone disease
- **Computerized tomography (CT):** Gives accurate definition of bone structure and can demonstrate even slight changes
- **Dual-energy X-ray absorptiometry (Dexa):** The most accurate way to evaluate bone density in screening for osteopenia and osteoporosis
- **Fluoroscopy:** Examination using a fluoroscope, a device used to examine deep body structures by means of x-rays

- **Magnetic resonant imaging (MRI):** Evaluates all soft tissues and is especially useful for assessing the ligaments, tendons, muscles, spinal stenosis, and degenerative disk changes; great for anything that doesn't show up on an x-ray
- **Positron emission tomography (PET):** A nuclear medicine imaging technique that produces a 3-D image of a body process
- **Quantitative computerized tomography (QCT):** Used to measure bone density in hip and spine
- **Single-photon emission computerized tomography (SPECT):** A very sensitive nuclear method for detecting bone abnormalities

Paging Dr. Terminology: Skeletal Surgeries and Procedures

Both bones and joints can be repaired with surgery. Joints can be surgically fixed with *arthrodesis* or surgically repaired with *arthroplasty*. Arthroscopic and arthroscopic assisted procedures will continue to be done on an outpatient basis as methodologies continue to streamline. Spine and joint procedures will still be performed on an inpatient basis but with new approaches, devices, instruments like robotics, and bone substitutions, which all will lead to less invasive surgical intervention over time.

Types of arthroplasties include:

- **Total hip replacement arthroplasty** is performed for degenerative joint disease or arthritis. The surgery involves replacement of the head of the femur of the hip joint with a prosthetic (artificial) metallic femoral head and a plastic-coated replacement *acetabulum* (a cup that the femoral head fits into).
- **Total knee joint replacement arthroplasty** is performed (largely by robots these days) to replace worn surfaces of the knee joint. Various prostheses are used in this procedure.
- **Unicompartmental hip/knee resurfacing** is performed when only one area of the knee or hip is damaged. The area is shaved down and remodeled rather than replaced, often on patients ages 20–50.
- **Core decompression** is performed by coring out a defective or diseased area of bone, with repair by filling the cored area with a bone graft.

- **Metatarsal arthroplasty** is performed to treat deformities associated with rheumatoid arthritis or *hallux valgus* (a deformity of the big toe), and to treat painful or unstable joints.
- **Nerve ablation** is performed to treat lower back pain.

TECHNICAL STUFF

Remember the root *arthro* when discussing joints. Arthritis is the inflammation of a joint, and most of the surgical procedures for joints use the same root *arthro*.

WARNING

The lone exception to the *arthro* rule is *synovectomy*, which is the excision of the synovial membrane of a joint.

The head and spine have several surgical options. A *craniotomy*, an incision into the skull, allows access to the brain for surgery. A *diskectomy* is an excision of an intervertebral disk. On the other hand, a *percutaneous diskectomy* is a procedure that uses fluoroscopy to guide insertion of a Nucleotome into a spinal disk, to remove the thick, sticky nucleus of the disk. *Nucleotome* is a registered brand name for instruments and protocol used to perform an automated percutaneous lumbar diskectomy. This allows the disk to soften and contract, relieving the lower back and leg pain. The excision of a lamina relieves symptoms of a ruptured disk, and a *spondylosyndesis* is the fusing together of the vertebrae (spinal fusion). A *lamina* is a part of the posterior (back) portion of a vertebra.

TECHNICAL STUFF

Most common bone diseases are treated with NSAIDs (nonsteroidal anti-inflammatory drugs) to lessen pain caused by inflammation. Antiresorptive medications (drugs that prevent bone breakdown) and anabolic therapy for osteoporotic fracture prevention are also used as treatment management.

Don't forget about fixing the appendicular skeleton (remember those good old appendages?). Fixing an arm or leg bone is about more than wrapping it in a cast. Consider these surgical options:

- **Meniscectomy:** Excision of a meniscus for a torn cartilage in the knee
- **Meniscopexy:** Surgical fixation of a meniscus
- **Ostealgia** or **osteodynia:** Pain in a bone
- **Osteoclasis:** Surgical breaking of a bone to correct a deformity
- **Osteoplasty:** Surgical repair of a bone
- **Osteotomy:** Incision into a bone
- **Patellectomy:** Excision of the patella
- **Phalangectomy:** Excision of a finger or a toe
- **Tenorrhaphy:** Suturing of a tendon
- **Tenotomy:** Incision of a tendon

IN THIS CHAPTER

- Finding out how your muscular system works
- Determining root words, prefixes, and suffixes appropriate to this system
- Using terminology of the muscular system to discuss common conditions and diseases
- Finding the right terms to use when diagnosing problems

Chapter 13

Getting Ripped: The Muscular System

Think about this the next time you hit the gym: Your body is the proud owner of more than 600 muscles! Luckily, you don't have to pump a different weight machine to work every single one. The beauty of the muscular system is that it is, in fact, a system in which different major muscle groups work together at the same time.

So relax and don't stress too much about that rowing machine. You're using muscles right now reading this book.

How the Muscular System Works

The *musculoskeletal* system is made up of muscles and joints. The muscles — all 600 of them and more — are responsible for movement. The skeleton provides attachment points and support for muscles, but it's the muscle tissue's ability to extend and contract that makes movement happen. So, for every climb of the elliptical machine, you can thank muscular tissue for making it possible.

Muscles make up the major part of fleshy portions of the body and account for one half of body weight. Muscles vary in proportion to body size, and the shape of the body is determined by muscles covering bones.

TECHNICAL STUFF

Muscles account for 40 percent of our total body weight; the skeleton accounts for only about 18 percent.

Muscular expanding and contracting doesn't just happen in your biceps. It happens all over the body. Muscles support and maintain posture and produce body heat. They help form many internal organs and regulate the work those organs do behind the scenes (such as the heart, uterus, lungs, and intestines) even when the body is not moving. The muscles of arteries, intestines, heart, and stomach, for example, are always at work even when we aren't thinking of them. However, the silent work muscles do inside your body is wholly different from more obvious muscular work done by your arms and legs, for example.

Internal movement involves the contraction and relaxation of involuntary muscles, muscles that we cannot consciously control. For example, heartbeats are performed by cardiac muscles. Breathing and digestion are facilitated by muscles called *visceral* (involuntary) muscles, whereas external movement is accomplished by contraction and relaxation of muscles that are attached to bones. The muscles that provide this external movement are known as voluntary muscles, as they perform movements on command.

All bodily movement, whether lifting of an arm, or the beating of the heart, involves the contraction and relaxation of voluntary or involuntary muscles.

Classes of muscles

The class system is alive and well, at least as far as your muscles are concerned. There are three classes of muscles: skeletal, visceral, and cardiac.

- **Cardiac** (involuntary striated) muscle has branching fibers and forms most of the wall of the heart. Its contraction produces the heartbeat.
- **Skeletal** (voluntary *striated,* meaning striped) muscles, are attached to the skeleton. They are called voluntary, of course, because they are controlled by your will. This type of muscle can be easily seen by flexing the forearm, which makes the biceps muscle become hard and thick.
- **Visceral** (involuntary smooth) muscle is found in the stomach, intestines, and blood vessels, and cannot be controlled at will.

TECHNICAL STUFF

Unlike other muscle, cardiac (heart) muscle keeps beating even when removed from the body, as in a heart transplant. And even if it stops beating, it can be jump-started with an external electrical charge. Not so with the other muscles.

Types of muscles

Oh, if it were only that easy. But there are also *types* of muscles. At first glance, the types of muscles are the same as the classes of muscle. But pay close attention and you'll see there are subtle differences. There are three *types* of muscles in the body.

Striated muscle

Striated muscles are also called skeletal or voluntary muscles. These are the muscles that move all the bones, as well as the face and the eyes. The body is able to consciously control the activity of a striated muscle.

Smooth muscle

The second type of muscle is *smooth muscle,* also known as visceral, involuntary or unstriated muscle. The body has no conscious control over smooth muscles, which move the internal organs such as the digestive tract. The smooth muscles are also found in blood vessels and secretory ducts leading from glands.

TECHNICAL STUFF

Skeletal muscle fibers are arranged in bundles, but smooth muscles form sheets of fibers that wrap around tubes and vessels.

Cardiac muscles

The third type of muscle is *cardiac muscle.* It is striated in appearance but is like smooth muscle in its actions. Movement of cardiac muscle cannot be consciously controlled. Cardiac muscle has branching fibers forming most of the wall of the heart and controlling the contractions producing the heartbeat.

Muscles and tendons

Now that you know the classes and types of muscles, let's take a more in-depth look at how they work. You already know that skeletal muscles, or striated muscles, are the muscles that move the bones of the body. Now get ready for the scoop on what makes it possible.

When a muscle *contracts,* one of the attached bones remains stationary, as a result of other muscles holding it in place. The point of attachment of the muscle to the stationary bone is called the *origin* or beginning of that muscle. When the muscle contracts, another bone to which it is attached, does move. The junction of the muscle to the bone that moves is called the *insertion* of the muscle. Near the point of insertion, the muscle narrows and is connected to the bone by a tendon. One type of tendon that helps attach bone to muscles is called an *aponeurosis.*

TECHNICAL STUFF

It takes 200 muscles working together to take a step.

Roundup of the superficial muscles

Sometimes, being superficial isn't a bad thing. Take, for example, your *superficial* muscles, so named because these are the ones you're most likely to see with the naked eye. These workhorses of the muscular system help make you unique. Though they all have complicated-sounding names, they help your body perform everyday functions like picking up objects and smiling.

Figures 13-1 through 13-4 illustrate four major muscle groups.

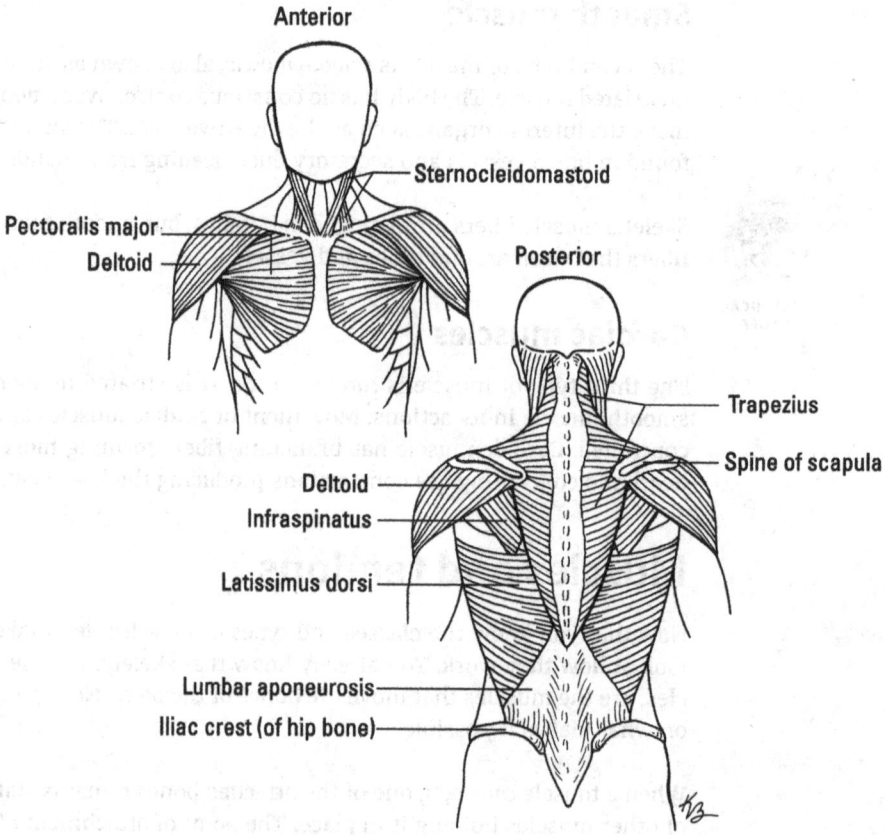

FIGURE 13-1: Posterior view of the neck and shoulder muscles.

Illustration by Kathryn Born

- **Arm muscles** consist of the upper arm muscles, *biceps brachii* and *triceps brachii.* In the forearm (lower arm) are the *flexor* and *extensor muscles* of the hands and fingers.
- **Head and face muscles** include the *frontalis, temporalis, orbicularis oculi, orbicularis oris, occipitalis, mentalis, buccinator, zygomatic major* and *minor,* and the *masseter* muscle.
- **Shoulder and neck muscles** include the *sternocleidomastoid, pectoralis major, latissimus dorsi,* and *trapezius* muscle, leading to the *deltoid* muscle of the shoulder.
- **The major chest and abdominal muscles** consist of the *diaphragm, pectoralis major,* the *rectus abdominis,* and the *external oblique.* Also associated with this region is the linea alba. The *linea alba* (meaning "white line") is a vertical band of connective muscular tissue that begins at the *xiphoid process* (sternum) and ends at the *symphysis pubis* (where the iliac bones join at the front of the pelvis).
- **The major muscles of the back** include the seventh cervical vertebral muscle, infraspinatus, supraspinatus, latissimus dorsi, and the rhomboid major muscle.

WARNING

The seventh cervical vertebra muscle is a muscle, whereas the seventh vertebra is a bone. Many muscles, tendons, and ligaments have the same name but don't have the same function. In this case, the seventh cervical muscle is a point of attachment aiding in support and movement of head and neck.

- **The pelvis and anterior thigh muscles** include the *tensor fascia lata,* the *adductors* of the thigh, the *vastus lateralis* and *vastus medialis,* the *rectus femoris,* and the *quadriceps.*
- **The lower leg muscles** from the knee to the ankle includes the *gastrocnemius,* which makes up a large portion of the calf muscles, the *tibialis anterior, soleus, peroneus longus,* and *peroneus brevis.* By the way, things aren't always what they seem: The *Achilles tendon* is technically classified as a muscle.
- **From the back, the buttocks** are composed of the *gluteus maximus* and *gluteus medius.* In the thigh are the *adductor magnus, vastus lateralis,* and *gracilis,* whereas the *biceps femoris, semitendinosus,* and *semimembranosus* combined comprise the hamstrings.

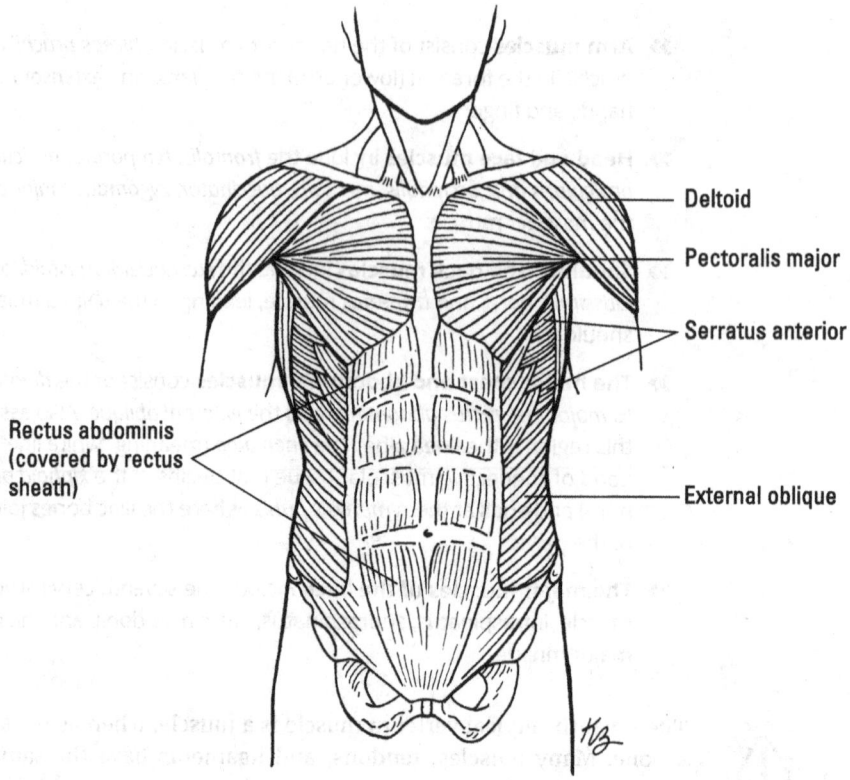

FIGURE 13-2: Anterior muscles of the chest and abdomen.

Illustration by Kathryn Born

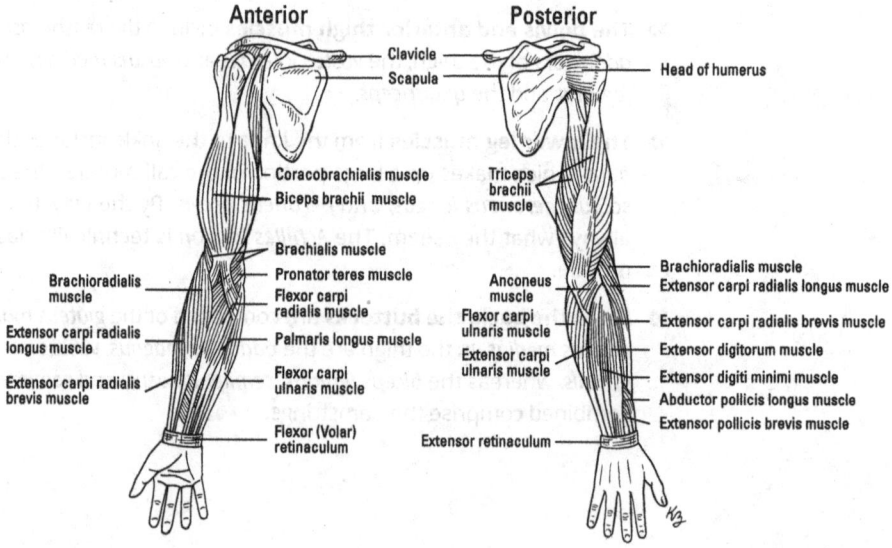

FIGURE 13-3: The muscles of the upper limb, anterior (A) and posterior (B).

Illustration by Kathryn Born

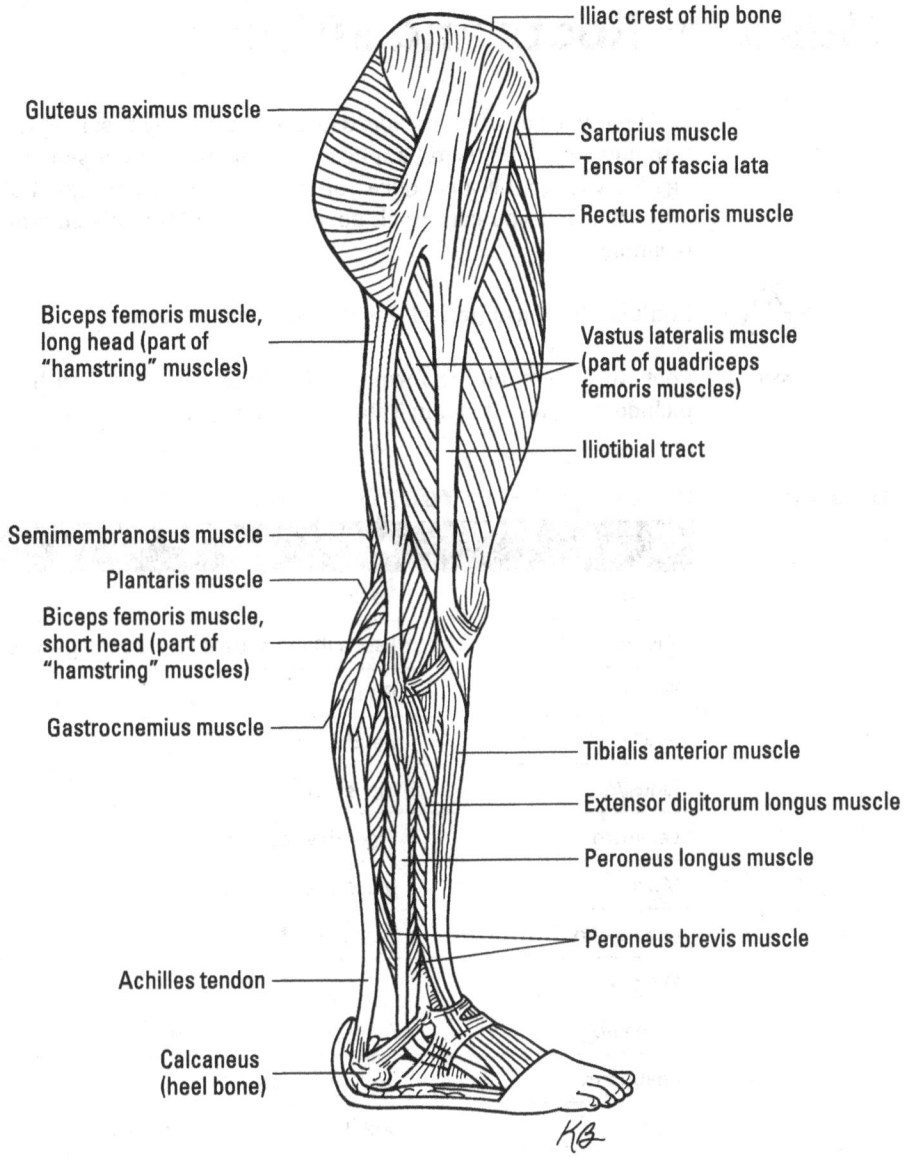

FIGURE 13-4: The muscles of the lower limb.

Illustration by Kathryn Born

So, the moral of our muscle story is teamwork. Bones cannot move alone without being attached to muscle. Muscles cannot move alone, without being attached to stationary bones to allow support for that movement. Neither bones nor muscles could function without the attachments provided by the tendons and ligaments. Body movement then, is made possible by the bones and skeletal muscles working together in addition to the visceral and cardiac muscles that function to maintain the muscular rhythm of our vital organs. It's all one big, happy family of muscles.

Muscular Roots and Suffixes

Let's put your newfound expertise into practice by breaking down the root words into meanings and useful applications. The roots are essential medical terminology knowledge, because once you master these roots (good ol' Greek and Latin ones, that is), you can break down any muscular-related word and discover its meaning.

WARNING

Don't confuse *myo* (muscle) with *myelo* (bone marrow).

Root words, combining forms, and suffixes associated with the skeletal system include the ones shown in Tables 13-1 and 13-2.

TABLE 13-1

Breaking Down Your Muscular Roots

Root Word	What It Means
Duct/o	To draw
Fasci/o	Fascia (band of tissue surrounding muscle)
Fibr/o	Fibers
Flex/o	Bend
Kinesi/o	Movement
Leiomy/o	Smooth visceral muscle
My/o	Muscle
Myocardi/o	Heart muscle
Myos/o	Muscle
Pronati/o	Facing down or backward
Rhabdomy/o	Skeletal or striated muscle
Sarc/o	Soft, fleshy, or connective tissue
Supinati/o	Facing up or forward
Tens/o	Stretch

UNOFFICIALOMA

Unofficial but not uncommon slang includes *incidentaloma,* which refers to something found in a study, which is not particularly important or else not relevant to the study at hand, but still worth noting. There's also *fascinoma,* something weird and noteworthy: "Hey, check this out, it's a real fascinoma."

TABLE 13-2 **Muscular Suffixes**

Suffix	What It Means
-algia	Pain in fibrous tissue
-desis	Surgical fixation
-dynia	Pain
-ectomy	Surgical removal or excision
-gram	Record
-graph	Instrument used to record
-graphy	The process of recording
-itis	Inflammation
-lysis	Breakdown
-ology	Study of, process of study
-oma	Tumor or mass
-otomy	To cut into
-pathy	Disease
-plasty	Surgical reconstruction, or shaping of
-rrhaphy	Suture repair

Action Item: The Movement of Your Muscles

Your muscles do a serious amount of work every single hour of every day. Though you may be reading this book propped up on some pillows while munching corn chips, your muscles are at work — muscles are moving your eyes across the words so you can read and comprehend, smooth muscles are working your organs, and superficial muscles are helping keep your body upright. Turns out, for every muscular action, luckily for you, there is a word to describe it. Here are just a few muscular action words to remember:

- **Abduction:** Movement of drawing away from the center of the body (such as fingers spread apart)
- **Adduction:** Movement of drawing toward the middle of the body (for example, fingers held together)
- **Eversion:** Turning outward
- **Inversion:** Turning inward
- **Extension:** Movement in which a limb is placed in a straight position
- **Flexion:** Movement in which a limb is bent
- **Rotation:** Turning around on its own axis
- **Pronation:** Movement that turns the palm of the hand downward
- **Supination:** Movement that turns the palm of the hand upward

TIP

To remember the difference between *-ectomy* and *-otomy*, remember *-ectomy* with *e for exit or excision* and *-otomy* for *o to open only.*

Common Muscular Conditions

Muscular conditions are fairly common in people of all ages and backgrounds. From tennis elbow to the enigmatic fibromyalgia, the muscular system can take a real beating. Here are the most common muscular conditions:

- **Bursitis:** Inflammation of the bursa sac, which lines the joint and provides smooth joint movement
- **Fibromyalgia:** Pain in fibrous tissues of muscles, tendons, or ligaments
- **Myoparalysis:** Paralysis of a muscle
- **Myotonia:** Muscles react slowly after contraction or stimulation
- **Polymyositis:** Inflammation of "many muscles"
- **Tendinitis or tendonitis:** Inflammation of a tendon

- **Tendinopathy:** Any disease involving a tendon
- **Tennis elbow:** The tendon that connects the arm muscle to elbow becomes inflamed due to the repetitive use of the arm

  The actual medical term for this is *lateral* or *medial epicondylitis* (*lateral* if referring to the bump on the outside of the elbow, *medial* to the bump on the inside).
- **Tenosynovitis:** Inflammation of the tendon and the sheath around it, often in a finger or the wrist

Finding the Culprit: Muscular Diseases and Pathology

Some of the most serious diseases affect the muscular system. From diseases that affect facial movement to the full-body atrophy of Lou Gehrig's disease, these diseases are all challenging:

- **Amyotrophic lateral sclerosis (ALS):** Movement disorder or muscle atrophy with degeneration of nerves in the spinal cord and lower region of the brain, also known as Lou Gehrig's disease
- **Dermatomyositis:** Polymyositis with inflammatory skin changes of face, neck, trunk, and arms
- **Dupuytren's contracture:** Disease affecting the *palmar fascia* of the hand, causing the ring finger and little finger to contract toward the palm
- **Isaacs Syndrome:** Progressive muscle stiffness and spasm
- **Leiomyoma:** Benign tumor of smooth muscle
- **Leiomyosarcoma:** Malignant tumor of smooth muscle
- **Mitochondrial myopathy:** Mitochondria, the power units of cells, are damaged, causing muscle weakness
- **Myasthenia gravis:** Lack of muscle strength with paralysis, characterized by weakness of muscles of the face and jaw, with difficulty swallowing
- **Myofascial pain syndrome:** Chronic disorder affecting one or more muscle groups

- **Myosarcoma:** Malignant tumor of muscle tissue
- **Myositis ossificans progressiva:** Progressive disease that begins in early life in which muscles gradually convert into bony tissue
- **Muscular dystrophy:** Inherited disease characterized by progressive weakness and degeneration of muscle fibers without involvement of the nervous system
- **Polymyalgia rheumatica:** Muscle pain, common in shoulder or pelvis, without arthritis or signs of muscle distress
- **Rotator cuff disease:** Inflammation of tendons and muscles in the shoulder; if they fuse you have a larger problem, a condition called *frozen shoulder* or *adhesive capsulitis*
- **Torticollis:** Acute myositis of the cervical muscles (wryneck)

Testing, Testing: Muscular Radiology and Diagnostic Tests

Though the list of muscular conditions and diseases is quite long, there are some simple diagnostic tests doctors can perform to diagnose most muscular ailments.

- **Elastograghy:** New image modality to map the elastic properties of soft tissues, used in conjunction with ultrasound and MRI.
- **Electromyogram (EMG)** is a record of electric activity in a muscle. This procedure is done to diagnose carpal tunnel syndrome. *Electromyography* is an electrical recording of activity in a muscle.
- **Isokinetic dynamometry:** A test to measuring the degree of muscular power using an instrument called a dynamometer.
- **MRI (magnetic resonance imaging):** The gold standard for making pictures of soft tissue such as fascia, tendons, ligaments, and muscle.
- **Ultrasound:** Safe and painless diagnostic procedure that produces images of inside the body using sound waves. Can be used to diagnose early rheumatoid arthritis, inflammation, sprains, and tears.

Paging Dr. Terminology: Muscular Surgeries and Procedures

Now that your muscles have been poked, prodded, tested, and diagnosed, it's time to fix what's broken. Most of these procedures are surgical in nature.

TECHNICAL STUFF

Many surgeries are performed arthroscopically, through a scope inserted into or near a joint space, with one lone endoscope, *Palmar uniportal endoscopic carpal tunnel release*. This is also called a *Mirza technique*, an endoscopic method for release of carpal tunnel, previously accomplished by open surgery.

The surgical players are

- **Fasciectomy:** Excision of fascia (fibrous band or membrane of tissue surrounding muscle)
- **Fasciodesis:** Surgical fusion or binding of muscle fascia
- **Fasciotomy:** Surgical cutting into muscle fascia
- **Myolysis:** Surgical breaking down or separation of a muscle
- **Myoplasty:** Surgical repair of a muscle
- **Myorrhaphy:** Suturing of a muscle
- **Tenodesis:** Surgical fixation of a tendon
- **Tenomyoplasty:** Surgical repair of a tendon and muscle
- **Tenorrhaphy:** Suturing of a tendon
- **Tenotomy:** Incision of a tendon

It's All Related: More Muscular Terms

While the makeup of the muscular system is pretty straightforward, there are still all sorts of useful terms you need to know in order to communicate about your muscles. Try a few of the words from Table 13-3 on for size.

TABLE 13-3 **Common Muscular Vocabulary**

Word	What It Means
Articulation	Joint
Atrophy	Without development, wasting away of a muscle
Bradykinesia	Slow body movement
Diathermy	Heat applied to deep tissues
Dyskinesia	Difficult body movement
Dystrophy	Abnormal development
Fascia	Band of tissue surrounding muscle
Fasciitis	Inflammation of fascia
Hyperkinesia	Excessive body movement or overactivity
Kinesiology	The study of movement
Ligament	Binds bone to bone
Myalgia	Muscle pain
Myasthenia	Muscle weakness
Myoclonus	Muscle relaxation and contraction in rapid succession
Myology	The study of muscles
Myopathy	Any muscular disease
Myorrhexis	Rupture or breaking away of muscle tissue
Tendon	Connective tissue binding muscles to bones
Tenodynia	Pain in a tendon
Tenosynovitis	Inflammation of the tendon and synovial membrane

IN THIS CHAPTER

- Finding out how your integumentary system works
- Determining root words, prefixes, and suffixes appropriate to this system
- Using terminology of the integumentary system to discuss common conditions and diseases
- Discovering the right terms to use when diagnosing problems

Chapter 14

Skin Deep: Skin, Glands, Nails, and Hair

Your skin (the body's largest organ), glands, nails, and hair — also known as the *integumentary* system — serve as the "public face" of your body. Consider it your marketing team, letting the world know by their condition how healthy the rest of your body is. Healthy skin, along with accessory organs glands, hair, and nails, are the hallmarks of healthy insides, so care for them accordingly.

Layers of Skin

Like an onion, your skin has several layers, and there is much more to it than what you see with the naked eye. The skin is a system of specialized tissue, containing glands that secrete fluids, nerves that carry impulses, and blood vessels that assist in the regulation of body temperature.

Integumentum means "covering." This system is the body's covering, made up mostly of skin, but with the help of the accessory organs.

The skin has almost as many jobs as it has layers. The skin acts as a protective membrane that is a barrier against microorganisms, and it protects organs from injury. Skin helps maintain and regulate body temperature and acts as a receptor for sensation (hot, cold, touch, and pain). The skin helps rid the body of waste products. It also guards deeper tissues of the body against excessive loss of water, salts, and heat. Secretions from the skin are somewhat acidic in nature and contribute to its ability to fight off bacterial invasion.

The skin has the large responsibility of keeping you cool. The many different tissues in the skin help maintain the body temperature. Nerve fibers coordinate this *thermoregulation* by carrying messages to the skin from heat centers in the brain that are sensitive to changes in the body temperature. Nerve impulses cause blood vessels to dilate to bring blood to the surface where the heat can dissipate and cause sweat glands to produce the watery secretion that evaporates, thereby acting as your cooling system.

The skin is the most important player in the integumentary system, and is made up of three layers. The outer layer is the epidermis, a thin, cellular membrane layer. The second layer is the dermis, dense fibrous connective tissue. The third layer is the subcutaneous tissue, fat-containing tissue that joins the skin to underlying muscle.

The structure of skin varies throughout the body. It is stretchable and tough and has different thicknesses. It is thick on the palms of the hands and soles of the feet, but thin on the eyelids. The skin is initially firm and elastic, but with age, becomes wrinkled, drier, and saggy, especially around the eyes, mouth, and neck. The skin covering palms of the hand and soles of the feet is different from that covering the rest of the body. The skin on fingers and toes has patterns of ridges that never change and are unique for each individual, and, as you know from crime dramas, provide a basis for the use of fingerprints as a means of positive identification.

In addition, the skin has various colors and tones, which are all denoted with — surprise, surprise! — medical terms and roots. Table 14-1 gives you a quick look at what those colorful root words look like.

TABLE 14-1 Skin Color Root Words

Root Word	What It Means
Cyan/o	Blue
Erythr/o	Red
Leuk/o	White
Melan/o	Black
Xanth/o	Yellow

Epidermis

The *epidermis* is the outer, totally cellular layer of skin. It is composed of epithelium. *Epithelium* covers both internal and external surfaces of the body. The epidermis has no blood vessels, lymphatic vessels, connective tissue, cartilage, or fat. It depends on the deeper dermis, or corium, layer and its network of capillaries for nourishment. Oxygen and nutrients from the capillaries in the dermis pass through tissue fluid, supplying nourishment to the deeper levels of the epidermis.

The deepest layer of the epidermis is called the *basal layer.* Cells in the basal layer are always growing and multiplying. As the basal layer cells divide, they are pushed upwards and away from the blood supply of the dermis layer by a steady stream of younger cells. These cells shrink, lose their nuclei, die, and become filled with a hard protein called *keratin.* They are then called *horny cells,* reflecting their composition of keratin. Within a three-to-four week period after living as a basal cell in the deepest part of the epidermis, the horny keratinized cell is sloughed off from the surface of the skin. The epidermis, then, is constantly renewing itself.

Cells die at the same rate at which they are born. The basal layer of the epidermis contains cells called melanocytes. *Melanocytes* contain a black pigment called *melanin.* The amount of melanin accounts for the color differences in skin. Darker skin possesses more active melanocytes, not a greater number of melanocytes. Melanin in the epidermis is vital for protection against harmful ultraviolet radiation, which can manifest as skin cancers.

Individuals, who through a flaw in their chemical make-up are incapable of forming melanin, are called *albino,* meaning white. Their skin and hair are white and their eyes are red (because of the absence of pigment, the tiny blood vessels are visible in the iris).

Dermis

The *dermis,* the second layer, below the epidermis, is also called the *corium.* The dermis differs from the epidermis in that it is living tissue composed of blood, lymph vessels, and nerve fibers, as well as the accessory organs of the skin. These accessories include the hair follicles, sweat glands, and oil glands.

To support this system of nerves, vessels, and glands, the dermis contains connective tissue cells and fibers. The dermis is composed of different types of connective tissue cells: fibroblasts, histiocytes, and mast cells. *Fibroblast* cells act to repair an injury to the skin. *Histiocytes* protect the body by surrounding foreign materials. *Mast cells* contain histamine, a substance released in allergies that causes itching.

Fibers in the dermis are composed of collagen. *Collagen,* meaning "glue," is a fibrous protein material found in bone, cartilage, tendons, and ligaments as well as the skin. It is tough, but also flexible. In an infant, collagen is loose and delicate but it becomes harder as the body ages. Collagen fibers support and protect the blood and nerve networks that pass through the dermis.

TECHNICAL STUFF

Hair shafts in the dermis have bundles of involuntary muscle called *arrector pili* attached to hair follicles. When you are frightened or cold, these muscles contract, the hair stands up, and "goosebumps" appear on the skin.

Subcutaneous layer

The subcutaneous layer of the skin is made up of connective tissue that specializes in the formation of fat. *Lipocytes,* plentiful in the subcutaneous layer, manufacture and store large amounts of fat. Areas of the body vary as far as fat deposition is concerned. This layer of skin is important in protecting deeper tissues of the body and also acts as a heat insulator. The subcutaneous layer connects the dermis to the muscles and organs below it. Its fat tissue insulates inner structures from temperature extremes.

Glands, Both Sebaceous and Sudoriferous

The skin has two types of glands that, as accessory organs, produce important secretions. These glands under the skin's surface are called the sebaceous (oil) glands and the sudoriferous (sweat) glands.

The *sebaceous* glands produce an oily secretion called *sebum*, whereas the *sudoriferous* glands produce a watery secretion called *sweat*. Sebum and sweat are carried to the outer edges of the skin by ducts and excreted through openings in the skin called *pores*. Sebum helps lubricate the skin. Sebaceous glands are closely associated with hair follicles, and their ducts open into the hair follicle through which the sebum is released.

Sebaceous glands are influenced by sex hormones. This causes them to be overactive at puberty and underactive in old age. This explains the excess oil production of the skin at puberty and gradual drying of the skin as we age.

Sudoriferous (sweat) glands are tiny coiled glands found on almost all body surfaces. You have about 2 million of them in your body. There are many more in the palms of the hands, and you'd find approximately 3,000 glands per square inch on the sole of your foot. The tiny openings on the surface are called *pores*. Sweat helps cool the body as it evaporates from the skin surface. Nerve fibers under the skin detect pain, temperature, pressure, and touch. The adjustment of the body to its environment depends on the sensory messages relayed to the brain and spinal cord by the sensitive nerve endings in the skin.

Diaphoresis comes from the Greek *dia*, meaning "through," and *phoreo*, meaning "I carry." Translated, it means "the carrying through of perspiration."

Figure 14-1 illustrates the layers of the skin and some of its structures.

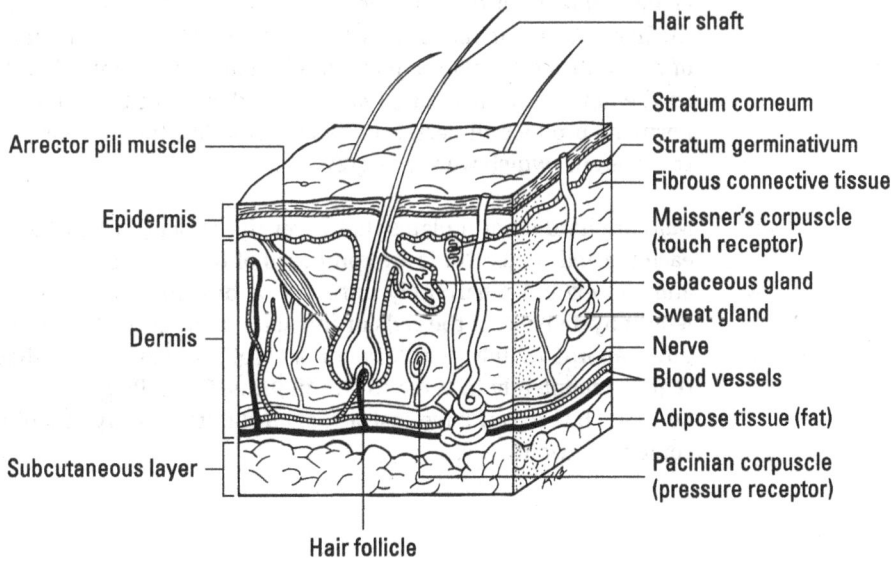

FIGURE 14-1: Cross section of the skin showing layers and some specialized structures.

Illustration by Kathryn Born

STINKING IT UP: YOUR SWEAT GLANDS

Sweat gets a bad rap for being smelly when, in fact, it's not your fault. Your body's smell is caused by bacteria. Sweat or perspiration is almost pure water, with dissolved materials such as salt making up less than 1 percent of its total composition. Sweat is actually colorless and odorless. The odor produced when sweat accumulates is due to the action of bacteria on it.

Certain sweat glands, active only from puberty onward and larger than ordinary sweat glands, are concentrated near the reproductive organs and in the *axillae* (armpits). These glands secrete an odorless sweat that contains substances that are easily broken down by skin bacteria. The breakdown products are responsible for the characteristic "human body odor." So the next time someone tells you your sweat stinks, you can say, "I beg to differ. My bacteria are the culprits."

The *ceruminous glands* are classified as modified sweat glands and are found in the ear canal. These glands produce a yellow waxy substance called *cerumen* (ear wax).

Hair and Nails

A *hair fiber* is composed of a network of horny cells (hold your giggles, please) filled with hard protein called *keratin*. Hair growth is similar to the growth of the epidermal layer of the skin. Deep-lying cells in hair roots move forward through the hair *follicles*, or shafts, that hold the hair fiber. *Melanocytes* located at the root of hair follicles supply the melanin pigment for the hair fiber. Hair color depends on the amount of melanin present, as it does with the color of the skin. Because hormone production decreases as we get older, the hair loses color and becomes transparent (which we see as gray).

Nails are hard keratin plates that cover the *dorsal* (top) surface of the last bone of each toe and finger. Nails are composed of horny cells that are cemented together and can extend indefinitely until cut or broken. A nail grows in thickness and length by division of the cells of the nerve root, at the base of the nail plate. Nails grow approximately 1 millimeter a week, which means that fingernails may regrow completely in three to five months. Toenails grow more slowly than fingernails, but if you have lost a toenail due to a nasty stubbing incident, it will come back eventually.

Integumentary Root Words

Now that you've gotten to know the specific parts of the integumentary system a bit better, it's time to put your expertise into practice by tracking down the meaning of root words and checking out their useful applications. The roots are essential medical terminology knowledge, because once you master these roots (good ol' Greek and Latin ones, that is), you can break down any hair/skin/nail/gland-related word and discover its meaning. Table 14-2 lists integumentary root words.

TABLE 14-2 **Breaking Down Your Integumentary Roots**

Root Word	What It Means
Aden/o	Gland
Adip/o	Fat
Albin/o	White
Aut/o	Self
Bi/o	Life
Blephar/o	Eyelid
Carcin/o	Carcinoma (cancer)
Cutane/o	Skin
Cry/o	Cold
Cyan/o	Blue
Derm/o, Derm/a, Dermat/o	Skin
Diaphor/o	Profuse sweating
Erythem/o	Red
Hidr/o	Sweat
Histi/o	Tissue
Icthy/o	Dry, scaly
Kerat/o	Hard, horny
Leuk/o	White
Lip/o, Lipid/o	Fat
Melan/o	Black

(continued)

TABLE 14-2 *(continued)*

Root Word	What It Means
Myc/o	Fungus
Necr/o	Death (cell or body)
Onych/o	Nail
Papill/o	Nipplelike
Papul/o	Papule, pimple
Pil/o	Hair
Py/o	Pus
Rhytid/o	Wrinkle
Sclera/o	Hardening
Seb/o	Sebum (fat)
Squam/o	Scale
Steat/o	Fat, sebum
Sud/o, sudor/o	Sweat
Trich/o	Hair
Ungu/o	Nails
Xer/o	Dry
Xanth/o	Yellow

TIP

Herpes comes from the Greek word *herpo*, meaning "to creep along." It is descriptive of the course and type of skin lesion as with herpes zoster (shingles).

Table 14-3 lists prefixes and suffixes pertaining to your hair, nails, skin, and glands.

TABLE 14-3 **Common Integumentary Prefixes and Suffixes**

Prefix	What It Means
Epi-	On, over, upon
Para-	Beside, beyond, around
Per	Through
Sub-	Under, below

Suffix	What It Means
-itis	Inflammation
-malacia	Softening
-opsy	View of, viewing
-orrhea	Flow, excessive discharge
-phagia	Eating or swallowing
-plasty	Surgical repair

Common Integumentary Conditions

Of all the conditions that plague the integumentary system, ones affecting the skin tend to be the most obvious and troublesome. From that odd, discolored freckle on your arm to run-of-the-mill acne, the list of unsavory and often embarrassing lesions is long. Take a look:

- **Acne:** Inflammatory pustular eruption of skin (*acne vulgaris* is the common variety)
- **Bulla:** Large vesicle or blister (plural: *bullae*), also called a bleb
- **Carbuncle:** A pyogenic (pus) infection of the skin usually arising from a hair follicle, causing a tender, pus-filled lump
- **Comedo:** Common blackhead caused by a buildup of sebum and keratin in a skin pore (plural: *comedones*)
- **Cyst:** Small sac or pouch containing fluid or semisolid fluid
- **Decubitus ulcer:** Bedsore
- **Fissure:** Groove or cracklike sore
- **Furuncle:** Similar to a carbuncle (commonly called a "boil")
- **Lichen planus:** Common skin disease with eruptions on skin and in mouth — and affecting appearance of finger and toenails
- **Macule:** A discolored lesion that lies flush with the skin (freckles, tattoo marks, and moles)
- **Papule:** Solid elevation of the skin
- **Polyp:** Mushroomlike growth extending on a stalk
- **Pustule:** Discrete raised area of pus on the skin

- **Ulcer:** Open sore or erosion of the skin
- **Vesicle:** Collection of clear fluid (blister)
- **Wheal:** Smooth elevated area that is red and itchy (such as *hives*).

Lesions aren't alone, though. A host of conditions affect the entire integumentary system. The majority of them, however, still affect the skin more than other parts of the system:

- **Alopecia:** Hair loss. Can result normally from aging process or be drug or illness induced
- **Cicatrix:** Scar left by a healed wound
- **Ecchymosis:** Purplish macular bruise, caused by hemorrhage into the skin
- **Keloid:** Abnormally raised, thickened scar
- **Petechia:** Small pinpoint hemorrhage (plural: *petechiae*)
- **Pruritus:** Itching, associated with forms of *dermatitis*
- **Purpura:** Merging ecchymoses with petechiae
- **Urticaria:** Hives with localized swelling with itching
- **Vitiligo:** Loss of pigment in area of skin or milk-white patch

Another important one is *burn:* injury to tissues caused by heat, flame, electricity, chemicals, or radiation contact. A *first-degree burn* is superficial with no blister and superficial damage in epidermis. A *second-degree burn*, or *partial thickness burn*, blisters and causes damage to epidermis and dermis. A *third-degree burn* is full-thickness, damaging the epidermis, dermis, and subcutaneous layer.

Finding the Culprit: Integumentary Diseases and Pathology

Once again, the skin is the major player when it comes to ailments. Surely the hair, nails, and glands won't feel too left out of this motley group of pathological conditions and diseases. These pathological conditions include the following:

- **Acne:** Inflammatory pustular eruption of skin (*acne vulgaris* is the common variety)
- **Athlete's foot:** Ringworm of the foot *(tinea pedis)* — a fungal infection with scaling and itching of the skin of the foot

- **Cutis laxa:** Rare connective tissue disorder — skin becomes very lax and hangs loosely in folds
- **Diaper rash:** Diaper dermatitis — red, shiny rash not caused by the diaper but by what is collected in the diaper (feces)
- **Ecthyma**: Ulcerative skin condition caused by bacteria, often from an insect bite
- **Eczema:** Inflammatory skin disease with reddened papular lesions; a common allergic reaction in children
- **Erysipelas:** Acute infection of upper dermis usually caused by streptococcus bacteria (Greek — erisipeles — "red skin")
- **Gangrene:** Death of tissue associated with loss of blood supply
- **Ichthyosis vulgaris:** Disorder of the skin causing dry, scaly skin; usually inherited
- **Impetigo:** Bacterial inflammatory skin disease presenting with vesicles, pustules, and crusted lesions; caused by bacteria
- **Melasma:** "Mask of pregnancy" tan or dark skin discoloration, hormone-related condition causing stimulation of melanocytes
- **Necrotizing Fasciitis:** Rare infection of the deep layers of the skin (also known as "flesh-eating disease")
- **Pemphigoid:** Rare autoimmune skin blistering disease, most common in women over 60
- **Pityriasis Rosea:** Common benign skin rash that is uncomfortable and lasts from six to eight weeks, not fungal and not allergenic
- **Psoriasis:** Chronic (ongoing) skin ailment with silver-gray scales covering red patches
- **Rosacea:** Chronic vascular dilatation of skin on nose and cheeks with papules and pustules
- **Roseola:** *(exanthema subitum)* Sudden rash (also called rose rash of infants); also known as *sixth disease* because it is the sixth rash-causing childhood disease
- **Scabies:** (known as the seven-year itch) Contagious skin infection caused by the mite *Sarcoptes scabiei* burrowing under the skin
- **Scleroderma:** Disorder affecting all connective tissue that causes abnormal tissue thickening usually on fingers, hands, or face
- **Telangiectasis:** Dilatation of small capillaries on the skin
- **Tinea:** Infection of the skin caused by a fungus (ringworm)

TECHNICAL STUFF

Scabies is a very common skin disorder, especially in children. It is estimated to affect 1.5 percent of the world's population.

There are also viral diseases that result in eruptions of skin from the infection. These include

- **Molluscum contagiosum:** "Water warts"
- **Rubella:** German measles
- **Rubeola:** Measles
- **Varicella:** Chickenpox

Sometimes, the skin experiences skin *neoplasms*, also known as "new growth." These are often benign and can include the following:

- **Hemangioma:** A cluster of blood vessels that make an abnormal but benign growth, often protruding from the skin; some birthmarks are hemangiomas
- **Keratosis:** Thickened area of the epidermis (wart, callus)
- **Nevus:** Mole (plural: *nevi*)
- **Seborrheic keratosis:** Thick, flattened, beige/brown plaques that appear commonly on hands and face with age; sometimes called senile warts.
- **Verruca:** Warts

Unfortunately, the news from the dermatologist can often be serious enough to warrant further testing and may involve the "Big C" — cancer. *Basal cell carcinoma*, for example, is a malignant tumor of the basal cell layer of epidermis. It is the most common type of skin cancer and is slow growing, usually occurring on the upper half of the face near the nose. It does not spread. *Squamous cell carcinoma* is a malignant tumor of the *squamous epithelial* cells of the epidermis. This tumor may arise from actinic or sun-related keratoses and may metastasize to lymph nodes. *Merkel cell (aka trabecular or neuroendocrine) carcinoma* is a rare skin cancer on or just beneath the skin. It is flesh colored or bluish-red in color and is most commonly found in Caucasian people between the ages of 40 to 60.

Malignant melanoma is a cancerous tumor composed of melanocytes. Tumors often metastasize or spread to liver, lung, and brain. Finally, *mycoses fungoides* is a rare chronic skin disease caused by the infiltration of malignant *lymphocytes*. It is characterized by large red raised areas that spread and ulcerate; malignant cells may involve lymph nodes.

TECHNICAL STUFF

Breslow's depth — a classification or staging of a malignant melanoma to determine the prognosis factor, measuring the depth of invasion — is named after Dr. Alexander Breslow, an American pathologist. This classification is now included in the AJCC (American Joint Committee on Cancer) guidelines for melanoma treatment.

Testing, Testing: Integumentary Radiology and Diagnostic Tests

There are two major ways that dermatologists and their colleagues diagnose issues with the integumentary system by taking a tissue sample from the body. These two types of tests involve the winning combination of bacteria and fungus. Bacterial analysis and fungal testing are laboratory tests in which the doctor takes cultures or swabs and then examines them in the lab.

- **Bacterial analysis** is performed by taking a sample of a purulent or pus-filled material or exudates (fluid that accumulates in the space or passes out of tissue). The sample is then sent for examination to determine what type of bacteria is present.
- **Fungal testing** occurs when scrapings from skin lesion are placed on a growth medium for several weeks and then examined for evidence of fungal growth.

Paging Dr. Terminology: Integumentary Surgeries and Procedures

Many of the more common, everyday integumentary conditions can be fixed or improved via in-office or outpatient procedures. These procedures aren't necessarily pretty, but they sure do get the job done. They are as follows:

- **Debridement** is the removal of dirt, foreign material, or damaged tissue from a wound to prevent infection and promote healing.
- **Incision and drainage** involve cutting open a lesion such as an abscess to remove or drain contents.
- **Intradermal test** is performed by injection of a reactive substance between layers of the skin to observe for a reaction. This test is used to detect sensitivity

to infectious agents such as *tuberculosis* (the Mantoux test) or PPD (purified protein derivative) test, or the test for diphtheria (the Schick test). Strong reactions indicate ongoing infection, or previous exposure.

- **Patch skin test** is performed by applying a piece of gauze or paper to the skin, on which has been placed an allergy-causing substance. If area becomes red and swollen, the result is positive.
- **Punch biopsy** is used to obtain tissue in cases in which complete excision is not necessary or possible. Involves using a surgical instrument that removes a core of tissue by rotation of its sharp edge.
- **Sclerotherapy** is used in the treatment of varicose veins. Injecting the vein with a *sclerosing solution* irritates the tissue, causes swelling, and closes off the vein.
- **Skin biopsy** is removal of living tissue for microscopic examination. Skin lesions that might be in danger of producing a malignant change are removed and sent for pathologic examination.
- **Skin scratch test** involves making several scratches in the skin and injecting a very minimal amount of test material into the scratches; a test is considered negative if no reaction occurs.

We Americans are a vain people, no doubt. Cosmetic surgery is practically a pastime in the United States. But consider that this type of surgical procedure can be about more than looking and feeling younger. Cosmetic surgery is a vital field that helps people recover from all sorts of serious wounds. For example, cosmetic surgery helps the person with the scarred face caused in an auto accident, the woman mourning the loss of a breast to cancer, or the child born with a facial deformity. The following includes both surgical and non-invasive procedures, to complete the plastic/cosmetic picture:

- **Abdominoplasty** is a surgical "tummy-tuck."
- **Blepharoplasty** is surgical reduction of the upper and lower eyelids.
- **Brachioplasty** is surgical removal of excessive, aging skin from the upper arms (also known as "bingo wings" surgery).
- **CoolSculpting** is a non-invasive procedure similar to liposuction where fat cells are frozen, liquefied, picked up by the circulatory system, and eliminated.
- **Cryotherapy** involves destruction of tissue by freezing with liquid nitrogen.
- **Dermabrasion** means scraping away of the top layer of skin using sandpaper or wire brushes to remove tattoos or disfigured skin.

- **Dermatoplasty** is surgical reconstruction of the skin. Typically, the surgical replacement of injured or diseased skin.
- **Electrolysis** is destruction of tissue by electricity and is used to remove unwanted body hair.
- **Face lift, non-surgical** is a non-invasive procedure using one or a combination of dermal fillers, Botox, and chemical facial peels to enhance and improve the appearance of facial skin.
- **Laser therapy** involves removal of skin lesions such as *papillomas* and *hemangiomas* using an intense beam of light. This can also be used to remove tattoos or warts from around the nails or on the soles of feet.
- **Laser hair removal therapy** destroys the base of a hair follicle (the source of new growth).
- **Liposuction** is surgical removal of fat from subcutaneous tissue by means of suction.
- **Lipotripsy** is a non-invasive method to treat arms, legs, and abdomen by stimulating fat breakdown and collagen synthesis.
- **Rhytidectomy** means removal of wrinkles by removal of excess facial skin. Also known as a facelift.

More Integumentary Terms

The integumentary system involves many different components that are not necessarily outwardly similar, from skin and hair to nails and glands. As such, there are tons of vocabulary words for this system. Table 14-4 shows a sampling.

TABLE 14-4 Common Integumentary Vocabulary

Word	What It Means
Abrasion	Scraping away of superficial layer of injured skin
Adenoma	Glandular tumor
Albinism	Lack of pigment in skin, hair, and eyes
Albino	Person with skin deficient in pigment or melanin
Adipose	Pertaining to fat

(continued)

TABLE 14-4 *(continued)*

Word	What It Means
Anhidrosis	Lack of sweat
Collagen	Structural protein found in skin and connective tissues
Cuticle	Band of epidermis extending from nail wall to nail surface
Dermatitis	Inflammation of the skin
Dermatologist	Physician who specializes in skin and its diseases
Dermatology	Study of the skin and its diseases
Diaphoresis	Profuse sweating
Epithelium	Layer of skin forming the outer and inner surfaces of body
Erythema	Red discoloration of the skin
Histiotoma	Fatty tumor of sebaceous gland
Hypodermic	Under the skin
Hyperhidrosis	Excessive secretion of sweat
Hyperkeratosis	Excessive growth of the outer layer of skin
Keratin	Hard protein material found in epidermis, hair, and nails
Lipocyte	Fat cell
Lipoma	Tissue or mass containing fat
Lunula	The half-moon shaped white area at base of the nail
Melanin	Black pigment formed by melanocytes
Onychomycosis	Fungal infection of nail
Pyogenic	Pus forming, or related to pus formation
Seborrhea	Increased discharge of sebum from glands

IN THIS CHAPTER

- Seeing how your sensory system works
- Ferreting out root words, prefixes, and suffixes appropriate to this system
- Using terminology of the sensory system to discuss common conditions and diseases
- Sensing the right terms to use when diagnosing problems

Chapter 15

It Depends on Your Perception: The Sensory Systems

You can thank your sensory systems for all the fun you get to have in life. While your other, also very important, systems handle the background work that keeps you running, the senses let your body have a little fun. What you see, hear, smell, touch, and taste makes life the enjoyable experience it is. So the next time you're smelling some truly fantastic barbecue or watching a dazzling fireworks display, be grateful for your senses.

The Eye

For humans, the eye is the most important sense organ — the Big Kahuna of the senses. Sight provides the most information for us, for what we see, of course, but that includes what we can read. The eye is located in the *orbit* (the bony protective cavity of the skull). The eye lets light in, focuses it, transforms it into nerve impulses, and sends these impulses to the brain.

Here's how: Light rays enter the eye via an adjustable opening, the dark center of the eye, called the *pupil*, which regulates the amount of light allowed in. Behind the pupil is the *lens*, which focuses the light. The lens is not rigid and it can adjust its shape in order to adapt to near and far objects. The light is focused by the lens into the back of the eye, where it strikes the *retina*. The retina transforms the focused image into nerve impulses that travel along the optic nerve to the *occipital lobe* of the brain for processing.

Figure 15-1 gives you a peek inside the eye.

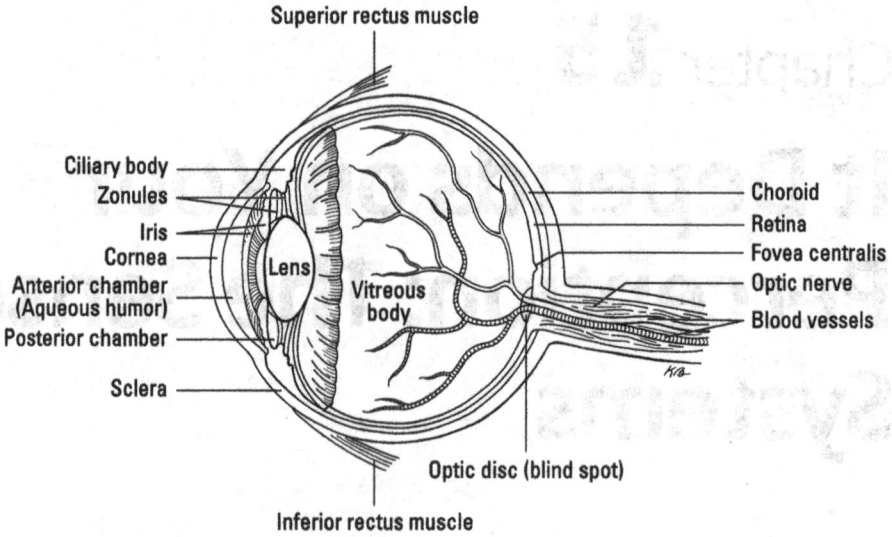

FIGURE 15-1: Internal structures of the eye.

Illustration by Kathryn Born

The eye consists of the *inner eye* (the eyeball) and the *outer eye* (the facial structures and eye muscles surrounding the eye).

Inner eye

The inner eye is made up of three layers.

The outer layer contains the cornea and the sclera. The *cornea* is the transparent anterior portion of the eye. It allows light in and aids in the focusing of light onto the back of the eye. The *sclera* is the white of the eye, providing a protective covering for the eyeball.

EYE LIKE IT SHORT

Here are some common abbreviations for the eye. You might hear these in conversation or see them on medical charts.

- **OD:** Right eye (oculus dexter)
- **OS:** Left eye (oculus sinister)
- **OU:** Each eye (oculus uterque)
- **PERRLA:** Pupils equal, round, and reactive to light and accommodation
- **VA:** Visual acuity
- **VF:** Visual field

The middle layer, the *uvea,* consists of the choroids, the ciliary body, and the iris. The *choroids,* the inner lining of the sclera, contain blood vessels that nourish the eye. The *ciliary body* consists of the ciliary muscles and the ciliary process. The muscles adjust the shape of the lens for focusing, and the process produces a watery substance, *aqueous humor,* bathing the anterior region of the eye. The *iris* is the circular colored portion of the eye. The opening in the iris, the pupil, regulates the amount of light that enters the eye. In bright light, muscle fibers in the iris contract the pupil. These muscles relax in dimmer light, and the pupil resumes its normal size. Radial muscles in the iris enlarge the pupil beyond normal size when a person is stressed or excited, called *dilation.*

The inner layer is the *retina,* which has layers of nervous tissue called *cones* and *rods.* Each of your eyes has approximately 6 million cones and 120 million rods in the retina. The cones are more sensitive in light than the rods. Color and sharpness of vision depend on the cone cells. Rods function better in dim light and are helpful in night vision. One small area of the retina has no cones or rods and doesn't produce a visual image. Called the *optic disc* or *blind spot,* it's the entry point for the major blood vessels of the eye and where the optic nerve crosses from the brain into the eye.

In front of and in back of the lens are two cavities. The *anterior (front) cavity* contains *aqueous humor* produced by the ciliary processes. This watery fluid flows freely from the posterior chamber, through the pupil, to the anterior chamber. Inability to drain aqueous humor causes increased *intraocular pressure.* This condition, known as *glaucoma,* can result in blindness because of damage caused to the retina and optic nerve, by the extra pressure. Equal production and drainage maintains the equilibrium of the intraocular pressure. The *posterior (back) cavity* of the eye is filled with clear, jellylike material called *vitreous humor.* This preserves the spherical shape of the eyeball, holding the retina firmly against the choroid. Both the aqueous and vitreous humors function to further refract light rays.

CHECK YOUR LENSES

As light passes through the lens of the eye, the light is bent in a process called *refraction*. The refracted light must be focused on the retina for a clear image. In order to focus light, the lens changes shape. The ciliary muscles change its shape to allow for clear vision of far and near objects. This lens changing is called *accommodation*. When a person reaches his or her 40s, the lens loses some of its elasticity, causing difficulty focusing light from near objects. Reading glasses provide the refraction that the lens can no longer perform. The lens loses its transparent quality with age, becoming thick and dense and sometimes opaque and cloudy and interfering with the refraction of light rays. This results in a common condition, cataracts. Cataracts, once a leading cause of serious vision loss, are now routinely removed surgically.

Outer eye

The outer eye consists of the orbital cavity, the ocular muscles, the eyelids, conjunctival membrane, and lacrimal apparatus. The *orbital cavity* is the bony depression that the eyeball fits. *Ocular muscles* attach to the sclera and move the eye. *Eyelids* shield the eye from light, dust, and trauma. The *conjunctival membrane* lining the eyelids and the anterior part of the eye exposed to the air provides protection and lubrication.

The *lacrimal apparatus* produces, delivers, and drains tears from the eye, providing cleaning and lubricating. The *lacrimal glands* produce the tears, which are continuously delivered to the eyes by the *lacrimal ducts*. Small openings called *punctae* drain tears from the eyes into channels in the nose. This is the reason you nose runs when you cry. Tears clean and lubricate the eye as well as fight infectious microorganisms.

Cataract comes from the Greek *kato*, meaning "down," and *raktos*, meaning "precipice." Combined, they can be interpreted as "waterfall." Through a cataract, sight is like a waterfall or misty. *Glaucoma* — Greek *glaukos* — means "blue-grey," and *oma* means "a condition." In glaucoma, a gray color replaces the black pupil.

The Ear

The ear has two functions: to hear and to help provide the body's balance or equilibrium. We can hear because sound waves vibrate through the ear where they are transformed into nerve impulses that are then carried to the brain. The sensations of sound are heard within the nerve fibers of the cerebral cortex.

Figure 15-2 shows the different parts of the ear.

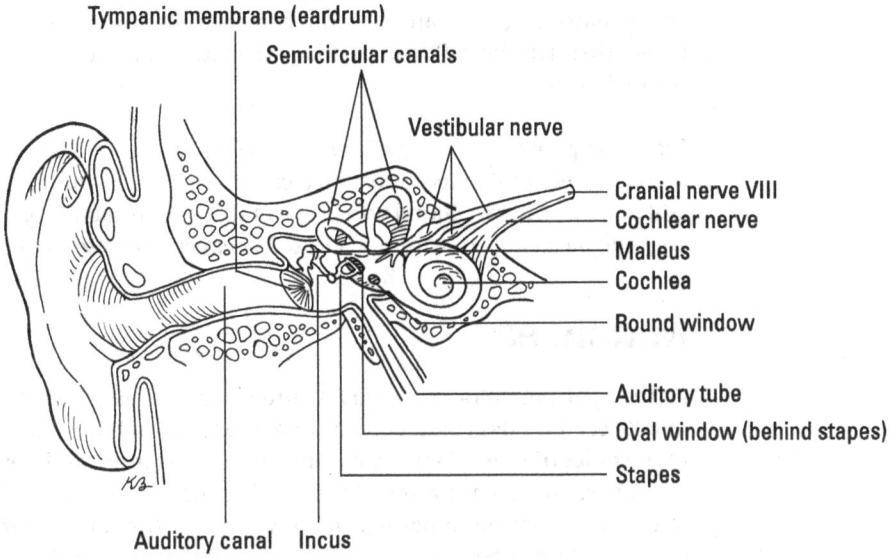

FIGURE 15-2: Anatomy of the ear.

Illustration by Kathryn Born

The ear is divided into three separate regions: the outer, middle, and inner ear. The outer and middle ears look after the conduction of sound waves through the ear. The inner ear contains the structures that carry the waves to the brain.

THE SHORT VERSION OF YOUR EARS

Some of the most common ear-related abbreviations include

- **AC:** Air conduction
- **AD:** Right ear (auris dextra)
- **AS:** Left ear (auris sinistra)
- **AU:** Both ears (aures unitas)
- **BC:** Bone conduction
- **HD:** Hearing distance
- **ENT:** Ear, nose, and throat
- **OM:** Otitis media

Outer ear

Sound waves are encouraged toward the ear canal by the *auricle*, or *pinna*, the visible outer ear, the hard, arching cartilage that forms the outer ear curve, the *tragus*, that hard little flap of cartilage that sticks out in front of the ear canal, and the earlobe.

From the pinna, the *external auditory meatus* is lined with numerous glands that secrete a yellowish waxy substance called *cerumen*. Cerumen (earwax) lubricates and protects the ear. Sound waves travel through the auditory canal and strike the *tympanic membrane* or *eardrum*, located between the outer and middle ear.

Middle ear

As the eardrum vibrates, it moves three small bones or *ossicles* that make up the middle ear. Ossicles conduct the sound waves through the middle ear. These bones in the order of their vibration are the *malleus*, the *incus*, and the *stapes*. As the stapes moves, it touches a membrane called the *oval window*, which separates the middle ear from the inner ear. Another part of the middle ear is the *auditory* or *eustachian tube*, a canal leading from the middle ear to the pharynx. The eustachian tube equalizes air pressure on both sides of the eardrum.

Inner ear

The inner ear is also called the *labyrinth* because of its circular, mazelike structure. The part of the labyrinth that leads from the oval window is a bony, snail-shaped structure called the *cochlea*. The cochlea contains auditory liquids that the vibrations travel through. In the cochlea is a sensitive auditory receptor called the *organ of Corti*. Tiny hair cells in the organ of Corti receive vibrations from the auditory liquids and relay the sound waves to auditory nerve fibers, which end in the auditory center of the cerebral cortex. It is there that these impulses are interpreted and "heard."

Tympanic membrane comes from the Greek *tympanon*, meaning "drum," because it resembles a drum (hence *eardrum*). *Stapes*, Latin for "stirrup," was named, not surprisingly, for its stirrup like shape.

The ear is also an organ of *equilibrium* or balance. The three organs within the inner ear responsible for equilibrium are the *semicircular canals*, the *saccule*, and *utricle*. These organs contain a fluid called *endolymph*, as well as sensitive hair cells. The fluid and hair cells fluctuate with movement of the head and transmit impulses in nerve fibers leading to the brain. Messages are then sent to muscles throughout the body so that equilibrium (balance) is maintained.

DEMYSTIFYING DEAFNESS

Deafness is diminished or total loss of hearing, and there are two types.

Conductive hearing loss is caused by obstruction of the path travelled by the sound waves from the external ear to the inner ear. Examples could be build-up of earwax (cerumen), or a foreign body lodged in the external auditory meatus. Conductive deafness can be treated by removal of the obstruction.

Sensorineural deafness results from the damage to the auditory nerve or cochlea, preventing nerve stimuli from reaching the brain from the inner ear. This can occur with age but also can be caused by loud noises from machinery, music, tremors, infection, or injury. Hearing aids can help in treating sensorineural deafness. However, if a hearing aid is not successful, cochlear implants may be needed to have hearing restored.

The Nose

Our sense of smell, though not as important to humans as it is to animals, basically performs the same purpose. An animal's sense of smell is acute, as it warns of danger and acts as a guide in finding food. We aren't so different, more in degree than in kind — we can smell smoke before we see fire, and we all know about smelling good food.

The *olfactory epithelium* of the nose is the organ of smell. Olfactory (*olfact* refers to smell) receptors in the *root* (area between eyes) of the nose are stimulated by odor, and chemical messages are transmitted to the *olfactory bulb* and sent to the olfactory centers of the brain. We can smell six basic odors: fruity, flowery, spicy, burned, putrid, and resin. The sense of smell acts to complement the taste sense, which is why a clogged nose with a head cold interferes with smelling, and food loses its flavors.

Because this chapter is about the special senses, we're really dealing with the nose's sense of smell. The mucus, hairs, and septum (the part separating the nostrils) have nothing to do with smelling. But, if you're so inclined to know more about them, check out Chapter 17.

TECHNICAL STUFF

You have 60 million olfactory epithelium cells in your nose. Way to go!

The Mouth

The organs of taste are the *taste buds*, found on the tongue and in the mucous membranes lining the soft palate of the mouth.

We can distinguish only four primary tastes: sweet, sour, salty, and bitter; the variety of tastes we experience are mixtures of the four, much as the colors we see are mixtures of the three primary colors. For food to initiate the sensation of taste, it must be dissolved by saliva, which is why taste buds are in a moist area. Much that we think we taste is really smelled, and the taste depends on the odor. Our senses of taste and smell work together in this way.

TECHNICAL STUFF

You have 10,000 taste bud *papillae* on surface of your tongue.

The Touch Receptor

The skin (the body's largest organ) is our only *touch receptor*. Touch sensation, often referred to as *light pressure*, varies in different parts of the body. The sensitive areas are those that provide the most information about ourselves and the external environment. Lips and fingers have the most receptors, in a concentrated area, which is why we use them more than, say, our elbows, to touch and identify objects.

The *dermis* of the skin has nerve endings that act as the receptors. They sense hot and cold, pain, pressure, and touch. The nervous system carries messages to the brain when changes to temperature, injury, or pressure occurs. For more information on your skin, see Chapter 14.

Sensory Root Words

Get ready. The sensory systems use a *lot* of root words, prefixes, and suffixes, and with good reason. Consider that this set of systems includes some delicate and sophisticated body parts: eyes, ears, nose, mouth, and skin. It's no wonder that we need a lot of combining forms and roots to fully describe the wonders of the senses.

We'll start small with taste, smell, and touch in Table 15-1. Then you can move on to the eyes and ears, which are slightly more complicated.

TABLE 15-1

Forms of Taste, Smell, and Touch

Word or Word Part	What It Means
A- or an-	Without, or lack of
Dys-	Difficult or uncomfortable
Geusia	Taste
Hyper-	Excess — more than normal
Hypo-	Less than normal
-itis	Inflammation
Osmia	Smell

See, that wasn't so hard! Now that you have your feet wet (or nose, as it may be), you can move on to the eye, which has about a gazillion (okay, maybe that's an exaggeration) root words and combining forms. Check it out in Table 15-2.

TABLE 15-2

Visual Roots

Root Word	What It Means
Aque/o	Water
Blephar/o	Eyelid
Conjunctiv/o	Conjunctiva (membrane lining eyelids)
Core/o, cor/o	Pupil
Corne/o	Cornea
Dacry/o	Tear, tear duct
Dipl/o	Double
Emmetr/o	In due measure
Glauc/o	Gray
Ir/o, irid/o	Iris (colored portion of the eye)
Is/o	Equal
Kerat/o	Cornea
Lacrim/o	Tear, tear duct
Logad/o	White of the eye
Mi/o	Smaller, les

(continued)

TABLE 15-2 *(continued)*

Root Word	What It Means
Mydri/o	Wide
Ocul/o	Eye
Ophry/o	Eyebrow
Ophthalm/o	Eye (ophthalmologist, specialist in eye disorders)
Opt/o	Eye, vision
Phac/o, phak/o	Crystalline lens
Phot/o	Light
Presby/o	Old age
Pupill/o	Pupil
Retin/o	Retina
Scler/o	Sclera (white of the eye)
Uve/o	Iris, ciliary body, and choroids
Vitre/o	Glassy
Xer/o	Dry

A prefix and a few suffixes associated with sight include the ones in Table 15-3.

TABLE 15-3

Visual Prefix and Suffixes

Prefix or Suffix	What It Means
Bi- or bin-	Two
-chalasis	Relaxation
-ician	One who
-metrist	Specialist in the measurement of
-opia or -opsia	Vision (condition)
-ory	Pertaining to
-oscopy	Visual examination of internal cavity using a scope
-plasty	Surgical repair or reconstruction
-tropia	To turn

The labyrinth of your ear is a complicated place with twists, turns, and many working parts. As such, medical professionals have a lot of words to use when describing what goes on in there. Thankfully, though, the list of root words and suffixes (no prefixes here) is fairly compact. Listen up to Tables 15-4 and 15-5.

TABLE 15-4

Listening to Your Roots

Root Word	What It Means
Acous/o, Acou/o, Acoust/o	Hearing
Audi/o, Audit/o	Hearing
Aur/o, Aur/i	Ear
Bar/o	Pressure, weight
Cerumin/o	Cerumen (earwax)
Cochle/o	Cochlea
Mastoid/o	Mastoid process (process of temporal bone behind the ear)
Myring/o	Eardrum, tympanic membrane
Ot/o	Ear
Son/o	Sound
Staped/o	Stapes (third ossicle of middle ear)
Tympan/o	Eardrum, middle ear

Strangely, as we mention, there really aren't any ear-related prefixes to discuss. There are, however, several suffixes to keep you busy in Table 15-5.

TABLE 15-5

Hearing Suffixes

Suffix	What It Means
-cusis	Hearing
-gram	Record
-itis	Inflammation
-metry	Process of measuring
-otomy	Process of cutting into
-phonia	Sound
-rrhea	Discharge or flow
-scope	Instrument used to visually examine

It's All Related: More Anatomical Terms

Holy lists and sidebars, Batman! As you can see, this chapter is chock-full of words you need to know about the senses. What can you say? There is a lot of ground to cover with these, but very important, parts of your body. Just the eye alone gets its own list of extra vocabulary words here (see Table 15-6). Get your flashcards and markers ready to rock.

TABLE 15-6

Sight Words, Literally

Word	What It Means
Accommodation	Adjustment of the lens to focus on the retina
Astigmatism	Defective curvature of the refractive surface of the eye
Binocular	Pertaining to two or both eyes
Blepharitis	Inflammation of the eyelid
Corneal	Pertaining to the cornea
Conjunctivitis	Inflammation of the conjunctiva
Diplopia	Double vision
Hyperopia	Farsightedness
Keratitis	Inflammation of the cornea
Keratoconus	Noninflammatory protrusion of the cornea
Keratometer	Instrument used to measure the curvature of the cornea, used when fitting contact lenses
Myopia	Nearsightedness
Nyctalopia	Poor vision at night or in faint light
Ophthalmalgia	Pain in the eye
Ophthalmic	Pertaining to the eye
Ophthalmologist	Physician who specializes in ophthalmology
Ophthalmology	The study of diseases and treatment of the eye
Ophthalmoscope	Instrument used for visual examination of the interior of eye
Optician	One who is skilled in filling prescriptions for lenses

Word	What It Means
Optometer	Instrument used to measure power and range of vision
Optometrist	A health professional who prescribes corrective lenses
Optometry	Measurement of visual acuity and prescribing of corrective lenses
Presbyopia	Impaired vision as a result of aging

Hopefully your head isn't spinning from vocabulary overload at this point. If so, take a breather before continuing on to the next big list of words, which is a big ol' bunch of aural word salad (see Table 15-7).

TABLE 15-7

An Earful of Vocabulary

Word	What It Means
Acoumeter	Instrument used to measure hearing
Audiologist	One who specializes in audiology
Audiology	The study of hearing
Aural	Pertaining to the ear
Otologist	A physician who studies and treats diseases of the ear
Otology	The study of the ear
Otorhinolaryngology (ENT)	The study and treatment of diseases and disorders of ear, nose, and throat
Otorhinolaryngologist	A physician specialized in otorhinolaryngology
Otorrhea	Discharge from the ear
Otoscope	Instrument used for visual examination of the ear
Purulent otitis media	Inflammation of the middle ear, resulting in the build-up of pus
Serous otitis media	Inflammation of inner ear, resulting in a build-up of watery fluid
Tympanometer	Instrument to measure middle ear function
Tympanometry	Measurement of the movement of the tympanic membrane

Common Sensory Conditions

Though it may seem obvious, it deserves being said. Most of the conditions associated with smell and taste involve the body's inability to perform those sensory tasks. Having trouble smelling your spring flowers? Can't taste your famous five-alarm chili? Chances are that it's dues to one of these conditions:

- **Ageusia:** Lack of or impairment of taste
- **Anosmia:** Absence of sense of smell
- **Dysgeusia:** Abnormal or perverted sense of taste
- **Dysosmia:** Impaired sense of smell
- **Hypergeusia:** Excessive or acute sense of taste
- **Osmesis:** The process of smelling

As usual, the eye is infinitely more complicated than, say, your tongue. So it stands to reason that there are many more possible conditions associated with your sense of sight. Though common, all these conditions are serious and should not be taken lightly. They are

- **Chalazion:** Small, hard mass on the eyelid due to oil gland enlargement
- **Esotropia:** A type of strabismus (one eye turns inward, cross-eyed)
- **Exotropia:** A type of strabismus (one eye turns outward)
- **Glaucoma:** Increased intraocular pressure
- **Hemianopia (hemianopsia):** Loss of one half of the visual field (the space of vision of eye)
- **Hordeolum (sty or stye):** An infection of the oil gland of the eyelid
- **Nystagmus:** Involuntary, rapid movements of the eyeball
- **Retinal detachment:** The retina, or part of it, becomes separated from the choroid layer
- **Strabismus:** Abnormal deviation of the eye; also called a squint

Moving on to the other complicated sense organ, the ear, you can see that quite a few of these conditions result in some form of hearing loss. Some are unavoidable, but thankfully, some of these can be avoided by exercising good hygiene and staying away from rock concerts (or at least wearing ear plugs).

- **Macrotia:** Abnormal enlargement of the pinna (excessively large ears)
- **Microtia:** Abnormally small pinna (excessively small ears)

- **Myringitis:** Inflammation of tympanic membrane
- **Otalgia:** Pain in the ear (earache)
- **Otitis externa:** Inflammation of the outer ear; also known as swimmer's ear
- **Otitis media:** Infection of the middle ear
- **Tympanitis:** Inflammation of the middle ear (otitis media)
- **Serous otitis media:** Inflammation of the inner ear without infection
- **Suppurative otitis media:** Bacterial infection of middle ear
- **Tinnitus:** Ringing sound in ears; cause unknown, may be associated with chronic otitis, myringitis, or labyrinthitis
- **Vertigo:** Sensation of irregular or whirling motion, of body or external objects, due to severe disturbance of equilibrium organs in the labyrinth

Finding the Culprit: Sensory Diseases and Pathology

Once again, the eyes and ears rule. These two areas are just as susceptible to pathological diseases as any other site on the body. Some of the greatest hits include

- **Acoustic neuroma:** Benign tumor in acoustic nerve in the brain causing tinnitus, vertigo, and decreased hearing
- **Cataract:** Clouding of the lens, causing decreased vision
- **Cholesteatoma:** Collection of skin cells and cholesterol in a sac in the middle ear
- **Diabetic retinopathy:** Retinal effects of diabetic mellitus
- **Macular degeneration:** Deterioration of the *macula lutea* of the retina
- **Meniere's disease or syndrome:** Vertigo, hearing loss, nausea and tinnitus, leading to progressive deafness caused by rapid violent firing of the fibers of the auditory nerves
- **Otosclerosis:** Hardening of the bony tissue of the labyrinth causing hearing loss and progressive deafness
- **Presbycusis:** Hearing loss occurring with old age
- **Retinitis pigmentosa:** Progressive retinal sclerosis and atrophy; an inherited disease associated with decreased vision and night blindness (nyctalopia)

Testing, Testing: Sensory Radiology and Diagnostic Tests

Your physician will want to run a battery of tests if you ever encounter problems with any of your senses, particularly with the eyes and ears. There is no doubt that your body and brain get a huge percentage of incoming information from these two sense organs alone, and if you lose the capability for either, your entire world will change. These are tests to take very seriously:

- **Audiogram:** The graphed test results of audiometry
- **Audiometry:** An audiometer delivers acoustic stimuli of specific frequencies to determine hearing for each frequency using an instrument to measure acuity of hearing
- **Diathermy:** The use of high-frequency electrical current to coagulate blood vessels within the eye
- **Gonioscopy:** Involves the examination of the angle of the anterior chamber of the eye to diagnose glaucoma
- **Laser photocoagulation:** Used to treat diabetic retinopathy and senile macular degeneration
- **Ophthalmoscopy:** Visual examination of the interior of the eye
- **Otoscopy:** Visual examination of the ear with an otoscope
- **Proetz test:** Test for acuity of smell
- **Slit lamp biomicroscopy:** A microscopic study of the cornea, conjunctiva, iris, lens, and vitreous humor
- **Tonometry:** Measurement of the tension or pressure within the eye
- **Tuning fork test (Weber's test):** A vibration source (tuning fork) is placed on forehead to note sound perception on right, left, or midline
- **Visual acuity:** Test of clarity or clearness of vision; reading the Snedden eye chart of black letters in decreasing size with the chart at a distance of 20 feet. 20/20 vision indicates that letters can be clearly seen at that distance. 20/50 vision indicates the eye is able to see at 20 feet what it is supposed to be able to see at 50 feet.
- **Visual field test:** Test measures the area within which objects can be seen when the eye is fixed and looking straight ahead

Paging Dr. Terminology: Surgeries and Procedures

Thankfully, there is something that can be done about a lot of those common eye conditions and diseases. Surgical procedures for the eye have improved dramatically over time and often involve less invasive procedures. Either way, though, you might want to call a cab afterwards.

- **Blepharoplasty:** Surgical repair of the eyelid
- **Cataract surgery:** To remove the lens when a cataract has formed
- **Cryoextraction of a cataract:** This method uses a cold probe to the anterior surface of the lens to lift the lens out as it adheres to the probe
- **CXL (Corneal collagen cross-linking):** To treat keratoconus — not intended to correct vision but is combined with PRK to improve refractive results
- **Enucleation:** Surgical removal of the eye
- **Keratoplasty:** This procedure, also called a *corneal transplant,* involves replacement of a section of an opaque cornea with a normal transparent cornea in an effort to restore vision.
- **LASIK (Laser-assisted in situ keratomileusis):** Commonly referred to as laser eye surgery or laser vision correction — to correct myopia, hyperopia, and astigmatism
- **Phacoemulsification:** Removal of cataract
- **Phacoemulsification of a cataract:** Involves using ultrasonic vibration to break up portions of the lens. The lens is aspirated through the ultrasonic probe.
- **PRK (Photoreactive keratectomy):** Laser surgery used to reshape the cornea to reduce the need for glasses or contact lenses
- **Scleroplasty:** Repair of the sclera
- **SMILE (Small incision lenticule extraction):** A laser procedure similar to LASIK to remove a small portion of the corneal tissue called a lenticule. This procedure reshapes the cornea and corrects vision.
- **Vitrectomy:** Diseased vitreous humor is removed and replaced with clear solution.

Procedures for the ear are a bit more invasive, obviously, because so much is going on within the labyrinth of canals inside your head. Some of the most common clinical and surgical procedures for the ear include

- **Fenestration:** Forming an opening into the labyrinth to restore hearing
- **Labyrinthectomy:** Excision of the labyrinth
- **Mastoidectomy:** Excision of the mastoid bone
- **Mastoidotomy:** Incision into the mastoid bone
- **Myringoplasty:** Surgical repair of the tympanic membrane
- **Myringotomy:** Incision of the tympanic membrane performed to release pus and relieve pressure in the middle ear
- **Stapedectomy:** Excision of the stapes
- **Tympanectomy:** Surgical removal of the eardrum
- **Tympanoplasty:** Surgical repair of the eardrum

Terminology RX: Sensory Pharmacology

Antibiotics, corticosteroids, and antivirals are often used to treat both ear and eye infections. Most eye infections are treated with *topical drugs* (ointments, liquids or creams, *topical* meaning applied directly to the area, eye drops, ear drops, and antibiotics). Most *ophthalmic antibiotics* are classified as topical applications, as are *corticosteroids* used to treat inflammation often after surgery, trauma, or chemical contact. Here are some other sensory meds to know:

- **Balanced salt solution** (BSS) is used during eye surgery to irrigate and wash the eye.

  Do not confuse BSS with *normal saline,* as they are not the same. BSS is a registered ophthalmic preparation used in eye surgeries, a slightly different compound than normal saline, which is a sterile salt solution.
- **Beta blockers** are used to treat glaucoma.
- **Mydriatic drugs** (drugs that dilate the pupil) are used at eye examinations.
- **Prostaglandin analogs** are used to treat glaucoma.
- **Silver nitrate** is commonly used as a topical anti-infective agent, administered to eyes of newborn infants to prevent infection.

4 Let's Get Some Physiology Terminology

IN THIS PART . . .

Keeping the beat moving with discussion of the cardiovascular system

Inhaling terms for the respiratory system

Ingesting terminology of the gastrointestinal system

Cleaning up with the endocrine system

Introducing the nervous system

IN THIS CHAPTER

- Discovering how your heart, blood vessels, and lymph nodes work together
- Memorizing root words, prefixes, and suffixes appropriate to these systems
- Familiarizing yourself with common cardiovascular and lymphatic conditions and diseases
- Getting to the heart of the correct terms to use when diagnosing problems
- Understanding how to communicate terms used in surgeries and procedures

Chapter 16

The Heart of the Matter: The Cardiovascular and Lymphatic Systems

Ever wonder how we have fresh, clean water to drink? A vast network of lakes, reservoirs, pumping and purification stations, and pipes ultimately bring us the life force that is water. We, in turn, use it for drinking, cooking, cleaning, and a multitude of tasks.

Your cardiovascular system is not so different. Consider your heart as the big central pumping station that supplies the rest of your body with valuable liquid — mainly, blood. Blood carries oxygen and nutrients to body tissues and collects carbon dioxide and waste materials to be eliminated. You can think of the complementary lymphatic system as the wastewater treatment facility that cleans and purifies what was once useless into clear, clean fluid.

How the Cardiovascular System Works

Let's try another metaphor. Although the heart is the main character in this sweeping drama called *Your Body,* it couldn't do its work without a strong cast of supporting characters: blood, blood cells, and vessels. The separate but complementary lymphatic system works like ushers at a play, guiding no-longer-useful folks out at the end of the show. None of these components can work alone. They are a merry band of players who must share the spotlight.

The main organ of the circulatory (another name for cardiovascular) system is the *heart,* of course, and its main job is making the blood flow freely through your veins. By pumping, the heart creates pressure that forces the blood to move throughout the body via a channel system of *arteries* and *veins.* That system reaches from the center of your chest out to the nether regions of your appendages and back again, ensuring that life-giving and sustaining blood cells are carried through your entire body.

The lymphatic system works to complement the actions of the cardiovascular system by carrying *lymph fluid* through the body via a system similar to veins. The lymph fluid flows forward through a grouping of *vessels, ducts,* and *nodes* that filter the fluid before it reenters the bloodstream. In this chapter, you find out more about the individual components of these two powerful systems and get to know the specific terminology associated with both.

TECHNICAL STUFF

An adult human's normal heart rate is 70–80 beats per minute. A child's is 100–120, an elephant's about 25, a mouse's 700, and a canary's heart beats about 1,000 times per minute. Your heart beats around 100,000 times a day, pumping 2½ ounces with each contraction. That's 5 quarts a minute, 75 gallons per hour, 1,800 gallons a day, and 657,000 gallons per year.

Greek plays a role in the roots of the word for heart, *cardium.* This word, which you'll get to know quite well in this chapter, is taken from the Greek word *kardia. Cardium* takes on other identities in the commonly known forms of *cardi* and *cardio.* But make no mistake, it's all the same root.

Now, meet the individual players responsible for the pumping of the red stuff that keeps you going every day. Each has its own special function and terminology to go along with it. If watching ER is your only entrée into the world of medical terminology, fear not and consider this section your crash course in all things cardiovascular.

The heart

To take a tour of the heart, consider three components: layers, chambers, and valves. Together, these elements form the most powerful muscle in the body. Located to the left of the midline of your chest's center, this muscle, about the size of your fist, pumps a continuous stream of life-giving blood through your blood vessels.

Figure 16-1 illustrates the heart.

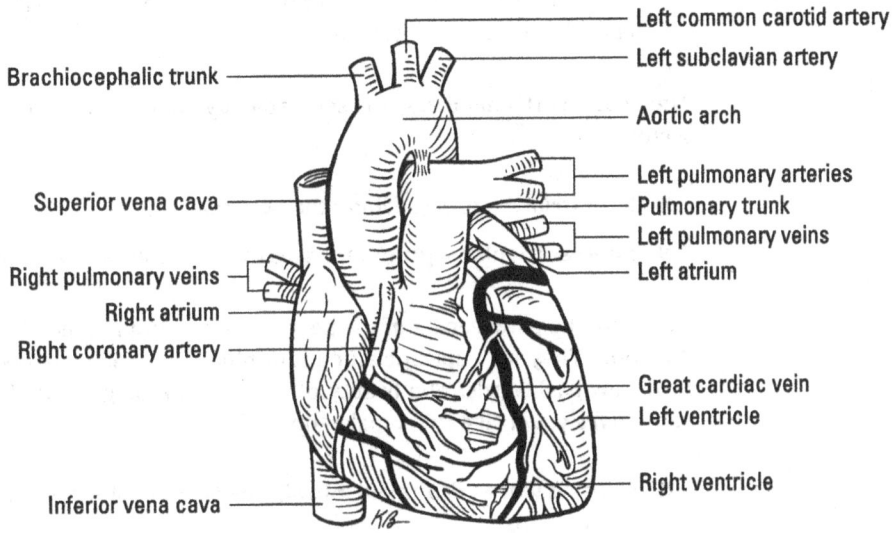

FIGURE 16-1: Anterior view of the heart.

Illustration by Kathryn Born

The heart is enclosed in a fluid-filled sac called the *pericardium*, located in the chest cavity just to the left of the midline. It consists of three major layers, each one performing a unique job in the day-to-day activities of your most vital organ.

- **Endocardium:** *Endo-* is the Greek prefix for "within." This is the inner layer of the heart, lining the chambers and covering the valves.
- **Epicardium:** *Epi-* is the Greek prefix for "on." This is the outer layer of the heart.
- **Myocardium:** *Myo-* is the Greek prefix meaning "muscle." This is the actual heart muscle and makes up the thick middle layer.

The four hollow places in the heart are called *chambers*. There are two types of chambers:

- **Atrium:** *Atrium* is taken from the Greek word *atrion,* meaning "hall." The right and left *atria* (*atrium* is the singular form) are the two upper heart chambers serving as receiving stations for blood. Valves connect each atrium to the ventricles below.
- **Ventricles:** *Ventricle* is taken from the Latin word *venter,* meaning "little belly." The right and left ventricles are thick, lower chambers and are responsible for pumping blood. The atria receive blood from the body, and the ventricles pump blood back out into the body.

The four heart chambers are separated by membranes called *septa* (plural of *septum*).

- **Interatrial septum** separates the two atria.
- **Interventricular septum** separates the two ventricle chambers.

Valves are the gatekeepers of the heart, making sure the blood flows in the correct direction. They let a specific amount of blood into each chamber and don't allow it to flow backwards. The beauty of valve terminology is that the name of each valve gives you a clue to its make-up.

- **Bicuspid valve (also called mitral):** The *bi-* prefix shows you that this valve has two flaps.
- **Pulmonary semilunar valve and aortic semilunar valve:** Both have a half-moon shape, thus being named from *semi* (part) and *lunar* (moon).
- **Tricuspid valve:** *Tri-* indicates this valve has three flaps, keeping blood moving forward.

Blood vessels

The vast network of blood vessels (made up of arteries and arterioles, veins and venules, and capillaries) begins at the heart and spans out through the entire body to the far reaches of the fingertips and toes. Together, these different types of vessels work to carry blood pumped by the heart through the body.

REMEMBER

Arteries take care of clean, oxygenated blood. *Veins* handle the movement of deoxygenated blood. Your little friends, the *capillaries*, serve as mini bridges between the two types of vessels.

Arterial system

The *arterial system* is composed of arteries and *arterioles* (smaller arteries). The Greek *aer* is the basis for the word *artery*, meaning "air." Combined with *terein*, meaning "to keep," you get the word *artery*. Starting with the largest artery, the *aorta*, the arteries carry oxygenated blood away from the heart to the arterioles, and then on to the capillaries, where the exchange of gases (oxygen and carbon dioxide) takes place.

WARNING

The *pulmonary artery*, with its two branches, is the exception of the arterial world. Instead of carrying oxygen-filled blood to other parts of the body, its branches carry oxygen-deprived blood to the right and left lungs.

Venous system

The venous system is made up of veins and *venules* (little veins). The veins are the workhorses of the vessel system, carrying oxygen-depleted blood back to the heart. The journey ends with the blood from the head and upper body being returned to the heart via the body's largest veins, the *superior vena cava*, and from the lower body via the *inferior vena cava*, received into the right atrium. The pulmonary veins carry oxygen-rich blood from the lungs back to the heart.

Capillaries

If you look at a map of the blood vessel system, you see that capillaries are incredibly small and look tiny, like hair. It's no accident, then, that the word *capillary* is Latin for "hairlike." These super-tiny vessels (one cell thick, to be exact) bridge the gap between arterioles and venules to keep blood flowing in a continuous motion.

Figure 16-2 illustrates capillary exchange.

Blood

There's more to the make-up of your blood than the obvious red blood cells. A large percentage of your blood is actually made up of *plasma*, which is, in turn, largely composed of water. The red and white cells, plus *platelets*, make up the rest of your ever-flowing life force. Here's a bit more about what makes up your blood:

- **Plasma:** Mostly water, a small percentage of plasma is composed of proteins, nutrients, waste, and gas. *Albumin, fibrinogen,* and *immunoglobulins* are all proteins found in plasma.

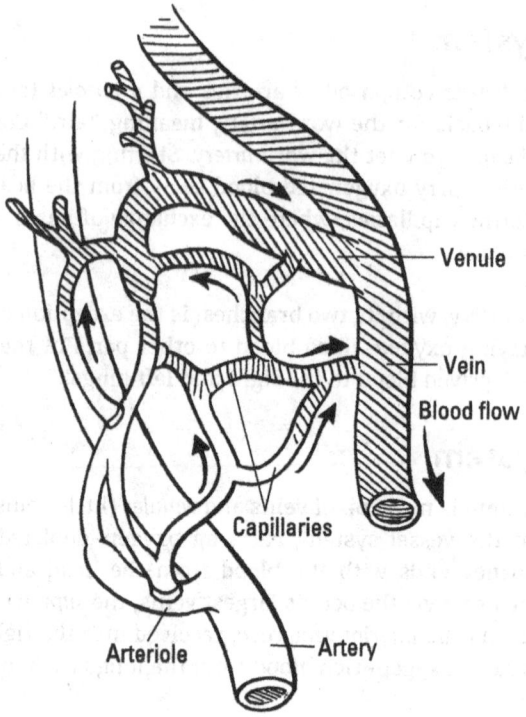

FIGURE 16-2: Artery, vein, and capillary exchange.

Illustration by Kathryn Born

FOLLOWING THE TRAIL OF BLOOD

A great way to remember much of the terminology associated with the heart is to think more about the path the blood takes each time it makes a trip through the vast muscle.

The *rule of two* will get you started. Remember that the heart has two different types of chambers: ventricles and atria, which both contract at the same time. Similarly, the blood travels through two paths: the arterial system for sending oxygen-rich blood out and the venous system for bringing oxygen-poor blood back.

Next, try to think of the blood's path as "The Hokey Pokey." Remember? "You put your right foot in. You put your right foot out," and so on. Think of where the blood goes in and out, and you can click through around 15 cardiovascular terms. Let's follow it:

Left ventricle > aorta > arteries > arterioles > capillaries of body tissues > back through venules > veins > superior/inferior venae cavae > right atrium > right ventricle > pulmonary artery > alveoli of the lungs > lung capillaries > pulmonary veins > left atrium > left ventricle . . . and it begins again. Feel free to put this path to the music of your choice and sing along!

- **Platelets:** The body's little firefighters. Platelets are always putting out "fires" in the body by beginning the clotting process and putting a stop to any blood escaping from a compromised vessel.
- **Red blood cells:** Also known as *erythrocytes,* these cells contain *hemoglobin,* an arrangement of proteins and iron composed of molecules. Red blood cells carry oxygenated blood throughout the body.
- **White blood cells:** Called *leukocytes,* these are the double agents of the cardiovascular system. They work as the body's homemade antibiotics, fighting germs in both the bloodstream and in tissue fluid and lymph fluid.

Path of the blood

Veins carry blood back to the heart via the superior and inferior venae cavae. The *superior* (meaning "near the top") *vena cava* takes blood from the upper body to the right atrium; the *inferior* (meaning situated below) *vena cava* carries blood from the lower body to the right atrium, which then empties the blood into the right ventricle. The ventricle contracts, expelling the blood into the pulmonary artery.

Pulmon is the Latin word for "lung." The pulmonary arteries carry the blood through to the lungs where it is *oxygenated.* From there, the pulmonary veins carry the oxygenated blood back to the left atrium, which then moves the blood into the left ventricle, which pumps the blood into the aorta.

Thank good old Aristotle for the word *aorta,* meaning "that which is hung." The philosopher named it so because of the upside-down, hanging curve of the artery.

Cardiac cycle

All this pumping and moving of blood comes down to rhythm. The *cardiac cycle* is controlled by the heart's natural pacemaker, the *sinoatrial (SA) node.* The rhythmic pulsations conduct through the *AV node,* down the *AV bundle* (also known as the *bundle of His*), through the *Purkinje fibers,* jump-starting contraction of the ventricles.

There are two phases in the cardiac cycle:

- **Diastole** is the resting period, when the heart rests and fills with blood.
- **Systole** is the period when ventricles contract and send blood out, causing pressure on the walls of the arteries during the heart's contraction.

Both words share a Greek root, *stole,* meaning "to send." The difference lies in the prefix. *Dia-* means "apart," whereas *sy-* means "together."

How the Lymphatic System Works

Most directly associated with immunity, we discuss the lymphatic system in the same chapter as the cardiovascular system due to the similar make-up of the system and the fact that, once cleaned by the lymph nodes, lymphatic fluid is released directly into the bloodstream. Lymph vessels are arranged in a similar pattern as the blood vessels, but work to clear the body of impurities.

Lymphatic vessels

Lymphatic vessels borrow their name from the fluid they pump, called, not surprisingly, *lymph fluid.* Curiously, at the heart of the word *lymph* is the Greek *nymph,* a term used to describe a beautiful maiden. The word eventually took on Latin roots, when the *n* was replaced with *l.* Because lymph fluid is a clear, clean fluid, and *lymph* rhymes with *nymph,* the transition was apparent to Latin wordsmiths.

The lymphatic vessels interlace with blood vessels to carry clean lymphatic fluid through the body. They collect the proteins and water, which continually filter out of the blood into tissue fluid, and return to the blood. The proteins and water filter out of the blood and escape into tissue fluid. The lymphatic vessels pick up the proteins and water from the tissues and return them to the blood.

Lymph nodes, also called "glands"

Shaped much like small beans, the *lymph nodes* are located throughout the body. We discuss what the nodes do later in the chapter, but here is the lowdown on the location of these helpful little guys. Lymph nodes are located in several regions of the body. Depending on where they are, lymph nodes are known by different names, including

- **Axillary:** Underarm and upper chest
- **Cervical:** Neck
- **Inguinal:** Groin

Figure 16-3 illustrates a lymph node.

Lymphatic System

The lymphatic system is largely responsible for creating an immunity barrier by developing and distributing *lymphocytes,* a type of WBC (white blood cell) throughout the body. Lymphocytes are our little buddies, which you read about earlier. The lymph nodes release these *lymphocytes* and remove or destroy *antigens* (foreign substances that invoke an immune response) that circulate through the blood and lymphatic vessels.

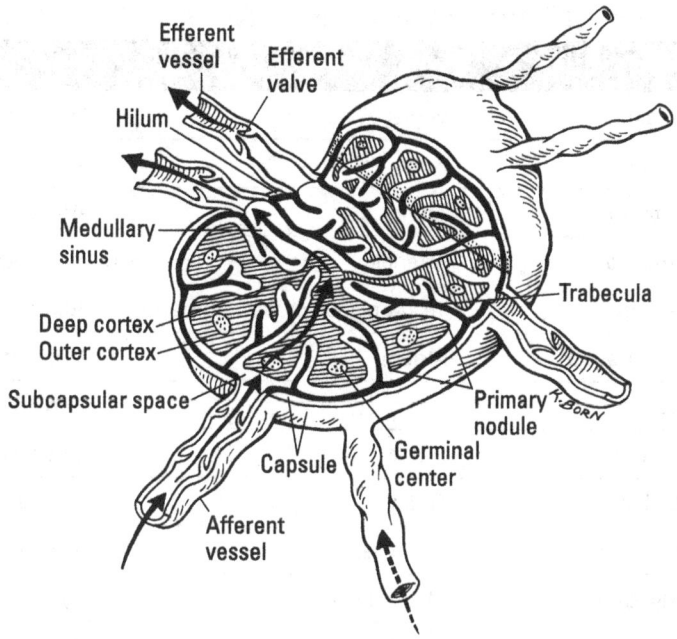

FIGURE 16-3: Anatomy of a lymph node, cross section.

Illustration by Kathryn Born

Lymph fluid enters the node, filters through *sinuses* within the node, and drains through a single exit vessel. Consider it a one-way ticket for lymph fluid to get into the bloodstream. This filter system cleans out all the yucky stuff: bacteria, foreign particles, and those naughty malignant cells. The lymph nodes also destroy invading cells and particles in a process known as *phagocytosis.* The *thoracic duct* (there is only one) is the largest vessel of the lymph system. It collects lymph from the body below the diaphragm and from left side of body above the diaphragm.

The spleen, tonsils, and thymus are accessory organs of this system. The *spleen* enlarges with infectious diseases and decreases in size in old age. Some phagocytosis takes place in the spleen. The *tonsils* filter out bacteria and foreign matter. The *thymus* produces cells that destroy foreign substances.

Cardiovascular and Lymphatic Root Words

Now that you've gotten to know the specific parts of the cardiovascular and lymphatic systems a bit better, it's time to put your expertise into practice. Table 16-1 lists cardio roots, prefixes, and suffixes. It also gives an example medical term for each.

TABLE 16-1 **Breaking Down Your Cardio Words**

Root Word	What It Means	Example
Angi/o	Vessel	Angiogram
Aort/o	Aorta	Aortic
Arteri/o	Artery	Arteriosclerosis
Arteriol/o	Arteriole	Arteriolitis
Ather/o	Yellow plaque or fatty substance	Atherosclerosis
Atri/o, atri/a	Atrium	Atrioventricular
Cardi/o	Heart	Cardiomegaly
Coron/o	Heart	Coronary
Embol/o	Embolus	Embolectomy
Hemangi/o	Blood vessel	Hemangioma
Myocardi/o	Myocardium	Myocarditis
Ox/o, ox/i	Oxygen	Oximeter
Phleb/o	Vein	Phlebitis
Pulmon/o	Lung	Pulmonary
Scler/o	Hardening	Sclerotherapy
Sphygm/o	Pulse	Sphygmomanometer
Thromb/o	Clot	Thrombus
Valv/o, valvul/o	Valve	Valvular
Vas/o	Vessel	Vasoconstriction
Ven/o	Vein	Venotomy
Venul/o	Venule	Venulitis
Ventricul/o	Ventricle	Ventricular
Prefix or Suffix	**What It Means**	**Example**
Brady	Slow	Bradycardia
Tachy	Fast	Tachycardia
-graph	Instrument used to record	Electrocardiograph
-graphy	Process of recording	Electrocardiography
-gram	Picture or finished record	Electrocardiogram

Table 16-2 lists lymphatic roots and suffixes.

TABLE 16-2

Breaking Down Your Lymphatic Roots

Root Word	What It Means
Aden/o	Gland
Bas/o	Base (opposite of acid)
Eosin/o	Red, rosy
Erythr/o	Red
Granul/o	Granules
Hem/o, Hemat/o	Blood
Immun/o	Safe, protection
Kary/o	Nucleus
Leuk/o	White
Lymph/o	Lymph
Lymphaden/o	Lymph gland
Lymphangi/o	Lymph vessels
Mon/o	One, single
Morph/o	Shape, form
Myel/o	Bone marrow
Necr/o	Death
Neutr/o	Neither, neutral
Nucle/o	Nucleus
Phleb/o	Vein
Sider/o	Iron
Spher/o	Globe or round
Splen/o	Spleen
Thromb/o	Clot
Thym/o	Thymus
Tonsill/o	Tonsil

(continued)

TABLE 16-2 *(continued)*

Suffix	What It Means
-apheresis	Removal
-blast	Immature
-cytosis	Condition of cells
-emia	Blood condition
-globin	Protein
-globulin	Protein
-megaly	Enlargement
-phoresis	Carrying, transmission
-poiesis	Formation
-stasis	Stop or control

Hundreds of medical terms can be created by using the roots, prefixes, and suffixes mentioned in the previous tables. Table 16-3 lists some common cardiovascular and lymphatic vocabulary words.

TABLE 16-3

Cardiovascular and Lymphatic Vocabulary Words

Word	What It Means
Anticoagulant	Agent or drug that slows the clotting process
Aorta	Largest artery in the body
Atrium, Atria	Upper chambers of the heart
Auscultation	Hearing sounds in the body through a stethoscope
Blood pressure	Pressure exerted by blood against the vessel walls
Capillary	Smallest blood vessel
Cardiac	Pertaining to the heart
Cardiologist	Physician who studies and treats diseases of the heart
Cardiology	Study of the heart and its diseases
Cardiopulmonary resuscitation:	(CPR) Emergency procedure consisting of artificial ventilation and external cardiac massage
Coronary arteries:	The blood vessels that branch from the aorta to carry oxygen-rich blood to the heart muscle

Word	What It Means
Diastole	The relaxation phase of the heart beat
Endocardium	Inner lining of the heart
Erythrocyte	Red blood cell
Hematologist	Physician who studies and treats diseases of the blood
Hematology	Study of the blood
Hemolysis	Breakdown of blood
Hemostasis	Stoppage of bleeding
Immunoglobulins	Antibodies secreted by plasma cells
Leukocyte	White blood cell
Manometer	Instrument used to measure pressure of fluid
Mitral valve	Valve between the left atrium and left ventricle
Myelogenous	Produced by the bone marrow
Occlude	To be closed tightly
Percussion	Tapping of the body surface with fingers to determine density of the part beneath
Peyer's patches	Lymphatic filters located in the small intestine
Pulmonary arteries	Arteries carrying oxygen-poor blood from the heart to lungs
Pulmonary circulation	Flow of blood from the heart to the lungs and back to the heart
Pulmonary veins	Veins carrying oxygenated blood from the lungs to the heart
Sinoatrial (S-A) node	Pacemaker of the heart
Sphygmomanometer	Instrument used to measure blood pressure
Systemic circulation	Flow of blood from body cells to the heart and then back out of the heart to the cells
Systole	Contracting phase of the heartbeat
Thrombocyte	Clotting cell or platelet
Venae cavae	The largest veins in the body; the superior and inferior bring blood into the right atrium

Common Cardiovascular and Lymphatic Conditions

Some cardiovascular conditions pertain specifically to the heart and surrounding system of veins and arteries. First, let's consider what can ail some of the individual parts of the heart. *Aortic stenosis* is the narrowing of the aorta. *Endocarditis* is the inflammation of the inner lining of the heart, whereas *pericarditis* is an inflammation of the pericardial sac (pericardium).

Then there are conditions that involve the entire heart muscle, including *cardiomegaly*, enlargement of the heart, and *cardiomyopathy*, disease of the heart muscle. *Myocarditis* is an inflammation of the muscle of the heart. The two big daddies are — no surprise here — a *myocardial infarction*, also known as a heart attack, and good old *cardiac arrest*, the sudden cessation or stoppage of cardiac output and effective circulation. Don't forget *congestive heart failure*, *angina*, and *atrial fibrillation*.

Our blood travels through the superhighway of our arterial and venous systems, and it carries a lot of passengers, from oxygen to lymph. Because it is so multifaceted, the blood and its cells can harbor all sorts of conditions. Here is a sampling:

- **Anemia:** Lack of red blood cells
- **Dyscrasia:** Abnormal or pathological condition of the blood
- **Embolism:** The blockage of an artery by foreign material in the bloodstream, most often a blood clot but could be fat, an air bubble, or a clot of bacteria. The foreign material is called an *embolus* (plural *emboli*).
- **Hemorrhage:** Rapid flow of blood
- **Hyperbilirubinemia:** Excessive amounts of bilirubin (a bile pigment excreted by the liver) in the blood
- **Hypercholesterolemia:** Excessive amounts of cholesterol (steroid alcohol that maintains membrane fluidity) in the blood
- **Hyperlipidemia:** Excessive amounts of fat in the blood
- **Hyperchromia:** Excessive pigmented red blood cells
- **Hypertension:** Blood pressure that is above normal range of 120/70
- **Hypotension:** Blood pressure that is below normal

- **Intermittent claudication:** Pain or discomfort in a body part caused by any activity which exerts the affected body part; often occurs in the calves while walking; a result of occlusive arterial disease
- **Leukocytosis:** Marked increased in the number of white blood cells
- **Thrombolysis:** Breakdown of a clot that has formed in the blood

The lymphatic system has its own fair share of health issues. *Lymphadenitis* is an inflammation of lymph nodes. *Lymphedema* is an accumulation of fluid due to obstruction of lymphatic structures. And *splenomegaly* is an enlargement of the spleen.

Finding the Culprit: Cardiovascular and Lymphatic Diseases and Pathology

Pathology is a scary word, and for good reason. *Pathology* is the study of disease as it affects body tissue and function. Some conditions of the heart and lymph system are more serious and more risky than others. Although all conditions and diseases should be considered serious, these heavy hitters are ones that often require more in-depth procedures and treatments.

Why not start at — literally — the heart of the matter. Some pathological conditions affecting the heart and blood vessels include

- **Aneurysm,** a local widening of an artery, may be due to weakness in the arterial wall or breakdown of the wall due to atherosclerosis.
- **Angina pectoris** is an episode of chest pain due to temporary difference between the supply and demand of oxygen to the heart muscle.
- **Arterial hypertension** refers to high blood pressure. There are two types of hypertension: essential and secondary. In *essential hypertension,* the cause of the increased pressure is unknown or idiopathic. In *secondary hypertension,* there is an associated lesion, such as *nephritis, pheochromocytoma, or adenoma of the adrenal cortex,* which can be responsible for the elevated blood pressure.
- **Bacterial endocarditis** is inflammation of the inner lining of the heart caused by bacteria.

  Keep the three types of cardiac arrhythmia straight. The *heart block* is a failure of proper conduction of impulses through the A-V node and can be overcome by implantation of an electric pacemaker. A *flutter* is rapid but regular contractions of the atria or ventricles, while *fibrillation* is rapid, random irregular contractions of the heart as high as 350+ beats per minute.

Damage to the heart valves can produce lesions called vegetations, which may break off in the bloodstream as emboli or floating clots. Vegetation is an overgrowth of bacteria that gains a foothold on an injured valve, becoming fruitful and multiplying.

- **Cardiac arrhythmia** is an abnormal heart rhythm. Some examples include heart block, flutter, and fibrillation.
- **Congenital heart disease** refers to abnormalities in the heart at birth, resulting from some failure in the development of the fetus. *Coarctation of the aorta* is a narrowing of the aorta. Surgical treatment consists of removal of the constricted area with *end-to-end anastomosis* or joining together of the aortic segments.
- **Congestive heart failure** is a condition where the heart is unable to pump its required amount of blood. Blood accumulates in the lungs and liver. In severe cases, fluid can collect in the abdomen and legs or in the pulmonary air sacs (known as *pulmonary edema*). Congestive heart failure often develops gradually over the years and can be treated with drugs to strengthen the heart and diuretics to promote loss of fluid.
- **Coronary artery disease (CAD)** is a disease of arteries supplying blood to the heart. This is usually the result of *atherosclerosis,* the deposition of fatty compounds on the inner lining of the coronary arteries.
- **Heart murmur** refers to an extra heart sound heard between normal heart sounds. Murmurs are heard with the aid of a stethoscope and are caused by a valvular defect or disease, which disrupts the smooth flow of blood in the heart.
- **Hypertensive heart disease** is high blood pressure affecting the heart.
- **Mitral valve prolapse** is improper closure of the mitral valve when the heart is pumping blood, often referred to as a "floppy valve."
- **Raynaud's phenomenon** is short episodes of discoloration and numbness in fingers and toes due to temporary constriction of arterioles. These may be triggered by cold temperature, stress, or smoking.
- **Rheumatic heart disease** is heart disease caused by rheumatic fever.
- **Varicose veins** are abnormally swollen veins usually occurring in the legs, due to damaged valves that fail to prevent the backflow of blood. The blood then collects in the veins, causing *distention.*

The blood itself can suffer from specific diseases and pathological conditions. Consider the diseases specific to both the red and white blood cells. *Anemia,* a common symptom, is a deficiency in erythrocytes or hemoglobin, can take several forms, including the following:

- **Aplastic anemia:** Failure of blood cell production due to absence of development and formation of bone marrow cells
- **Hemolytic anemia:** Reduction in red cells due to excessive destruction
- **Pernicious anemia:** Lack of mature erythrocytes due to inability to absorb vitamin B12
- **Sickle-cell anemia:** Hereditary condition in which distorted cells clump and block blood vessels

Other issues affecting the blood include *thalassemia,* an inherited defect in the ability to produce hemoglobin; *polycythemia vera,* a malignant condition associated with increased red blood cells; and *hemochromatosis,* excessive deposits of iron through the body. *Thalassemia* is usually found in patients of Mediterranean background.

The white blood cells often make people think of the "Big C," also known as cancer. This is for good reason, as the white cells have a lot to do with a very serious disease called *leukemia.* Leukemia, of course, is the kingpin of white blood cell pathology. It is, in simple terms, an excessive increase in white blood cells — a cancerous disease of the bone marrow with malignant leukocytes filling the marrow and bloodstream. Four forms of leukemia include:

- **Acute lymphocytic leukemia (ALL):** Seen most often in children and adolescents
- **Acute myelogenous leukemia (AML):** Derived from or originating in bone marrow; follows an aggressive course
- **Chronic lymphocytic leukemia (CLL):** Occurs late in life and follows a slow, progressive course
- **Chronic myelogenous leukemia (CML):** Slowly progressive

All types of leukemia are treated with chemotherapy, using drugs that prevent cell division and selectively injure rapidly dividing cells. Effective treatment can lead to *remission,* or disappearance of signs of the disease. *Relapse* occurs when leukemia cells reappear in the blood and bone marrow, necessitating further treatment. Watch out for leukemia's nasty cousin, *multiple myeloma.* This is a malignant tumor of bone marrow in which malignant cells invade bone marrow and destroy bony structures.

Keep these two blood-clotting health issues in mind:

- **Hemophilia** is excessive bleeding caused by a congenital lack of coagulation factor necessary for blood clotting.
- **Purpura** is a symptom caused by low platelets involving multiple pinpoint hemorrhages and accumulation of blood under the skin.

We couldn't leave our good friends in the lymphatic system out of the pathology discussion. Who knew that such small things like lymph nodes could be so prone to disease?

The lymph nodes themselves are the sites of many a showdown between good health and an extended hospital stay. *Hodgkin's disease* is a malignant tumor arising in lymphatic tissue such as lymph nodes and spleen. *Lymphosarcoma (lymphoma)* is a malignant tumor of lymph nodes that resembles Hodgkin's disease. Often referred to as *non-Hodgkin's lymphoma*, it affects lymph nodes, spleen, bone marrow, and other organs. *Burkitt's lymphoma* is a malignant tumor of lymph nodes usually affecting children and most common in central Africa.

Inflammation is another common trait of lymphatic system pathology. Sometimes those pesky lymph nodes just get too big for their britches in diseases like the following:

- **Lymphadenitis:** Inflammation of lymph nodes usually due to infection
- **Mononucleosis:** Acute infectious disease with enlarged lymph nodes and spleen due to increased numbers of lymphocytes and monocytes
- **Sarcoidosis:** Inflammatory disease in which small nodules form in lymph nodes and other organs

HIV AND AIDS

Perhaps the most serious diseases affecting the cardiovascular and lymphatic systems are HIV and AIDS.

HIV is also known as *human immunodeficiency virus*, the agent attacking the immune system and causing AIDS.

AIDS (acquired immunodeficiency syndrome) is a disease marked by a decrease in immune response in which the patient has severe depletion of *helper T-cell lymphocytes*.

Testing, Testing: Cardiovascular and Lymphatic Radiology and Diagnostic Tests

Confirming the diagnosis of a condition or disease is a full-time job. Think about the insurance claim notices you receive every time you get blood work or a urine sample done. There is a lab test to diagnose practically anything that might ail you.

Lab tests for issues affecting the heart include *serum enzyme test or studies,* more commonly known as *cardiac enzymes.* During a myocardial infarction (heart attack), enzymes are released into the bloodstream from the dying heart muscle. These enzymes can be measured and are useful as evidence of an infarction. *Lipid tests* measure the amount of these substances in a blood sample. High levels of triglycerides and cholesterol can be associated with a greater risk of coronary atherosclerosis.

The *blood test* is the most common of all diagnostic tests. Blood work can help reveal a plethora of problems that not only affect blood but also major systems and organs. Another gold standard test is the *cardiac catheterization,* which involves inserting a long, thin tube, or catheter, into a blood vessel in the arm, neck, or groin that is then threaded to the heart to monitor and record pressure and patterns and locate clots.

Lipoprotein electrophoresis is a process in which *lipoproteins* (fat and protein molecules bound together) are physically separated from a blood sample. High levels of *low-density lipoprotein* (LDL) are associated with cholesterol and triglyceride deposits in arteries. Having high levels of *high-density lipoprotein* (HDL), containing less lipids, is a positive factor in keeping the heart healthy.

TIP

Remember *HDL* is the "happy" cholesterol in the blood. So, just remember *H* for "happy." *LDL* is the "bad" cholesterol. Remember *L* for "lousy."

Other laboratory blood tests include the following:

- **Antiglobulin test (Coombs' test)** determines whether erythrocytes are coated with antibody and useful in determining the presence of antibodies in infants of Rh-negative mothers. (Rh-negative is a blood type in which all Rh factors are lacking.)
- **Bleeding time** is measurement of the time it takes for a small puncture wound to stop bleeding; normal time is 8 minutes or less.
- **Coagulation time** is the time required for blood to clot in a test tube; normal time is less than 15 minutes.

- **ESR (erythrocyte sedimentation rate)** measures the speed at which erythrocytes settle out of plasma. The rate is altered in disease conditions such as infection, joint inflammation, and tumor.
- **Hemoglobin test** is the measurement of the amount of hemoglobin in a blood sample.
- **Platelet count** is the number of platelets per cubic millimeter of blood. Platelets normally average between 200,000–500,000 per cubic millimeter.

TIP

A common diagnostic test counts the red blood cells and/or the white blood cells. To remember the normal range for each, remember *RBC(really big count)* for RBC (red blood cells). The normal number is about 5 million per cubic millimeter. The *WBC(white blood cell count)* is much smaller, averaging between 5,000–10,000 per cubic millimeter.

- **Prothrombin time (PT)** measures the ability of the blood to clot, used to follow patients taking blood thinners or anticoagulant drugs such as Coumadin.
- **White blood cell differential count** determines the number of different types of leukocytes, mature and immature, that are present in a blood sample.

ABBREVIATIONS: KEEP IT SHORT AND SIMPLE

You probably won't believe us, but saying all these terms over and over again can get tedious. Thankfully for those of you who must utter blood-related phrases on a daily basis, there are some handy-dandy abbreviations:

- **BP:** Blood pressure
- **CBC:** Complete blood count
- **DVT:** Deep vein thrombosis
- **Hct:** Hematocrit
- **Hgb or Hb:** Hemoglobin
- **PT:** Prothombin time
- **RBC:** Red blood cell count (erythrocytes)
- **WBC:** White blood cell count (leukocytes)

Paging Dr. Terminology: Cardiovascular and Lymphatic Surgeries and Procedures

So, what do you do about all these conditions and diseases? Thankfully, there are almost as many possible surgeries and procedures as there are conditions and diseases. The clinical procedures for the cardiovascular system are many, so hunker down. The great majority of these directly involve the old ticker.

Electrocardiography is a record of the electricity flowing through the heart. Speaking of electricity, *cardioversion* or *defibrillation* is a treatment procedure whereby short discharges of electricity are applied across the chest to stop cardiac arrhythmia.

Angiocardiography is a procedure involving injection of contrast dye into the bloodstream followed by chest x-ray to determine the dimensions of the heart and large vessels. This is often used to diagnose an enlarged heart. Similarly, *digital subtraction angiography* can be used to get a closer look at the vessels. Video equipment and computer are used to produce x-rays of the blood vessels.

Other procedures focus on finding out more about how efficiently the heart is working. In *cardiac catheterization*, a catheter is introduced into a vein or artery and guided into the heart for purposes of detecting pressure and patterns of blood flow. The *cardiac scan* is when a radioactive substance is injected intravenously and its accumulation in the heart muscle is measured with a scanner.

Cardiac ablation is a procedure used to destroy or scar heart tissue that triggers or sustains an abnormal heart rhythm. It is used to correct *heart arrhythmias* (atrial fibrillation).

The presence of areas of *ischemia* (deficiency of blood in a body part due to constriction or complete obstruction of a blood vessel) and myocardial infarction can be demonstrated on this scan. Everyone's favorite, the *stress test*, determines the body's response to physical exertion or stress. An *echocardiogram* and other measurements of blood pressure and breathing rate are taken while the patient is exercising, usually jogging on a treadmill.

Other fun and exciting procedures include the following:

- **Doppler flow study** uses ultrasound waves to determine the velocity of flow of blood within vessels.
- **Laser angioplasty** uses light amplification to stimulate emission of radiation or a laser beam to blocked arteries, especially in the legs.

- **Percutaneous transluminal coronary angioplasty (PTCA)** is when a balloon catheter is passed through a blood vessel to the area where plaque has formed. Inflation of the balloon flattens the plaque against the vessel wall and allows blood to circulate more freely. Also called a *balloon angioplasty.*
- **Stent Insertion:** Percutaneous coronary intervention often follows PTCA. In this procedure, a coronary stent is inserted in the diseased arteries that supply the heart — think of a stent as a meshlike straw — that keeps the artery open to allow adequate blood flow.
- **Venogram:** X-ray film of the veins taken after the injection of dye.

ZEN AND THE ART OF TICKER MAINTENANCE

Sometimes surgeons have to get down and dirty to fix a heart condition. This typically involves major surgery, a Skilsaw, and lots of time. Though it may be hard to believe that these surgeries are standard issue, remember that heart surgeons perform them every day with great success.

Angioplasty is the surgical repair of a vessel. An *endarterectomy* is an excision within an artery of a thickened interior, usually named for the artery that is being "cleaned out." More vein work includes *phlebotomy,* an incision into a vein to remove or give blood. This is also called *venipuncture.* These procedures can be done in a doctor's office but are commonly performed in an outpatient lab.

The big fun happens when surgeons get more involved with the heart. In *cardiac pacemaker insertion,* a battery-powered or nuclear-powered apparatus is implanted under the skin to regulate the heart rate.

Think bypasses are only for major cities with traffic issues? Not so. The *coronary artery bypass graft (CABG)* is a surgical technique to bring a new blood supply to heart muscles by detouring around blocked arteries, whereas a *femoropopliteal bypass* is surgery to establish an alternate route from the femoral artery to the popliteal artery in the leg, to bypass obstruction.

Bypass surgery can now be performed using MIDCAB (minimally invasive direct coronary artery bypass graft) and TECAB (totally endoscopic coronary artery bypass graft) with the help of the world's most advanced surgical robot, da Vinci Si. This robot has three arms and a 3D high-definition camera, and miniaturized surgical instruments are mounted on the arms. With the surgeon's guidance, the procedure that once required a 10- to 12-inch sternal incision can now be accomplished through small portals, allowing less trauma to the body, minimal scarring, and faster recovery time.

There certainly aren't as many clinical procedures for the lymphatic system, but they are equally important.

A *bone marrow biopsy* is just as serious as it sounds. A needle is introduced into the bone marrow cavity, and a small amount of marrow is *aspirated* (removed from the body) and examined under microscope. This procedure is helpful in the diagnosis of blood disorders such as anemia and leukemia.

Also in the category of "beyond serious" is the *bone marrow transplant.* Bone marrow cells from a donor, whose tissue and blood cells match those of the recipient, are infused into a patient with leukemia or aplastic anemia. The patient is first given aggressive chemotherapy to kill all diseased cells and then the donor's marrow is intravenously infused into the patient to repopulate the marrow with normal cells.

Taking a closer look at the lymphatic system's working parts involves the *lymphangiogram,* when dye is injected into lymph vessels in the foot and an x-ray is taken to show the path of lymph flow as it moves into the chest region. *Lymphadenography* is an x-ray of the lymph nodes and glands, after the injection of dye.

Terminology Rx: Cardiovascular and Lymphatic Pharmacology

Your friendly neighborhood pharmacist will know all the details of what to use for cardio and lymph-related ailments. In the meantime, you have us. This section lists the most common types of drugs used to correct cardiovascular and lymphatic conditions and diseases.

ACE (angiotensin-converting enzyme) inhibitors are medications that slow the activity of the enzyme ACE. These medications allow blood vessels to enlarge and dilate and blood pressure to reduce.

Aldosterone antagonists help the body get rid of salt and water, much like diuretic drugs (aka "water pills") do.

Antiarrhythmics correct cardiac arrhythmias (irregular heartbeat). Examples include digoxin (Lanoxin) and propranolol hydrochloride (Inderal).

Anticoagulants slow blood clotting. Examples include heparin calcium (Calcilean) and warfarin sodium (Coumadin).

Antihypertensives prevent or control high blood pressure. Examples include nadolol (Corgard), furosemide (Lasix), and diltiazem hydrochloride (Cardizem, Cardizem CD).

Beta blockers treat hypertension, angina, and other abnormal heart rhythms. Metoprolol tartrate (Lopressor) and carteolol hydrochloride (Ocupress, Cartrol) are popular examples.

Calcium channel blockers treat hypertension, angina, and various abnormal heart rhythms. Typical ones are nicardipine hydrochloride (Cardene) and bepridil hydrochloride (Vascor).

Lipid-lowering agents reduce blood lipid (fat) levels, such as niacin (Nicobid), lovastatin (Mevacor), and atorvastatin (Lipitor).

IN THIS CHAPTER

- Finding out how your respiratory system works
- Determining root words, prefixes, and suffixes appropriate to this system
- Using terminology of the respiratory system to discuss common conditions and diseases
- Finding the right terms to use when diagnosing problems

Chapter 17

Just Breathe: The Respiratory System

As you go about your day, you probably don't think to yourself, "Breathe in, now, breathe out," over and over. Perhaps the only time you are conscious of what your respiratory system does is when it is working overtime — during your workout or at the top of stairs you just climbed.

Because the cycle of breathing is continuous and constant, it's easy to take it for granted sometimes. Breathing is something we don't give much thought to because it looks after itself automatically. The body's trillions of cells need oxygen and need to get rid of carbon monoxide, and this exchange of gases is accomplished by the respiratory system.

How the Respiratory System Works

Air contains about 21 percent oxygen that is inhaled through the nose, finds its way to the lungs, into the lungs' air spaces, and passes into tiny capillary blood vessels surrounding the air spaces. At the same time, carbon dioxide — the gas produced when oxygen and food combine in cells — passes from the capillary blood vessels into the air spaces of the lungs to be exhaled. Exhaled air contains about 16 percent oxygen.

External respiration occurs between the outside environment and the capillary blood stream of the lungs, whereas another method of respiration is happening between the body cells and capillary blood vessels that surround them. This process is called *internal* or *cellular respiration.* Internal respiration is the exchange of gases not in the lungs, but in cells of all body organs. Oxygen passes out of the bloodstream and into the tissue cells. At the same time, carbon dioxide passes from the tissue cells into the bloodstream and is carried by the blood back to the lungs to be exhaled.

Capnia comes from the Greek *kapnos,* meaning "smoke." The word now refers to carbon dioxide.

TECHNICAL STUFF

The normal adult cycle of inhaling and exhaling, including a short rest between, takes place about 16–18 times per minute. This is known as the *respiratory rate.*

Figure 17-1 illustrates the respiratory system.

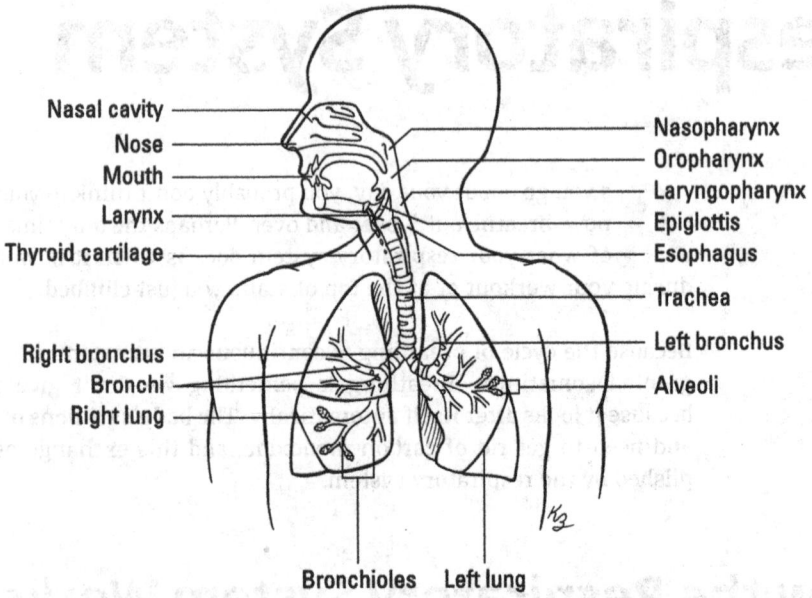

Illustration by Kathryn Born

FIGURE 17-1: Anatomic structures of the respiratory system.

Nose

When we inhale, or *inspire*, air enters the body through the nose via the external *nasal nares* (nostrils) and passes through the nasal cavity. This cavity is lined with a mucous membrane and fine hairs called *cilia* that filter out foreign bodies (such as dust and pollen) and warm and moisten the air. The *paranasal sinuses* are hollow, air spaces in the skull that join up with the nasal cavity. Paranasal sinuses have a mucous membrane lining and secrete mucus. They make the bones of the skull lighter and help in the production of sound (which is why you sound different when your sinuses are clogged). They connect with the nasal cavity and are named for the bones they are located in: the *frontal, ethmoid, sphenoid,* and *maxillary.* The singular form of nostrils, or nares, is *naris.*

TECHNICAL STUFF

Five hundred cubic feet of air passes through the nasal cavities every 24 hours.

Pharynx and larynx

After passing through the nasal cavity, air reaches the *pharynx* (the throat), which is made up of three parts. The *nasopharynx* is nearest the nasal cavity and contains the *adenoids,* which are masses of lymphatic tissue, which, in children, if enlarged, can obstruct the airway passage. Below the nasopharynx, closer to the mouth, is the *oropharynx,* where the *tonsils,* two rounded masses of lymphatic tissue, are located. The third part of the pharynx is the *hypopharynx,* where the pharynx serves as a common passageway for food from the mouth and air from the nose. This area is divided into two branches, the *larynx* (voice box) and the *esophagus* (passage to stomach). The larynx leads downward to the trachea, where the air goes down to the lungs. The vocal cords have a slit between them called the *glottis.* Sound is produced as air moves out of the lungs, through the glottis, causing vibration. As food enters from the mouth and air enters from the nose, they both come together in the pharynx.

Adenoid comes from the Greek *aden,* meaning "gland," and *cidos,* meaning "like." The term was once used for the prostate gland. The first adenoid surgery took place in 1868.

TECHNICAL STUFF

What stops food from going into the trachea and respiratory system after it's swallowed? The *epiglottis* is a flap of cartilage attached to the roof of the tongue that acts like a lid over the larynx. When swallowing food, the epiglottis closes off the larynx so that food can't enter.

Trachea

On its way to the lungs, air passes from the larynx to the *trachea* (windpipe), a tube 4½ inches long and about 1 inch in diameter. The trachea is kept open by

16–20 rings of cartilage that stiffen the front and sides of the tube. Some of these rings make up the thyroid cartilage forming the projection called the *Adam's apple.*

TECHNICAL STUFF

The Adam's apple is the largest cartilage ring in the larynx. The name is thought to come from the story that Adam sinned when he ate the forbidden fruit and was unable to swallow the apple stuck in his throat.

Bronchi

The trachea divides into two branches called the *bronchi.* Each *bronchus* (the singular form of *bronchi*) goes to a separate lung and subdivides into smaller and finer tubes, like the branches of a tree. The smallest of the bronchial branches are called *bronchioles.* At the end of the bronchioles are clusters of air sacs called *alveoli.* Each *alveolus* (singular of *alveoli*) is made up of a layer of *epithelium.* This very thin wall permits exchange of gases between the alveolus and capillaries that surround and come in close contact with it. The blood that flows through the capillaries takes the oxygen from the alveolus and leaves behind carbon dioxide to be exhaled. The oxygenated blood then carries the oxygen to all parts of the body.

Bronchi comes from Greek *brecho,* meaning "to pour" or "wet." The ancient Greeks believed that the esophagus carried solid food to stomach and the bronchi carried liquids (which it doesn't, and not to the stomach, for sure).

Lungs

Each lung is covered by a membrane called the *pleura.* The outer layer nearest to the ribs is *parietal pleura.* The inner layer closest to the lungs is the *visceral pleura.* The pleura is moistened with a watery fluid that assists in the movement of the lungs in the chest cavity. The two lungs are in the *thoracic* or *chest cavity.* The right lung is slightly larger than the left, divided into three *lobes,* the right upper, middle, and lower lobes. The left lung has two lobes, the left upper and lower lobes. To remember how many lobes each lung has, remember that the heart resides on the left side of the chest, thus taking up more room and hence leaving room for only two lobes.

TIP

One lobe of a lung can be surgically removed without damaging remaining lobes, which continue to function.

The lungs extend from the collarbone to the diaphragm in the chest cavity. The *diaphragm* is the muscular partition that separates the chest/thoracic cavity from the *abdominal* cavity. This muscle aids in the process of breathing. The diaphragm contracts and descends with each inhalation. The downward movement of the muscle enlarges the thoracic cavity area, allowing air to flow into the lungs to equalize pressure. When the lungs are full, the diaphragm relaxes and elevates, making the thoracic cavity smaller, increasing the air pressure in the thorax. Air is then expelled out of the lungs to equalize the pressure. This is called *exhalation* or *expiration*.

Atelectasis, from the Greek *ateles*, means "not perfect." *Ektasis*, "expansion," is an incomplete expansion of the lung, in particular at birth. Incomplete expansion can also occur after surgery when the patient avoids or cannot take deep breaths. This can cause the lungs to remain uninflated long enough for the air sacs to collapse into each other and create dead spaces in the lungs.

SHORT BREATHS: RESPIRATORY ABBREVIATIONS

The respiratory system is known for having some, um, long-winded words. Here are some of the more common abbreviations that you can memorize to make communicating about the nose, pharynx, larynx, trachea, bronchi, and lungs a little bit easier. You'll be sounding like a cast member of a medical drama in no time.

- **A&P:** Auscultation and percussion
- **ABG:** Arterial blood gases, to determine oxygen and CO_2 levels dissolved into the arteries
- **ARDS:** Adult respiratory distress syndrome caused by injury or illness
- **COPD:** Chronic obstructive pulmonary disease
- **CPR:** Cardiopulmonary resuscitation
- **CXR:** Chest x-ray
- **ENT:** Ears, nose, and throat
- **PE:** Pulmonary embolus
- **PFT:** Pulmonary function tests, to determine lung function
- **SIDS:** Sudden infant death syndrome
- **SOB:** Shortness of breath
- **TB:** Tuberculosis
- **URI:** Upper respiratory infection
- **VPS:** Ventilation perfusion scan, to diagnose pulmonary embolism, or to evaluate circulation of air and blood in the lungs (also called lung scan or V-Q scan)

Respiratory Root Words

You just got to know about all the individual parts of the respiratory system. Each one is equally important. The nose without the pharynx or the lungs without the bronchi would be nothing more than spare parts, like on an old junker in a garage. Similarly, the parts of medical terms must coexist and work together to help us understand their meanings. Prefixes, suffixes, and root words work in harmony to bring the world of the respiratory system into focus. Let's start at the beginning, in Table 17-1, with prefixes.

TABLE 17-1

Start Your Engine with Prefixes

Prefix	What It Means
An-, a-	Without, absent
Endo-	Within
Inter-	Between
Intra-	Within

That was simple enough, right? Suffixes outnumber prefixes by more than half, but you should find the list in Table 17-2 still quite manageable.

TABLE 17-2

Exhale with Respiratory Suffixes

Suffix	What It Means
-ar, -ary	Pertaining to
-capnia	Carbon dioxide
-centesis	Surgical puncture with needle to aspirate fluid
-ectasis	Stretching or expansion
-gram	Record
-graphy	Process of recording
-itis	Inflammation
-osmia	Smell
-ostomy	Creation of an artificial opening
-oxia	Oxygen

Suffix	What It Means
-phasia	Speech
-phonia	Voice, sound
-pnea	Breathing
-scope	Instrument used to visually examine
-scopy	Visual examination
-sphyxia	Pulse
-stenosis	Narrowing or constricting
-thorax	Chest

Root words and combining forms associated with the respiratory system include the ones listed in Table 17-3.

TABLE 17-3

Breaking Down Your Respiratory Roots

Suffix	What It Means
Adenoid/o	Adenoids
Alveol/o	Alveolus, air sac
Atel/o	Imperfect, incomplete
Bronch/o	Bronchus
Bronchi/o	Bronchial tubes
Bronchiol/o	Bronchioles
Capn/o	Carbon dioxide
Coni/o	Dust
Cyan/o	Blue
Epiglott/o	Epiglottis
Laryng/o	Larynx (voice box)
Lob/o	Lobes
Mediastin/o	Mediastinum
Nas/o	Nose

(continued)

TABLE 17-3 *(continued)*

Suffix	What It Means
Ox/o, Ox/i	Oxygen
Pector/o	Chest
Pharyng/o	Throat
Phas/o	Speech
Phon/o	Voice, sound
Phren/o	Diaphragm
Pleur/o	Pleura
Pneum/o	Lung, air
Pulmon/o	Lung
Py/o	Pus
Respir/o, respirat/o	Breathe, breathing
Rhin/o	Nose
Sept/o	Partition
Spir/o	To breathe
Steth/o	Chest
Thorac/o	Chest
Tonsill/o	Tonsils
Trache/o	Trachea (windpipe)

It's All Related: More Anatomical Terms

But that's not all! We still have all sorts of great respiratory words for you to consider. For example, *respirology* is the study of respiratory diseases and respiratory system, and a *respirologist* is a physician specializing in disorders and treatment of respiratory systems.

Getting in and around your body are two gases with which you should be familiar: oxygen and carbon dioxide. Good old *oxygen* is the gas that passes into the bloodstream in the lungs and travels to all body cells. Conversely, carbon dioxide (CO_2) is the gas produced by cells that is exhaled through the lungs. *Internal respiration* is the exchange of gases at the tissue cells. Sometimes, however, these gases are missing. *Acapnia* is the absence or less than normal level of carbon dioxide in blood, whereas *anoxia* is the absence of oxygen in the blood. Some other respiratory-related health issues include

- **Aphonia:** Absence of voice
- **Apnea:** Absence of breathing
- **Bronchospasm:** Sporadic contraction of the bronchi
- **Dysphonia:** Difficulty in speaking
- **Dypsnea:** Difficulty breathing
- **Eupnea:** Normal breathing
- **Hemoptysis:** Coughing up blood from the lung
- **Hyperventilation:** Ventilation of lungs beyond normal body needs
- **Hypoxemia:** Deficient oxygen content in blood
- **Hypoxia:** Deficient oxygen to body tissue
- **Mucoid:** Resembling mucus
- **Mucous:** Pertaining to mucus
- **Mucus:** Secretion (slime) from the mucous membranes
- **Orthopnea:** Able to breathe only in upright or sitting position
- **Nasopharyngeal:** Referring to the nose and throat
- **Rhinorrhea:** Discharge from the nose

Next we have some terms specifically related to descriptions of respiratory body parts and functions. Get to know the following individual components of the system a bit better:

- **Adenoids:** A collection of lymph tissue in the nasopharynx
- **Alveolus:** An air sac in the lung
- **Apex:** Upper portion of the lung
- **Apical:** Pertaining to the apex
- **Base:** The lower portion of the lung
- **Bronchus:** The branch of the trachea that acts as the passageway into the air spaces of the lung
- **Bronchioles:** Smallest branches of the bronchi

- **Bronchodilator:** Agent causing the bronchi to widen or open up
- **Cilia:** Tiny hairs in the mucous membranes lining the respiratory tract
- **Hilum:** Middle portion of lung where bronchi, blood vessels, and nerves enter and exit the lungs
- **Lobes:** Divisions of the lungs. The right lung has three lobes and the left has two. Want an easy way to remember that? The left lobe only has two to make room for the heart.
- **Mediastinum:** Region between lungs in the chest cavity containing heart, aorta, esophagus, and bronchial tubes

Now for the potpourri, the mishmash, and everything but the kitchen sink. Table 17-4 is a grouping of additional vocabulary words that you need to know in order to relate to the respiratory system.

TABLE 17-4

A Mixed Bag of Respiratory Vocabulary

Word	What It Means
Bronchoconstrictor	Agent causing narrowing of the bronchial airways
Bronchodilator	Agent causing widening or clearing of bronchial airways
Hyperventilation	Ventilation of the lungs beyond normal body needs
Mucopurulent	Containing both mucus and pus
Nebulizer	Device creating a fine spray for giving respiratory treatments
Oximeter	Instrument used to measure oxygen in blood
Paroxysm	Periodic or sudden attack
Patent	Open
Pulmonary	Pertaining to the lungs
Rales	Abnormal rattling sounds heard on auscultation
Sputum	Secretion from lungs, bronchi, and trachea coughed up and ejected through the mouth
Ventilator	Mechanical device used to assist with or substitute for breathing when patient cannot breathe unassisted

Common Respiratory Conditions

Of all the most common respiratory conditions, the bronchial tubes get the big daddy: asthma. *Asthma* is attacks of *paroxysmal dyspnea* (sudden onset of wheezing and difficulty breathing) with airway inflammation and wheezing due to contraction of the bronchi, leading to airway obstruction if severe enough. The condition affects millions of people of all ages.

Asthma comes from the Greek *astma*, meaning "to pant."

The lungs have all sorts of wild and wacky conditions associated with them. *Atelectasis*, for example, is the imperfect expansion of air sacs of the lungs. *Emphysema* is the distention of the alveoli with swelling and inflammation of lung tissue. Often seen in heavy smokers, this condition is marked by loss of elasticity of the lungs. *Pneumonia* is the acute inflammation and infection of the alveoli. A couple of different varieties exist: *Lobar pneumonia* involves distribution of infection in one or more lobes of a lung, whereas *pneumocystis carinii pneumonia (PCP)* is an infectious disease caused by P. carinii, the infectious agent. It is fungal in origin and is common in AIDS patients.

Pneumonia can be distributed in different ways, for example, confining itself to only one lobe, as is often the case with a viral infection, versus presenting a "cotton-wool" appearance on x-ray, with scattered white spots throughout the lungs, as with PCP. It can be caused by many different infectious agents such as viruses, bacteria, and what are known as *atypical agents*, such as *Mycoplasma*, a common cause of pneumonia in teenagers and young adults.

TECHNICAL STUFF

Before 1980, PCP was rare. Sixty to 80 percent of AIDS patients develop PCP.

When we breathe, we don't just breathe in air. Sometimes foreign particles sneak in, like crashers at your respiratory party. Dust is the most common culprit. *Pneumoconiosis* is an abnormal condition of dust in the lungs. Differing types of pneumoconiosis include the following:

- **Anthracosis:** Coal dust (black lung disease)
- **Asbestosis:** Asbestos particles in lungs
- **Silicosis:** Silica dust or glass (grinder's disease)

Speaking of foreign matter hanging out in the lungs, the pleura (that membrane that covers the lungs) can also be affected by foreign matter, namely fluid. *Pleurisy* is an inflammation of the pleura. *Pleural effusion* is the escape of fluid into the pleural cavity. Examples of a pleural effusion include *empyema* (that pus in the pleural cavity you read about earlier) and *Hemothorax*, which is blood in the pleural cavity typically caused by a trauma, and is not quite as common but obviously a serious problem — just ask anyone who works in the ER. Other greatest hits of pleural effusion include lung malignancy and congestive heart failure, due to the increased pressure of blood backing up in the pulmonary vessels.

But wait! There's more fluid and pus! It can be a pusapalooza in those lungs, and can often develop into very serious conditions, like these three:

- **Pulmonary abscess:** Localized area of pus formation in the lungs
- **Pulmonary edema:** Swelling and fluid in the air sacs and bronchioles, caused by poor blood supply to the heart muscle
- **Pulmonary embolism:** Floating clot or other material blocking the blood vessels of the lung

If you thought that was all that could possibly affect your breathing, think again. Because there is such a great chance for foreign particles, dust, or communicable disease (from the common cold to more serious conditions), the lungs and its buddies are susceptible to a wide range of conditions. Here are some more examples:

- **Adenoiditis:** Inflammation of the adenoids
- **Atelectasis:** Incomplete expansion of the lungs
- **Bronchiectasis:** Dilatation of the bronchi
- **Bronchitis:** Inflammation of the bronchi
- **Laryngitis:** Inflammation of the larynx
- **Laryngotracheobronchitis:** Croup
- **Pneumothorax:** Air between the lung and chest wall
- **Pulmonary neoplasm:** A new growth in the lung, which can be malignant or benign depending on the composition
- **Rhinitis:** Inflammation of mucous membranes of nose
- **Tonsillitis:** Inflammation of the tonsils
- **Tracheitis:** Inflammation of the trachea

Finding the Culprit: Respiratory Diseases and Pathology

Now for the really serious, land-you-in-the-hospital sort of stuff: diseases and pathological disorders. One of the most frightening respiratory diseases is *tuberculosis*, also known as *TB*. Because of its communicable nature, this infectious disease, which is caused by *acid-fast bacilli* spread by inhalation of infected droplets, always causes a commotion when reported to health officials. So much so, in fact, that before antibiotics, hospitals built solely for the treatment of TB were quite common. TB is a bit more under control today and is treated with a specific antibiotic regime, usually over a long-term (6-month) period. There are still many cases reported, though, particularly in the Global South.

Diphtheria is another infectious disease of the upper respiratory tract, affecting the throat. *Influenza*, that pesky *flu*, is a highly infectious respiratory disease that is viral in origin. Though for most people nowadays it involves some time off work and chicken soup, the flu can be deadly if not treated, or in high-risk groups like small children and the elderly. *Legionnaires' disease* is a form of *lobar pneumonia* caused by the bacterium Legionella pneumophilia.

TECHNICAL STUFF

Legionnaires' disease gained notoriety after a highly publicized epidemic of it occurred at the American Legion convention in 1976.

Tired yet? Hang in there. There are a few more respiratory diseases you should know. Here's the lowdown:

- **Adult respiratory distress syndrome (ARDS)** is respiratory failure in an adult as a result of disease or injury.
- **Bronchogenic carcinoma** is a cancerous tumor arising from the bronchus. This tumor can *metastasize* (spread) to brain, liver, and other organs.
- **Chronic obstructive pulmonary disease (COPD)** refers to any persistent lung disease that obstructs the bronchial airflow. Examples include asthma, chronic bronchitis, and emphysema.
- **Cor pulmonale** is a serious cardiac disease associated with chronic lung disorders such as emphysema.
- **OSA,** or obstructive sleep apnea, occurs when the pharynx collapses during sleep leading to absence of breathing.
- **Pulmonary edema** means fluid accumulation in the alveoli and bronchioles.

WATCH THOSE KIDDOS

Some diseases present in infancy or develop more predominantly in children. One that is commonly associated with children is *pertussis,* more commonly known as *whooping cough.* This is a contagious bacterial infection of the upper respiratory tract (the pharynx, larynx, and trachea). *Croup* (laryngotracheobronchitis) is another respiratory disease affecting children. It is an acute respiratory syndrome in children and infants marked by an obstruction of the larynx, hoarseness, and cough.

On a whole other level are those diseases that can be inherited. *Cystic fibrosis* is one to watch. This is an inherited disease of infants and children in which there is excess mucus production in the respiratory tract. It is a dysfunction of the exocrine glands with chronic (longstanding) lung disease due to excessive mucus secretion in the respiratory tract, pancreatic deficiency, and sometimes liver cirrhosis. It is a multitude of dysfunctions, but the mucus production is the main problem.

If you are pregnant, consult with your OB about prescreening for cystic fibrosis to determine if you or your partner is a carrier for the disease.

- **Pulmonary embolism** is a blood clot, fat clot, or air carried in blood circulation to pulmonary artery where it blocks the artery.
- **URI** is upper respiratory tract infection of pharynx, larynx, and trachea. LRI (lower respiratory infection) usually refers to an infection of everything that's left — bronchi and lungs. It's hard to have a LRI without the URI, but you can have the URI by itself.

Testing, Testing: Respiratory Radiology and Diagnostic Tests

Now that you have all these conditions and disease terms floating around in your head, you're probably wondering what, if anything, can be done about them? Thanks to the wonders of modern technology, there are all sorts of ways physicians and other medical professionals can diagnose what ails those airways.

To start, physicians rely on their senses to look and listen to what your lungs and associated respiratory parts are doing. Every time, for example, the doctor listens to your heart and lungs with a *stethoscope*, she is performing *auscultation*, which simply means . . . listening to sounds within the body using a stethoscope. This simple method allows doctors and nurses to hear the sounds of the lungs, pleura, heart, and abdomen. Another listening technique is *percussion*, in which the physician makes short, sharp blows (taps) to the surface of the body with a finger or instrument to determine density from sounds of the underlying tissue. A *laryngoscopy* occurs when the larynx is visualized with a laryngoscope. A *bronchoscopy* is the examination of the bronchus by passing a flexible fiber optic tube (endoscope) into the bronchus. A *tracheostomy* is cutting an opening into the trachea through the neck and inserting a tube to facilitate passage of air or removal of secretions.

TIP

IPPA stands for inspection, palpation, percussion, and auscultation. These are all part of a normal physical examination either in hospital or in physician's office.

Diagnostic tests are part of the respiratory physician's problem-solving bag of tricks. Some are more invasive than others, whereas some simply involve more looking and listening with the aid of medical equipment. Some of the most used tests are the following:

- **Arterial blood gases:** Blood test to measure levels of oxygen in blood.
- **Bronchial washing:** Specimens can be obtained for bacterial studies and *cytologic* or cell studies, by aspiration of bronchial secretions or by injecting fluid and retrieving it.
- **Chest x-ray (CXR):** Radiograph of chest to evaluate heart and lungs.
- **Endotracheal intubation** is when a tube is placed through the mouth, into the trachea, to establish an airway.
- **Lung biopsy:** Lung tissue is obtained by forceps or brush (bronchial brushing). Can also be accomplished through a catheter inserted under x-ray guidance.
- **Lung plethysmography:** Also known as pulmonary or body plethysmography, this test measures how much air you can hold in your lungs (lung capacity).
- **Lung scan:** Radioactive material is injected or inhaled and images are recorded of its distribution into lung tissue.
- **Pulmonary angiography:** X-ray image of the blood vessels of the lungs after injection of contrast material.
- **Pulmonary function tests** evaluate ventilation capacity of the lung. A *spirometer* measures the air taken in and out of the lungs to diagnose asthma and COPD.
- **Sputum culture:** Sputum is analyzed for presence of bacteria.

» **Thoracentesis:** Chest wall is punctured with a needle to obtain fluid from the pleural cavity for diagnostic studies or to relieve pressure in the lung.

» **Tuberculin test** is when an antigen is applied to the skin by multiple punctures or tines test, or intradermally by the Mantoux test. An inflammatory reaction is observed in 48-96 hours in an infected patient.

One very useful way to view what is going on in the respiratory system is to use x-ray and endoscopic procedures to take a closer look. Two major types of x-ray are used for this system: A *bronchogram* is an x-ray of the bronchi, and a *chest x-ray* is used to evaluate the lungs and heart. Another widely used diagnostic method is the *bronchoscopy*, a visual examination of the bronchus using a *bronchoscope*. A *chest CT* is also called *computerized axial tomography (CAT scan)*. This is when physicians and radiologists use computerized images of the chest cavity to diagnose tumors, abscesses, and pleural effusion.

Paging Dr. Terminology: Respiratory Surgeries and Procedures

Now you've got the tools to identify and diagnose conditions and diseases of the respiratory system, so get your instruments and scrub in, because it's time to operate.

Most of the terms regarding surgeries and procedures revolve around the actual incisions, excisions, and repairs used to treat a myriad of conditions and diseases. As such, these terms are fairly straightforward. You'll see a lot of *-otomy* and *-plasty* suffixes here, denoting the type of procedure.

Start at the top, with repairs made to the nose. *Rhinoplasty* (your standard beak job) is a surgical repair of the nose, while *septoplasty* is the surgical repair of the nasal septum.

Moving down to the throat region, you have the *adenoidectomy*, an excision of adenoids. Similarly, the *tonsillectomy* is an excision of the neighboring tonsils, as well as a sure method of obtaining ice cream.

Two terms relate directly to the larynx. *Laryngectomy* is the excision of larynx, while *laryngoplasty* is the surgical repair of the larynx. Moving on to the trachea, we have the *tracheotomy*, often popularized in television and movies using some non-medical character who must perform one with a bottle of vodka and a Swiss Army knife or ball point pen. But let's leave it to the professionals, shall we?

This procedure involves an incision into the trachea. A *tracheoplasty* is a surgical repair of the trachea.

The lungs and chest cavity are next. Here are some of the most common surgeries and procedures pertaining to that area of the respiratory system:

- **Bullectomy:** Removal of large bullae (a.k.a. blisters, vesicles, and blebs) from the lungs with COPD
- **Decortication of lung:** Surgical removal of surface layer of lung, when thick outer layer restricts lung expansion
- **Lobectomy:** Excision of a lobe of a lung
- **Lung transplantation:** Partial or total surgical removal of diseased lungs, replaced by lungs from a donor
- **LVRS (lung volume reduction surgery):** An invasive open-chest surgery to remove diseased emphysematous lung tissue, allowing expansion and growth of the remaining, more functioning lung
- **Pleurocentesis:** Surgical puncture to aspirate fluid from pleural space
- **Pneumonectomy:** Excision of a lung
- **Thoracocentesis:** Surgical puncture to aspirate fluid from the chest cavity
- **Thoracotomy:** Incision into the chest cavity
- **Valve surgery:** By means of bronchoscopy, a one-way valve is inserted into the airway to provide air entry control with an over-expanded lung, typical in patients with severe emphysema

Terminology RX: Respiratory Pharmacology

Several kinds of medicines are used to treat the respiratory system. Many are used for other systems as well, but they are worth repeating so you will know what is safe to use with direct relation to the lungs. *Bronchodilators* are used to treat asthma, COPD, and exercise-induced bronchospasm. They relax muscles around the bronchi, increasing air flow. They are usually given orally, intravenously, or by nebulizer or aerochamber (inhaler) administered in puffs. *Corticosteroids* are used to control inflammatory responses. *Diuretics* (water pills) are used to treat pulmonary edema. *LABAs (long acting beta-2 agonists)* and *LAMAs (long acting muscarinic antagonists)* can be administered together to offer COPD sufferers relief of symptoms. LABAs can be given with a corticosteroid as another option.

When you are feeling the effects of a cold or bronchial infection, you probably take one of these next four drug types: *Decongestants* help reduce swelling in mucous membranes of the nose, to relieve stuffiness and allow secretions to drain. *Antihistamines* help dry up secretions. They are effective in treating allergic reactions, but not effective on the common cold. *Antitussives* decrease coughing by suppressing the cough center in the brain. *Expectorants* reduce the thickness of sputum so it can be coughed up more easily. If over-the-counter meds just won't cut it, a prescription may be in order. *Antibiotics* are used to treat respiratory infections, tuberculosis, and pneumonias. *Silver nitrate* can be used to cauterize superficial blood vessels that cause nosebleeds.

IN THIS CHAPTER

- Discovering how your gastrointestinal system works
- Determining root words, prefixes, and suffixes appropriate to this system
- Using terminology of the gastrointestinal system to discuss common conditions and diseases
- Finding the right terms to use when diagnosing problems

Chapter 18

Feeding Time: The Gastrointestinal System

That big steak dinner leaves you feeling like you need elastic pants for a reason. Your *gastrointestinal* (sometimes abbreviated *GI*) system has to work hard to make all that meat and potatoes into a useful substance that your body can use as energy, and it can only hold so much at one time.

Imagine the local swimming pool at the height of summer. Only so many kids can jump in, because otherwise the water overflows and makes a big mess. It's the same with the gastrointestinal system. If you put too many things in, something's bound to overflow. So, take small bites and try to digest everything there is to know about that full feeling you have after dinner. Elastic pants are optional.

The *gastrointestinal system*, also called the *alimentary* or *digestive tract*, provides a tubelike passage through a maze of organs and body cavities, beginning at the mouth, the food entrance into the body, and ending at the anus, where solid waste material exits the body.

This system and its organs perform three primary functions:

- Carrying food for digestion
- Preparing it for absorption
- Transporting waste products for elimination

How the Gastrointestinal System Works

Digestion begins with our help. Food is put in the mouth. It has to be broken down and digested both mechanically and chemically, as it makes its way through the gastrointestinal tract. Digestive enzymes help speed up the chemical reaction and assist in the breakdown or digestion of complex nutrients from the food.

During the digestive process, proteins break down to *amino acids*, complicated sugars reduce to simple sugars, such as glucose, and large fat molecules are broken down into *fatty acids* and *triglycerides*.

Absorption takes place when the digested food is absorbed into the bloodstream, by going through the walls of the small intestine. By this process, nutrients like sugar and amino acids travel to all cells in the body. Fatty acids and triglycerides are also absorbed through the wall of the small intestine, but enter lymphatic vessels rather than blood vessels.

The third stage is elimination of solid waste materials that cannot be absorbed into the bloodstream. This solid waste, called *feces*, collects in the large bowel and finally exits the body you know where.

You can follow the merry route taken through the various passages and organs that make up the digestive system, as shown in Figure 18-1.

Mouth and pharynx

The digestive tract begins with the *oral cavity* or the *mouth*. The lips provide the opening and the cheeks form the walls. The *hard palate* is the roof of the mouth, and the *muscular soft palate* lies behind it, horizontally separating the mouth from the *nasopharynx*, or posterior nasal cavity. Then everything blends in together. The mouth, or *oropharynx*, shades subtly into the *hypopharynx*, or the back of the mouth/top of the throat, and then the pharynx proper, or upper throat, which then becomes the esophagus. And that concludes our discovery tour of the pharynx.

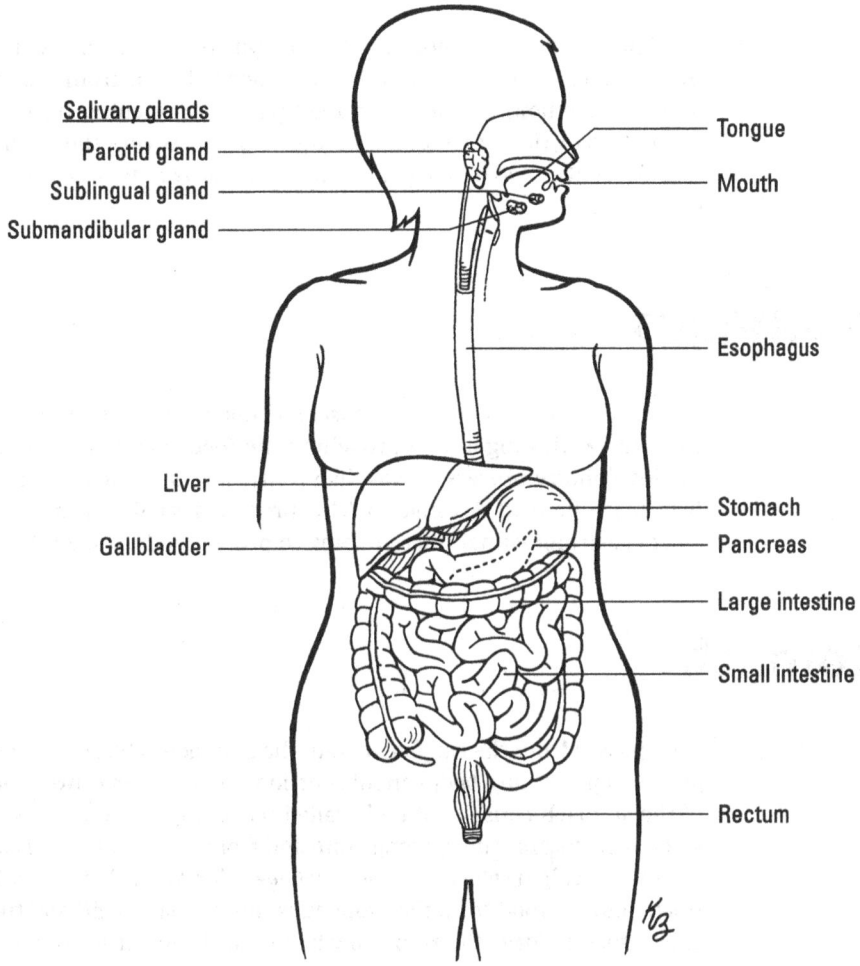

FIGURE 18-1: The organs of the digestive system.

Illustration by Kathryn Born

Hanging from the soft palate is a tiny piece of soft tissue called the *uvula*, which means "little grape." The tongue extends from the floor of the mouth and is attached by muscles to the lower jawbone. It moves food around during chewing *(mastication)* and swallowing *(deglutition)*. The tongue is covered with tiny projections called *papillae*, which contain taste buds that are sensitive to the chemical nature of foods.

The teeth are important because, during the chewing process, they break down food into smaller pieces to make the swallowing process easier. Around the oral cavity are three pairs of *salivary glands*. These glands produce *saliva*, which contains digestive enzymes. Saliva is released from the *parotid gland*, the *submandibular gland*, and the *sublingual gland*, on each side of the mouth. Narrow salivary ducts carry the saliva into the oral cavity.

Food passes from the mouth to the *pharynx* (throat), a muscular tube lined with mucous membrane. It acts as the passageway for air from the nasal cavity to the *larynx* (voice box) but also as a food passageway going from the mouth to the esophagus. A flap of tissue called the *epiglottis* covers the opening to the larynx and prevents food from going into the *trachea* (windpipe) when swallowing occurs.

Esophagus

The *esophagus* is a 9–10-inch muscular tube from the pharynx to the stomach. It aides in swallowing and in propelling the food toward the stomach. *Peristalsis* is the involuntary process of wavelike contractions in the esophagus that helps the food reach its next destination. This process actually takes place throughout the entire gastrointestinal tract, helping to propel food through the system.

Stomach

Food passes from the esophagus into the stomach. The stomach is made up of the *fundus* (top portion), *body* (middle portion), and *antrum* (lower portion). The lining of the stomach consists of folds called *rugae,* which allow the stomach to stretch when food enters. The openings into and from the stomach are controlled by rings of muscles called *sphincters.* The *esophageal* (or *cardiac*) *sphincter* relaxes and contracts moving food from the esophagus into the stomach, and the *pyloric sphincter* allows food to leave the stomach when it has been sufficiently broken down.

The function of the stomach is to prepare food chemically to be received in the small intestine for further digestion and absorption into the bloodstream. Food is churned and mixed with *gastric juices* to make a semiliquid called *chyme.* Food does not enter the bloodstream through the walls of the stomach. The stomach controls passage of food into the first part of the small intestine, so it proceeds only when it is chemically ready and in small amounts.

The liver, gallbladder, and pancreas are accessory organs of the digestive system. Food doesn't pass through these organs, but each plays a role in the proper digestion and absorption of nutrients.

Liver

The *liver* produces greenish fluid called *bile* that contains *cholesterol*, a fat substance, *bile acids*, and several *bile pigments*. Bile is continuously released from the liver and travels down the *hepatic duct* to the *cystic duct*. The cystic duct leads to the *gallbladder*, which stores and concentrates the bile for later use. After meals, the gallbladder contracts, forcing bile into the *common bile duct* joining with the *pancreatic duct*, just before the entrance of the duodenum. The *duodenum* receives a mixture of bile and pancreatic juices.

Pancreas

The *pancreas* produces juices filled with enzymes, *amylase* and *lipase*, to digest food. These pass into the duodenum through the *pancreatic duct*. An endocrine gland (see Chapter 19), the pancreas also secretes *insulin*. This hormone is needed to help regulate levels of glucose in the blood.

The *pancreas* is so named because of its fleshy appearance. Greek *pan* means "all," and *krea* means "flesh."

Gallbladder

The *gallbladder* is a sac-like structure 3–4 inches long tucked under the right lobe of the liver. It is part of the *biliary tract* (hepatic, cystic, and common bile ducts). It stores bile until needed in the duodenum to aid digestion.

TECHNICAL STUFF

You can live without a gallbladder. If inflamed or containing stones (a calcified pebble formed in the gallbladder), it is surgically removed. Bile can find another home in the biliary ducts, allowing the biliary process to function.

Intestines

The *small intestine*, or *small bowel*, extends from the pyloric sphincter to the first part of the large intestine. It is 21 feet long, 1 inch in diameter, and has three parts. The *duodenum*, a foot in length, receives the chyme from the stomach, as well as bile from the liver and gallbladder and pancreatic juices from the pancreas.

Duodenum is from the Latin *duodeni* meaning "twelve each," referring to its length.

Enzymes and bile help digest food before it passes into the second part of the small intestine, the *jejunum*. The jejunum is about 8 feet long and connects to the third portion, the *ileum*, which is 11 feet long. Most of the absorption process takes place in the ileum. In the wall of the small intestine are millions of tiny microscopic *villi*, fingerlike projections. Through tiny capillaries in the villi, digested nutrients pass through to enter the bloodstream and lymph vessels. At the lower end of the ileum is the *ileocecal valve*, the joining point of the small intestine to the large intestine.

Here's a quick look at two parts of the intestine. *Jejunum* (Latin *jejunas*) means "empty" and is so named because it was always found empty. *Ileum* (Greek *cilein*) means "to roll." This is a reference to the peristaltic waves that move food.

The *large intestine*, or *large bowel*, extends from the end of the ileum to the anus. It is made up of four parts: the *cecum*, *colon*, *sigmoid colon*, and *rectum*. It is 5 feet long and about 2½ inches in diameter. The *cecum* is a pouch that is connected to the ileum by the *ileocecal valve*.

The *appendix* hangs from the cecum. The appendix has no known function, which is why it's not a huge loss to your body if it must be removed. The colon has three divisions: the ascending, transverse, and descending colon. The sigmoid colon is S-shaped, at the end of the descending colon that leads into the *rectum*. The rectum terminates at the lower opening of the gastrointestinal tract at the anus. The entire large intestine receives fluid waste products of digestion that cannot be absorbed into the bloodstream and stores it until it is released from the body.

Gastrointestinal Root Words

A lot of players work together in the gastrointestinal tract. The good news, with regard to word building, is that the list of prefixes and suffixes is a lot less complicated than those of other large systems. The prefixes and suffixes listed in Table 18-1 will help you keep all the body parts, ailments, and procedures straight.

TABLE 18-1 **Food In, Food Out: Gastro Prefixes and Suffixes**

Prefix	What It Means
Exo-	Outside
Peri-	Surrounding
Pre-	Before or preceding
Post-	After or following
Re-	Back
Retro-	Backward, back
Suffix	**What It Means**
-ase	Enzyme
-chesia, -chezia	Defecation
-flux	Flow
-ectomy	Surgical removal, cutting out
-iasis	Abnormal condition
-itis	Inflammation
-lithiasis	Calculus or stone
-lysis	Destruction or breakdown
-pepsia	Digestion
-prandial	Meal
-orrhaphy	Surgical fixation or suturing
-ostomy	Creation of an artificial opening
-tresia	Opening, perforation
-tripsy	Crushing

REMEMBER

When in doubt, sound it out!

Now, in Table 18-2, it's time to find out what comes in between these word parts. Consider the combining forms and root words as you would the stomach — they break the word down into its most useful component. That root will, in turn, provide the nutritive content that gives the word its meaning.

TABLE 18-2 **The Meaty Part: Gastrointestinal Root Words**

Root Word	What It Means
Abdomin/o	Abdomen
An/o	Anus
Appendic/o	Appendix
Atel/o	Incomplete, imperfect
Bucc/o	Cheek (facial)
Cec/o	Cecum
Celi/o	Belly
Cheil/o, chil/o	Lips
Chol/e, bil/i	Gall, bile
Cholecyst/o	Gallbladder
Choledoch/o	Common bile duct
Col/o, colon/o	Colon
Dent/o, dent/I, odont/o	Teeth
Dips/o	Thirst
Duoden/o	Duodenum
Enter/o	Small intestine
Esophag/o	Esophagus
Gastr/o	Stomach
Gingiv/o	Gums
Gloss/o	Tongue
Gluc/o, glyc/o	Sugar
Hepat/o	Liver
Ile/o	Ileum
Jejun/o	Jejunum
Labi/o	Lips
Lapar/o	Abdomen

Root Word	What It Means
Lingu/o, gloss/o	Tongue
Lip/o	Fat, lipids
Lith/o	Stone
Odont/o	Teeth
Or/o	Mouth, oral
Orth/o	Straight, normal, correct
Palat/o	Palate
Pancreat/o	Pancreas
Peritone/o	Peritoneum
Phag/o, phagi/a	Eating, ingestion
Pharyng/o	Pharynx
Proct/o	Anus, rectum
Pylor/o	Pylorus
Pyr/o	Fever, heat
Rect/o	Rectum
Sialaden/o	Salivary gland
Sial/o	Saliva
Sigmoid/o	Sigmoid colon
Splen/o	Spleen
Steat/o	Fat
Stomat/o	Mouth
Submaxill/o	Lower jaw
Tonsill/o	Tonsil
Uran/o	Palate
Uvul/o	Uvula

Common Gastrointestinal Conditions

Because the gastrointestinal system is made of many parts, it shouldn't be a surprise that it can be prone to all sorts of ailments and maladies. Mouth conditions are some of the most obvious to the naked eye. Thankfully, two types of professionals can help find solutions to maladies of the mouth that affect mastication (chewing). Ask any parent about your friendly, neighborhood *orthodontist* — she or he specializes in the correction of deformed, crooked, or *maloccluded* (crooked or misaligned) teeth. The *periodontist* specializes in diseases of the tissue around the teeth. Don't forget the good old *dentist*, who takes care of dental issues; and the *oral* and *maxillofacial surgeons* who deal with dental and facial surgery to repair things like cleft palates and dental trauma.

Now, take a closer look at some of the conditions these specialists treat:

- **Aphthous stomatitis:** Canker sores in mouth
- **Bruxism:** Grinding teeth involuntarily, often while sleeping
- **Cleft palate:** Congenital split in the roof of the mouth or upper lip
- **Dental caries:** Cavities in the teeth (*caries* means "decay")
- **Dysphasia:** Difficulty speaking
- **Edentulous:** Without teeth
- **Gingivitis:** Inflammation of gums
- **Halitosis:** Bad breath
- **Herpes simplex:** Cold sore or fever blister on lip or nose due to herpes virus
- **Leukoplakia:** White plaques or patches of mouth mucosa
- **Sublingual:** Under the tongue

TECHNICAL STUFF

Your baby teeth are also called the *primary teeth.* Your first teeth (20 in all) include 8 incisors, 4 cuspids, and 8 molars. Your permanent teeth number 32, with 8 incisors, 8 premolars, 4 canines, and 12 molars.

The esophagus is the next stop on your tour of gastrointestinal conditions. Many of the following conditions result in discomfort both in swallowing (deglutition) and in the digestion process:

- **Aphagia:** Inability to swallow
- **Dysphagia:** Difficulty swallowing

- **Esophageal varices:** Just like varicose veins in the legs; boggy veins with inefficient valves that allow venous backflow, resulting in stagnant blood in bulging veins
- **Esophagitis:** Inflammation of the esophagus
- **Heartburn:** Burning sensation caused by reflux or flowing back of acid from the stomach into esophagus

REMEMBER

To keep *dysphasia* and *dysphagia* straight, remember the *s* in dysphasia for "speak," and the *g* in dysphagia for "gag."

Moving south, you find the stomach, an area full of possibility when it comes to conditions. *Gastroenterology* is the study of the stomach and intestines, and a *gastroenterologist* is the physician who treats conditions of the stomach and intestines.

Many of the conditions that eventually affect the esophagus or intestines start in the stomach. So, have your antacids ready for these:

- **Dyspepsia:** Difficult digestion
- **Emesis (vomiting):** Stomach contents expelled through the mouth
- **Eructation:** Act of belching or raising gas from stomach
- **Gastric ulcer:** Lesion on wall of stomach; also known as peptic ulcer
- **Gastritis:** Inflammation of the stomach
- **Gastrodynia:** Pain in the stomach
- **Hematemesis:** Vomiting of blood
- **Hiatal hernia:** Protrusion of part of the stomach through the esophageal opening into diaphragm
- **Hyperemesis:** Excessive vomiting
- **Nasogastric:** Pertaining to nose and stomach
- **Nausea:** Urge to vomit
- **Regurgitation:** Return of solids and fluids to mouth from stomach
- **Ulcer:** Sore or lesion of mucous membrane or skin

The liver, pancreas, and gallbladder all experience their own specific conditions, the most common of which is good, old-fashioned, often-painful *gallstones*.

- **Calculus** (plural is *calculi*): Stones
- **Cholelithiasis:** Condition of having gallstones
- **Duodenal ulcer:** Erosion or ulceration in the lining of the duodenum (first portion of the small intestine)
- **Gallstones:** Hard collections of bile that form in gallbladder and bile ducts
- **Hepatomegaly:** Enlargement of liver
- **Hepatoma:** Tumor of liver

All the twists and turns of both the large and small intestines can make for some interesting and often complicated conditions. The sheer length of these organs makes diagnosis and treatment a long and winding road. Start the journey with these intestinal conditions:

- **Ascites:** Abnormal accumulation of fluid in peritoneal cavity caused by cirrhosis, tumors, and infection
- **Borborygmus:** Rumbling, gurgling sound made by movement of gas in intestine
- **Cathartic:** Strong laxative
- **Colonic polyposis:** Polyps, small growths protruding from mucous membrane of colon
- **Constipation:** Difficult or delayed defecation caused by low peristalsis movement, over-absorption of water as contents sit too long in the intestine, or by dehydration
- **Diarrhea:** Frequent discharge of liquid stool (feces)
- **Diverticula:** Abnormal side pockets in hollow structure, such as intestine, sigmoid colon, and duodenum
- **Flatus:** Gas expelled through the anus
- **Hemorrhoids:** Swollen or twisted veins either outside or just inside the anus
- **Hernia:** A protrusion of an organ or part through the wall of the cavity that contains it
- **Ileus:** Intestinal obstruction that can be caused by failure of peristalsis following surgery, hernia, tumor, adhesions, and often by peritonitis
- **Inguinal hernia:** A small loop of bowel protruding through a weak place in the inguinal ring, an opening in the lower abdominal wall, which allows blood vessels to pass into the scrotum

- **Intussusception:** Telescoping of the intestine; common in children
- **Laxative:** Medication encouraging movement of feces
- **Melena:** Black stool; feces containing blood
- **Polyposis:** Condition of polyps in the intestinal wall
- **Pruritus ani:** Intense itching of the anal area
- **Steatorrhea:** Excessive fat in feces
- **Volvulus:** Twisting of intestine upon itself
- **Zenker's diverticulum:** A pouch at the junction of the pharynx and esophagus

Finding the Culprit: Gastrointestinal Diseases and Pathology

The gastrointestinal system can also play host to even more pathological diseases. Many of these involve inflammation of the various system components, which can cause major disruption to the work the system performs, as well as major discomfort.

- **Appendicitis:** Inflammation of the appendix
- **Cholecystitis:** Inflammation of the gallbladder
- **Crohn's disease:** Inflammation and ulceration of the intestinal tract of terminal or end portion of ileum
- **Diverticulitis:** Inflammation of diverticula (singular: diverticulum)
- **Enteritis:** Inflammation of the intestine
- **Gastroenteritis:** Inflammation of stomach and intestine
- **Hepatitis A:** Acute inflammation of the liver, spread by fecal-oral contact
- **Hepatitis B:** Inflammation of the liver due to a virus transmitted by blood and body fluids
- **Hepatitis C:** Virus affecting the liver spread through blood and body fluids. Like other forms of hepatitis, this can cause jaundice, a yellowish discoloration of the skin.
- **Hepatitis:** Inflammation of the liver caused by virus or damage to the liver

- **Pancreatitis:** Inflammation of pancreas
- **Periodontal disease:** Inflammation and degeneration of gums, teeth, and surrounding bone
- **Ulcerative colitis:** Chronic inflammation of colon with ulcers

As you can see, inflammation is a huge issue with the gastrointestinal system. Here are some other common diseases that can put a halt to this system's daily functions:

- **Anal fistula:** This is an abnormal tubelike passageway near the anus communicating with rectum.
- **Celiac disease:** Also known as *malabsorption syndrome,* this disease is thought to be precipitated by gluten-containing foods. The hairlike projections *(villi)* degenerate (or actually flatten) so they lose their absorption function. The disease can be hereditary and is common in people of Irish origin. Those with the disease must follow a gluten-free diet to control abdominal pain and diarrhea. Also known as *gluten enteropathy* or *nontropical sprue.*
- **Cirrhosis** is a scarring of the liver parenchyma, or tissue, due to damage from alcohol, drugs, and viruses like hepatitis.
- **GERD** means *gastroesophageal reflux disease.* It refers to the backward flow of gastrointestinal contents into the esophagus.
- **IBS:** *Irritable bowel syndrome* is a group of symptoms including diarrhea, abdominal bloating, cramping, and constipation associated with stress and tension (also known as *spastic colon*).

Testing, Testing: Gastrointestinal Radiology and Diagnostic Tests

Now that you know what can possibly be wrong with your gastrointestinal system, it's time to find out how medical professionals go about confirming their suspicions. There are three primary ways physicians diagnose digestive diseases and conditions: X-rays, ultrasounds, and blood tests. Check out these exciting x-ray methods:

- **Abdominal ultrasound:** Most common method to determine the presence of stones in gallbladder, can detect liver cysts, abscesses, gallstones, enlarged pancreas

- **Anorectal manometry:** To determine strength of muscles in rectum and anus, check for malformations, and to diagnose Hirschsprung's disease
- **Barium enema(lower GI series):** Series of x-rays taken of large intestine after the patient receives a barium enema
- **Cholangiogram:** X-ray film of bile duct, contrast medium is injected to outline the ducts
- **Cholecystogram:** X-ray of the gallbladder
- **Gastric emptying scan:** To view the rate at which the stomach empties, the patient is given food with a radioisotope (low radioactive substance) that allows radiologist to see food going into stomach and how quickly it leaves the stomach
- **Upper GI series:** Series of x-rays taken of stomach and duodenum after barium swallow or meal has been taken

A wide variety of blood tests can be done to diagnose gastrointestinal conditions and diseases, all of which look for varying levels of enzymes, proteins, and other blood elements. Some of the most common ones are as follows:

- **Alkaline phosphatase:** An enzyme which, when elevated, can indicate liver disease, certain kinds of cancer, bone disease, or a number of other problems. Is always elevated with bone activity, so it is always high in children who are still growing.
- **Amylase:** Pancreatic enzyme levels elevated in disease of pancreas
- **Bilirubin levels:** Present in liver and gallbladder disease
- **CBC (Complete blood count):** Measures types and levels of white blood cells (indicators of infection), red blood cells (measures of anemia), and platelets, or clotting factors
- **CMP (Complete metabolic profile):** Damaged organs release certain enzymes from their damaged tissue, and these elevated enzyme levels show up in the blood; nonfunctioning organs cannot clean waste products out of the blood the way they're supposed to, and elevated levels of these products also show up in the blood; CMP in particular looks at electrolytes, liver function, and kidney function
- **Helicobacter pylori antibody test:** Blood test to determine presence of H. pylori organisms, a bacteria that can be found in stomach lining, causing duodenal ulcer
- **Occult blood test:** Test to detect *occult* (hidden) blood in feces; also called *Hema-Check* and *Colo-Rec*
- **Protein:** Elevated in liver disease

Some diagnostic procedures are a bit more invasive, such as an *abdominocentesis* (also called *paracentesis*), a surgical puncture to remove fluid from abdominal cavity. Most of the other invasive procedures involve the use of an *endoscope*, an instrument used to visually examine internal organs and body parts. Almost every part of the digestive system can be viewed with the endoscope. The *fiberoptic (all one word) endoscope* has glass fibers in a flexible tube that allows light to be transmitted back to the examiner. The endoscope can be inserted into a body opening (mouth or anus) or through a small skin incision to view internal organs.

Some endoscopic procedures include the following:

- **Colonoscopy:** Visual examination of the colon using an instrument called a *colonoscope*
- **EGD (esophagogastroduodenoscopy):** Visual examination of esophagus, stomach, and duodenum
- **ERCP:** Also known as an *endoscopic retrograde cholangiopancreatography,* this involves an x-ray of bile and pancreatic ducts using contrast medium (like dye) and endoscopy
- **Gastroscopy:** Visual examination of the stomach using an instrument called a gastroscope
- **Laparoscopy:** Visual examination of any internal organ or cavity using an instrument called a *laparoscope*
- **Proctoscopy:** Visual examination of the rectum using an instrument called a *proctoscope*
- **Sigmoidoscopy:** Visual examination of the sigmoid colon using an instrument called a *sigmoidoscope*

Here a few more procedures that are now done without the need for the endoscope:

- **Capsule endoscopy:** A capsule containing a camera is swallowed by the patient to take pictures along portions of the digestive tract not reachable by other procedures (the capsule passes normally with stool). How cool is that?!?
- **MRCP (Magnetic resonance cholangiopancreatography):** Uses MRI technique to obtain images of the bile and pancreatic ducts.
- **Virtual colonoscopy:** Computer takes CT images of the colon and reconstructs a 3D model of the colon, to evaluate abnormalities.

Gastrointestinal Surgeries and Procedures

Luckily, many parts of the gastrointestinal system can be repaired using surgical methods such as surgical excision, repair, and suturing. You will likely be familiar with many of these terms, such as *appendectomy,* but some will be brand-spanking new to you. Let's start by taking a look at surgical excisions, or removals. Here are some of the most common:

- **Abdominoperineal resection:** Surgical excision of colon and rectum, by both abdominal and perineal approach
- **Appendectomy:** Surgical excision of appendix
- **Cholecystectomy:** Surgical excision of gallbladder
- **Colectomy:** Surgical excision of the colon or part of the colon
- **Gastrectomy:** Surgical excision of stomach
- **LAGB (Laparoscopic adjustable gastric band):** Inflatable device is placed around the top portion of the stomach to treat obesity
- **Polypectomy:** Surgical excision of a polyp
- **Transplantations (pancreas and liver):** Diseased pancreas or liver is removed or partially removed and replaced with a donor organ
- **Uvulectomy:** Surgical excision of uvula

Surgical repairs are next on the to-do list of procedures and surgeries. Gastrointestinal surgical repairs include

- **Anastomosis:** Surgical connection between two normally distinct structures
- **Anoplasty:** Surgical repair of anus
- **Choledocholithotomy:** Incision into common bile duct to remove stone
- **Laparotomy:** Surgical incision into abdomen
- **Palatoplasty:** Surgical repair of palate
- **Pyloroplasty:** Surgical repair of pylorus
- **UPPP (uvulopalatopharyngoplasty):** Surgical repair of uvula, palate, and pharynx to correct obstructive sleep apnea
- **Vagotomy:** Cutting of certain branches of vagus nerve performed during gastric surgery to reduce amount of gastric acid

One type of surgery that is more common today is *bariatric* surgery for weight loss. There are several kinds of procedures offered for weight loss surgery, but in general, they promote weight loss in one of two ways. First, bariatric surgery may accomplish a weight loss goal through diet *restriction*. This type of bariatric surgery helps limit the amount of food a stomach can hold, thus reducing caloric intake. Another method involves *malabsorption*. This type of surgery shortens or bypasses a portion of the small intestine, restricting the amount of calories and nutrients absorbed by the intestine.

Finally, surgeons use suturing and the creation of artificial openings to help treat conditions of the gastrointestinal tract. These are some of the most common:

- **Colostomy:** Artificial opening into the colon through abdominal wall
- **Gastrojejunostomy:** Artificial opening between stomach and jejunum
- **Gastrostomy:** Artificial opening into stomach through abdominal wall; this is a feeding method used when swallowing is not possible
- **Herniorrhaphy:** Suture of a hernia to repair
- **Ileostomy:** Creation of artificial opening into ileum through abdominal wall for passage of feces (used for Crohn's disease, ulcerative colitis, or cancer)
- **Jejunostomy:** Creation of artificial opening in the jejunum

Terminology RX: Gastrointestinal Pharmacology

Remember reading that you might need your antacids to get through this chapter? Well, we weren't kidding. *Antacids* are one of the most common and useful over-the-counter remedies for what ails your digestive tract. And most of them provide an added boost of calcium as well. Antacids with *simethicone* also relieve excess flatulence, if you need to avoid any embarrassing outbursts in public.

Another great OTC remedy is the *laxative*. This medication relieves constipation. Conversely, *antidiarrheals* relieve or stop diarrhea, and *stool softeners* allow fat and water in the stool to mix in order to soften hard stool.

A doctor may prescribe medications that provide a little more kick, so to speak:

- **Activated charcoal:** Used for its absorption powers; often used via *nasogastric tube* to assist with stomach pumping (drug overdose)
- **Antibiotics:** To treat Helicobacter pylori infections, diverticulosis, ulcerative colitis, and Crohn's exacerbations, and traveler's diarrhea
- **Anticholinergics:** To treat spasms of the GI system such as IBD, divericulitis, and even ulcers; effectively slow down peristalsis with a calming effect
- **Antiemetics:** Control nausea and vomiting; often prescribed when chemotherapy or radiation is administered
- **Bowel preparations and enemas:** Bowel cleansers taken before barium enema or bowel surgery
- **Emetics:** Used to induce vomiting; especially useful in cases of drug overdose or ingested poisons
- **H2 blocks (histamine 2 blockers):** Used to treat GERD and esophagitis by reducing the amount of acid that the stomach produces (includes products like Tagamet, for example)
- **Protein pump inhibitors (PPIs):** Prescribed for heartburn, stomach ulcers, or excessive stomach acid (omeprazole); reduces the amount of acid that the stomach produces

IN THIS CHAPTER

- Discovering how your endocrine system works
- Determining root words, prefixes, and suffixes appropriate to this system
- Using terminology of the endocrine system to discuss common conditions and diseases
- Choosing the right terms to use when diagnosing problems

Chapter 19

Gatekeepers of Health: The Endocrine System

Hormones — a word that strikes fear in the heart of every parent of a tween or teenage child, even the steeliest mom or dad chaperoning the middle school dance. But fear not, parents. It's a frequent misconception that hormones only affect teenagers who are finding their way to that first kiss. Hormones, as it turns out, are an important part of every person's physiology. They keep our systems running and send important signals to our major organs that dictate how they work.

Hormones don't just magically appear. They get a little help from their friends, the glands, who are kind enough to produce them, nurture them, and then send the little guys on their way to the appropriate organs.

How the Endocrine System Works

The *endocrine system* maintains the chemical balance of the body. It does this by sending chemical messengers called hormones throughout the body via the bloodstream. *Hormones* regulate and control the activity of specific cells or organs. Slowly released hormones control organs from a distance.

Endocrine glands are located in different parts of the body. They are called *ductless*, because they have no duct system to transport their secretions. Instead, hormones are released directly into the bloodstream. They regulate a variety of the functions of body organs. One can stimulate growth, another matures sex organs, and yet another controls metabolism.

TIP

Endocrine: Take *endo*, which means "within" or "inner," and add it to the Greek *krinein*, which means "to separate."

Endocrine glands, no matter which hormone they produce, secrete directly into the bloodstream to the target organ needing that hormone. They are unlike *exocrine glands* — such as the sebaceous glands in the skin — that deliver secretions via ducts directly to the body organ needing them. The endocrine system has two types of endocrine glands: central and peripheral.

The *central glands*, the *pituitary gland* and the *hypothalamus*, are located in the brain. The pituitary gland is referred to as the "master gland" because it produces a variety of hormones that travel via the bloodstream to regulate activities of other endocrine glands. The pituitary and hypothalamus glands work together to regulate body functions such as growth, salt and water balance, reproduction, and metabolism.

Peripheral glands include the *thyroid, parathyroids, adrenals, pineal,* and the *pancreas.* The thyroid, parathyroids, adrenals, and pineal glands have only one function: They produce hormones. The pancreas not only produces hormones but also performs important functions of the digestive system. The pancreas is similar to other mixed function organs, such as the heart, liver, kidneys, ovaries, and testes. In addition to their regular systemic functions, these organs also secrete hormones.

TECHNICAL STUFF

Believe it or not, the heart secretes hormones — as if it doesn't have enough to do already. The heart releases *ANP*, also known as *A-type natriuretic peptide* (or *polypeptide*), which helps to regulate renal and cardiovascular homeostasis. This hormone is released from the heart atria, whereas *BNP* (*B-type natriuretic peptide*) is released from the ventricles. Both help to lower blood pressure.

Figure 19-1 illustrates the endocrine system.

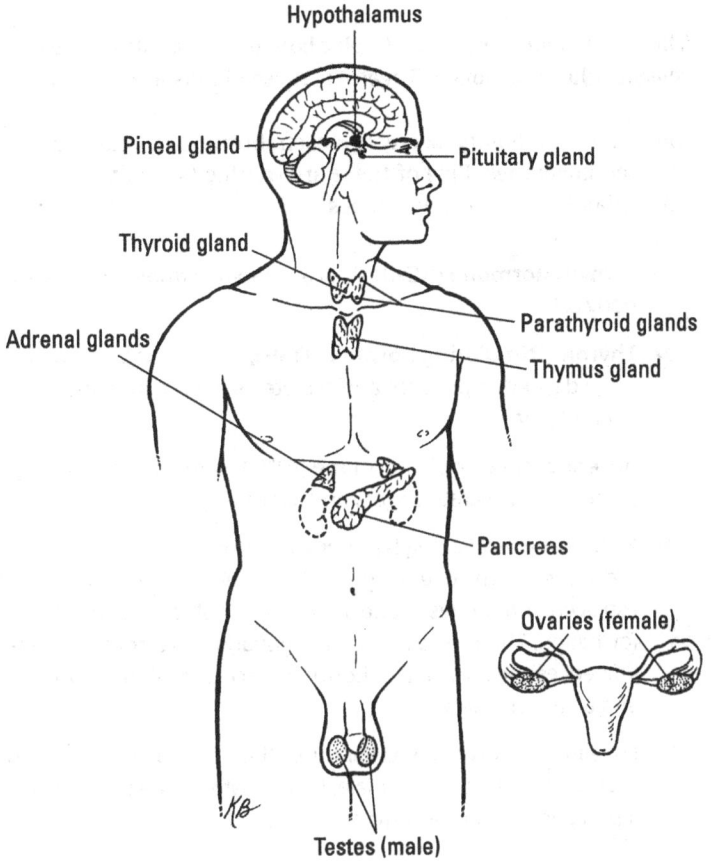

FIGURE 19-1: The endocrine system.

Illustration by Kathryn Born

Hormones

Before you get to know the endocrine glands better, take a second to say hello to their little friends, the *hormones.* These little messengers work like diplomatic peacekeepers, so to speak. They communicate with larger organs and systems to maintain chemical harmony and keep your body working. Because the individual parts of the endocrine system produce a variety of hormones, we discuss them in the context of their "home bases" — with each individual gland. Let's look at each of these glands, where they're located, their function, and what hormone they secrete.

Pituitary and hypothalamus

The *pituitary gland* — the grand master orchestra leader — is a pea-sized gland consisting of an *anterior* and *posterior lobe,* located at the base of the brain in a small depression of the skull called the *sella turcica,* just below the hypothalamus.

The *hypothalamus* secretes *trophic hormones* that stimulate the pituitary gland to release other hormones. Together, these glands are known as central glands.

The *anterior pituitary* secretes seven hormones, messaged by hypothalamus-released hormones. Five of these are trophic (stimulating) hormones that induce other glands to release hormones:

- **Growth hormone (hGH),** also called *somatotropin,* stimulates growth in body cells.
- **Thyroid-stimulating hormone (TSH),** also called *thyrotrophin,* stimulates the thyroid gland to produce and secrete its own hormones, *thyroxine* and *triiodothyronine.*
- **Adrenocorticotropic hormone (ACTH)** stimulates the adrenal cortex to produce and secrete *cortisol* and *aldosterone.*
- **Follicular-stimulating hormone (FSH)** in the female is responsible for the growth of the ovum (egg) in the ovaries and stimulates the secretion of estrogen and progesterone. In the male, FSH promotes sperm (spermatozoa) formation. This is also known as a gonadotropic hormone, one which influences the growth and hormone secretion of the ovaries in females and testes in males.
- **Luteinizing hormone (LH)** induces the secretion of progesterone and triggers ovulation. In the male, LH regulates testosterone secretion. This is also a gonadotropic hormone.

The remaining two hormones do not stimulate production of other hormones, so they are not tropic hormones. *Prolactin (PRL)* is the hormone that promotes the growth of breast tissue and sustains milk production after childbirth. *Melanocyte-stimulating hormone (MSH)* influences the formation of melanin and causes increased pigmentation in the skin.

THE PINEAL GLAND: ENDOCRINE GROUPIE

The pineal gland is a bit of a mystery, a sort of hanger-on to the endocrine system. It is included in the endocrine system because it is ductless. However, little is known about its endocrine function. It is located near the base of the brain and secretes a substance called *melatonin.* This is believed to increase the activity of the reproduction system and regulate the sleep cycle. Calcification of the pineal gland can occur and is used as a radiological marker when x-rays of the brain are examined.

The posterior lobe of the pituitary gland stores and secretes two hormones. *Antidiuretic hormone (ADH)*, also known as vasopressin, prevents excessive loss of water. *Oxytocin* stimulates uterine contractions in childbirth and maintains labor during childbirth. It also regulates the flow of milk from the mammary glands during breastfeeding.

Thyroid

The *thyroid gland* is composed of two pear-shaped lobes separated by a strip of tissue called the *isthmus*. It is located on either side of the trachea, just below a large piece of cartilage called the *thyroid cartilage*. This cartilage covers the larynx and is the prominence on the neck known as the Adam's apple. The thyroid is made up of tiny sacs filled with a jellylike fluid called *colloid*. The hormones secreted by the thyroid are stored in the colloid until passing into the bloodstream when required.

TECHNICAL STUFF

The thyroid weighs only about one ounce.

The two iodine-rich hormones secreted by the thyroid gland are *thyroxine (T4)* and *triiodothyronine (T3)*. These hormones are synthesized in the thyroid from iodine, which is picked up from the blood circulating through the gland. T3 and T4 are necessary to maintain a normal level of metabolism in the body. Thyroid hormone aids cells in the uptake of oxygen and supports the body's *basal metabolic rate (BMR)*. The BMR is the speed — or lack thereof — at which your body absorbs food, turns it into useful amino acids, fats, and sugars, uses these nutrients, and eliminates the waste. The BMR also refers to your overall energy level, temperature control, skin and hair condition, mood, energy level, and even the rate and effectiveness of your cognitive processes. Injections of thyroid hormone raise the metabolic rate, and removal of the gland diminishes the thyroid hormone content in the body. This results in a lower metabolic rate, heat loss, and poor physical and mental development. The gland also secretes *calcitonin*, which helps maintain the balance of calcium necessary for a variety of processes.

The *parathyroid glands* are four small (about ½-inch) oval bodies that lie on the back aspect of the thyroid gland, two on each side. These glands secrete the *parathyroid hormone (PTH)*. This hormone mobilizes calcium from bones into the bloodstream, where calcium is necessary for proper functioning of body tissue. Calcium in the food we eat is absorbed from the intestines and carried via the bloodstream to bones for storage.

TECHNICAL STUFF

The adjustment of levels of calcium in the blood is a good example of the way hormones control *homeostasis*, or equilibrium or consistency, of the body's internal environment.

Pancreas

The *pancreas* is located behind the stomach and functions as part of the gastrointestinal system. (We also discuss this gland in Chapter 18.) Consider it a jack of all trades and, as such, a member of more than one body system. As an endocrine gland, the pancreas produces hormones — that is, in this case, specialized cells in the pancreas produce hormones. The cells are called the *islets of Langerhans* and they secrete *insulin* and *glucagon*, both of which play roles in the proper metabolism of sugar and starch in the body. Insulin is necessary in the bloodstream for the use and storage of blood sugar and acts to decrease blood sugar levels, whereas glucagon acts to increase them by instructing the liver to synthesize new glucose in a process called *gluconeogenesis*.

Adrenals

The *adrenal glands* are two small glands, one on top of each kidney. Each gland consists of two parts, an outer portion called the *adrenal cortex* and an inner portion called the *adrenal medulla*. The cortex and medulla are two glands in one, each secreting its own hormone. The cortex secretes hormones called *steroids*, which are complex chemicals derived from cholesterol. The medulla secretes hormones called *catecholamines*, chemicals derived from amino acids.

The adrenal cortex also secretes *mineral corticoids*, also known as *mineralocorticoids*. These hormones regulate the amount of mineral sodium and potassium in the body. The main corticoid, *aldosterone*, is responsible for electrolyte and water balance, affecting blood sodium concentration and potassium. Aldosterone secretion increases in a severe sodium-restricted diet, enabling the body to hold needed salts. *Cortisol*, also called *hydrocortisone*, is a glucocorticoid hormone in that it increases the ability of cells to make new sugar out of fat. The adrenal cortex also secretes *androgens* that aid in the development of secondary male characteristics, such as growth of pubic and facial hair.

TECHNICAL STUFF

Addison's disease, a disease of the adrenal cortex, was named after Thomas Addison, an English pathologist.

The adrenal medulla secretes two hormones: *epinephrine* or *adrenalin* and *norepinephrine-noradrenalin*. Both hormones work in conjunction with the sympathetic nervous system. Under stress, these hormones are secreted by the adrenal medulla in response to nervous stimulation. They help the body respond to crisis situations by increasing the heart rate, blood pressure, blood glucose (sugar) level, and rate of blood clotting.

Gonads

The *gonads* (ovaries in the female, and testes in the male) are the gamete-producing glands. A *gamete* is a sex cell. Hormones that stimulate the gonads are known as *gonadotropins.*

Estrogen is secreted by the ovaries and is necessary in the development of secondary female sex characteristics (pubic hair and breast development, for example). It also regulates the menstrual cycle.

Progesterone is released in the second half of a menstrual cycle by the *corpus luteum* (empty egg sac) in the ovary. Its function is to prepare the uterus for pregnancy. If fertilization doesn't occur, secretion of progesterone stops, and the menstrual cycle follows. There are small levels of estrogen and progesterone present in males as well.

Human chorionic gonadotropin (HCG) is secreted by the placenta when a pregnancy occurs. This stimulates the ovary to keep producing estrogen and progesterone to maintain the pregnancy.

ENDOCRINE ABBREVIATIONS

Some common abbreviations associated with the endocrine system include:

- **ADA:** American Diabetes Association
- **BMR:** Basal metabolic rate
- **DI:** Diabetic ketoacidosis
- **DKA:** Diabetes insipidus
- **DM:** Diabetes mellitus
- **FBS:** Fasting blood sugar
- **GTT:** Glucose tolerance test
- **HCG:** Human chorionic gonadotropin
- **IDDM:** Insulin-dependent diabetes mellitus (more commonly known as Type 1 Diabetes)
- **NIDDM:** Non-insulin-dependent diabetes mellitus (More commonly known as Type 2 Diabetes)
- **PRL:** Prolactin
- **TSH:** Thyroid-stimulating hormone

Testosterone is secreted in the testes. It stimulates the development of secondary male sex characteristics (pubic and facial hair, deepening of voice). The hormone is also present in women to some degree, and some believe it increases female libido.

Endocrine Root Words

The glands of the endocrine system all produce different hormones that help keep the systems of the body running like clockwork. If you consider these glands the gatekeepers of the hormones they produce and send, you can consider prefixes and suffixes the gatekeepers of the root words. They both help tell you more about the meaning of the medical term. Table 19-1 shows some prefixes and suffixes associated with the endocrine system:

TABLE 19-1 **Coming and Going: Endocrine Prefixes and Suffixes**

Prefix	What It Means
Eu-	Normal
Ex-, exo-	Outside, outward
Hyper -	Excessive, above normal
Hypo-	Below normal
Pan-	All
Suffix	**What It Means**
-drome	Run, running
-emia	Blood condition
-genesis	Production
-ism	Condition
-tropin	Stimulating the function of

Next, in Table 19-2 we present the nitty-gritty of endocrine terminology. As always, the root words and combining forms let you know more about the condition or location involved with each term.

TABLE 19-2

Maintaining Balance: Endocrine Root Words

Suffix	What It Means
Acr/o	Extremities, height
Aden/o	Gland
Adren/o	Adrenal glands
Andr/o	Male
Calc/o	Calcium
Cortic/o	Cortex
Crin/o	To secrete
Dips/o	Thirst
Estr/o	Female
Galact/o	Milk
Gluc/o, glyc/o	Sugar
Gonad/o	Sex glands
Home/o	Sameness or unchanged
Immun/o	Safe
Kal/i	Potassium
Lact/o	Milk
Natr/o	Sodium
Pancreat/o	Pancreas
Parathyroid/o	Parathyroid gland
Pineal/o	Pineal gland
Pituitar/o	Pituitary gland
Radi/o	Radioactive
Somat/o	Body
Thym/o	Thymus gland
Thyr/o thyroid/o	Thyroid gland
Toxic/o	Poison
Ur/o	Urine

It's All Related: More Endocrine Anatomical Terms

It is, without a doubt, incredibly vital that the components of the endocrine system work in harmony because the system is a fairly complex collection of glands that produce a variety of hormones. The specialty study of this system of glands is known as *endocrinology*, with the physician in charge known as an *endocrinologist*.

Here's a closer look at even more aspects of this highly influential system. First, take a look at some hormone-related terms:

- **Adrenalin/epinephrine:** Adrenalin is a traditional trademark for the preparation of epinephrine (adrenaline) in the United States
- **Antidiuretic hormone (ADH):** Hormone secreted to stimulate water reabsorption
- **Cortisol:** Hormone secreted by adrenal cortex
- **Epinephrine:** Hormone produced by adrenal medulla
- **Glucagon:** Hormone produced by pancreas in islets of Langerhans that stimulates the release of sugar
- **Growth hormones (GH and hGH):** Secreted hormones stimulating the growth of long bones; also called somatotropin
- **Hydrocortisone:** Cortisol
- **Insulin:** Hormone secreted by islets of Langerhans; essential for the proper uptake and metabolism of sugar in cells
- **Islets of Langerhans:** Endocrine cells of the pancreas
- **Melatonin:** Hormone secreted by pineal gland
- **Oxytocin:** Hormone secreted to stimulate uterus to contract during labor
- **Renin:** Hormone secreted by kidneys to raise blood pressure
- **Somatotropin:** Growth hormone
- **Steroids:** Complex substance derived from cholesterol of which many hormones are made
- **Target tissue:** Cells toward which the effects of the hormone are directed
- **TSH:** Hormone secretion that stimulates the thyroid gland to produce thyroxine (T3) and triiodothyronine (T4)
- **Vasopressin:** Antidiuretic hormone ADH

Next, take a look at some of the other substances associated with the endocrine system. Though not hormones, these are vital products of this system, and help keep the body functioning properly.

- **Calcium:** Mineral substance necessary for proper functioning of body tissues and bones
- **Electrolytes:** Mineral salt found in blood and tissues; necessary for proper functioning of body cells; potassium, sodium, and calcium are examples of necessary electrolytes
- **Glucose:** Simple sugar
- **Glycogen:** Starch, a storage form of sugar
- **Iodine:** Chemical element composing a large part of thyroxine, produced by the thyroid gland

Protein comes from the Greek *protos*, meaning "first."

Common Endocrine Conditions

Most conditions associated with the endocrine system present more than just a common nuisance or annoyance. These conditions can really mess with the everyday function of your body and its organs. Effects like extreme weight gain or weight loss, extreme height issues, and even *renal* (kidney) *failure* are not uncommon when it comes to endocrine conditions.

You will notice that many of these common conditions are results of either glandular underactivity or overactivity. Many are also a result of a more serious endocrine disease, such as diabetes, covered in the next section.

Here are some pathological conditions that pertain to the pituitary gland:

- **Acromegaly:** Enlargement of the extremities due to hyperfunctioning of the pituitary gland after puberty
- **Dwarfism:** Congenital hyposecretion of growth hormone resulting in short stature and altered body proportions
- **Gigantism:** Hyperfunctioning of the pituitary gland before puberty, resulting in abnormal overgrowth of the body
- **Hypophysitis:** Inflammation of the hypophysis (stalk of the pituitary)
- **Panhypopituitarism:** Generalized insufficiency of pituitary hormones

Moving on to the thyroid, which is not without its own special issues, many of the following conditions involve both size of the gland as well as its output:

- **Cretinism:** Extreme hypothyroidism during infancy and childhood; results in decreased IQ, among other things
- **Euthyroid:** Condition of having a normal thyroid
- **Exophthalmos:** Abnormal protrusion of eyeballs
- **Goiter or thyromegaly:** Abnormal enlargement of thyroid
- **Graves' disease:** Autoimmune disorder that results in overproduction of thyroid hormones (hyperthyroidism)
- **Hashimoto's thyroiditis:** A progressive autoimmune *thyroiditis* (lymphocytic invasion of the thyroid gland) with developing goiter; leads to hypothyroidism and sometimes precedes Graves' disease; also called *chronic lymphocytic thyroiditis*
- **Hyperparathyroidism:** Excessive production of the parathyroid hormone
- **Hyperthyroidism:** Overactivity of the thyroid gland
- **Hypoparathyroidism:** Deficient production of parathyroid hormone
- **Hypothyroidism:** Underactivity of the thyroid gland
- **Myxedema:** Advanced hypothyroidism in adulthood
- **Thyroiditis:** Inflammation of the thyroid gland

Exophthalmos comes from the Greek *ex*, meaning "outwards," and *ophthalmos*, meaning "eye." Protrusion of the eyeball can be a symptom of hyperthyroidism, which was originally described by Robert James Graves, an Irish physician. Voila! We have Graves' disease.

Next is our old friend, the parathyroid, with an odd mix of conditions affecting calcium and, of all things, your wrists. Take a look:

- **Hypercalcemia:** Abnormally high levels of calcium
- **Hypocalcemia:** Abnormally low levels of calcium
- **Tetany:** A neurological disorder resulting in spasms (contractions) of a muscle; usually marked by sharp flexion of wrists or ankle joints, most often affects extremities

The adrenals are next on the checklist of conditions. Remember that these glands have one primary function: to produce hormones. So, if these are out of whack, so is your entire body.

- **Adrenal virilism:** Excessive output of adrenal androgens
- **Adrenopathy:** Disease of the adrenals

Now it's time to talk about the pancreas, that double-dipper gland that is involved in the inner workings of more than one system. In the case of the endocrine system, some common conditions can affect the performance of this gland of many talents. They are

- **Acidosis:** Abnormal condition characterized by reduced alkalinity of the blood and of the body tissues
- **Hyperglycemia:** Abnormally high sugar in the blood
- **Hypoglycemia:** Abnormally low sugar in the blood
- **Pancreatitis:** Inflammation of the pancreas

Conditions of the gonads can be troublesome and can cause some problematic side effects, such as heavy or irregular periods and ovarian cysts for women and erectile dysfunction for men. Discussing these conditions, in particular, requires a level of sensitivity.

- **Gynecomastia:** Excessive breast development in a male
- **Hypergonadism:** Excessive secretion of hormones by sex glands
- **Hypogonadism:** Deficient secretion of hormones by sex glands

Now, it's time for the potpourri of conditions. Many of these occur as a result of a more serious pathological disease, and some involve too much or too little of a specific substance in your body. It's an endocrine grab bag!

- **Diabetes insipidus:** Insufficient secretion of the antidiuretic hormone vasopressin; causes the kidney *tubules* to fail to reabsorb needed water and salt
- **Diabetic nephropathy:** Destruction of kidneys, causing renal insufficiency requiring hemodialysis or renal transplantation
- **Homeostasis:** Tendency in an organ to return to equilibrium or constant stable state

- **Hyperkalemia:** Excessive amounts of potassium in blood
- **Hyponatremia:** Deficient amount of sodium in the blood
- **Hyperparathyroidism:** A condition of excess parathyroid hormone secretion, whether from tumor, genetic condition, or medication
- **Ketoacidosis:** A primary complication of diabetes mellitus; fats are improperly burned leading to an accumulation of ketones in the body
- **Polyuria:** Excessive urination
- **Polydipsia:** Excessive thirst

Finding the Culprit: Endocrine Diseases and Pathology

While, admittedly, no condition of the endocrine system is simple or without side effects, the diseases we talk about in this section have especially serious consequences. One of the most common of these diseases is diabetes, which affects millions of people of all ages. Not only does diabetes affect the function of the body, it greatly affects a person's everyday habits. To manage the disease, one typically has to alter the diet and often take medications or insulin injections. Basically, the patient must learn a whole new lifestyle. Read on to find out more about this and other serious endocrine diseases.

The official name of diabetes is *Diabetes mellitus*, which means there is a lack of insulin secretion from the pancreas. Diabetes remains the seventh leading cause of death in the United States.

There are two major types of diabetes mellitus:

- **Type 1 diabetes** is also known as *insulin-dependent diabetes mellitus (IDDM)* or *juvenile* or *child onset diabetes;* it is often seen in children. It involves the destruction of the cells of the islets of Langerhans with complete deficiency of insulin in the body. Daily insulin injections are necessary.
- **Type 2 diabetes** is also called *non-insulin-dependent diabetes mellitus (NIDDM)* or *adult-onset diabetes;* are common factors. The islets of Langerhans are not destroyed, and there is deficiency of insulin secretion which causes insulin resistance in the body. Treatment includes diet, weight reduction, exercises, and if necessary, insulin or oral hypoglycemic drugs.

Some of the other serious pathological endocrine diseases affect the thyroid and the adrenal glands:

- **Addison's disease** is hypofunctioning of the adrenal cortex. Glucocorticoids are produced in deficient amounts. Hypoglycemia, excretions of large amounts of water and salt, weakness, and weight loss are symptoms of this condition. Treatment consists of daily cortisone administration and intake of salts.
- **Cushing's disease** involves hyperfunctioning of the adrenal cortex with increased glucocorticoid secretions. Hyperplasia of the adrenal cortex results from excessive stimulation of the gland by ACTH. Obesity, moon-like fullness of the face, excessive deposition of fat on the back called "buffalo hump," and high blood pressure are produced by excessive secretions of the adrenal steroid.
- **Thyroid carcinoma** is cancer of the thyroid gland.

Testing, Testing: Endocrine Radiology and Diagnostic Tests

That was quite a list of conditions and diseases, no? It would seem that the endocrine system has more potential conditions than Vegas has slot machines. Good thing physicians can use some relatively straightforward tests to evaluate the way the endocrine glands function.

Blood serum tests only require that you to give a few vials of blood at your local lab office. The professionals do the rest from there, running tests that measure the following levels (among many other things): calcium, cortisol, electrolytes, FSH, hGH, glucose, insulin, parathyroid hormones, T3, T4, testosterone, and TSH. All of these can be evaluated with blood serum tests.

Sometimes all the lab needs is a clean urine sample, so be prepared to pee in a cup. Urine testing can measure the following substances in the urine as indicators of endocrine disease: calcium, catecholamines, free cortisol, electrolytes, ketones, and glucose. *Glucose* comes from the Greek *gleukos*, meaning "sweetness."

Some other tests are a bit more complicated, such as the *glucose tolerance test (GTT)*, which requires both a blood test and urine sample. This test measures the glucose levels in the blood and urine in specimens taken 30 minutes, 1 hour, 2 hours, and 3 hours after ingestion of 100 g of glucose. The blood test portion measures levels of glucose in the blood, and the urine test measures for ketones in the urine, which is a symptom of uncontrolled diabetes. Other diagnostic tests for the endocrine system include the following:

- **Estrogen receptor test:** Determines whether hormonal treatment would be useful in cancer treatment by measuring the response of the cancer to estrogen
- **Goetsch's skin reaction:** Test for hyperthyroidism involving reaction to epinephrine injection, named for Emil Goetsch (1883–1963)
- **Radioactive iodine uptake:** Thyroid function evaluated by injecting radioactive iodine and then measuring how much is removed from the blood by the thyroid

Some clinical procedures associated with the endocrine system include:

- **CT scan:** Also known as *computerized tomography* or *CAT scan.* Here transverse views of the pituitary gland and other endocrine organs can diagnose pathological conditions.
- **Thyroid scan:** In a thyroid scan, a radioactive compound is given and localized in the thyroid gland. The gland is then visualized with the scanner to detect tumors or nodules.
- **Ultrasound:** Pictures obtained from ultrasound waves can identify pancreatic, adrenal, and thyroid masses. This procedure is also used to diagnose conditions and diseases of many other systems of the body.

Paging Dr. Terminology: Endocrine Surgeries and Procedures

The majority of the surgeries and procedures associated with the endocrine system involve either incision into or removal of a gland. It is important to note in this system that once an endocrine gland is surgically removed, usually for tumor or enlargement, hormone replacement is necessary. Whatever hormone is secreted by the removed gland must be artificially replaced in the body by drug administration.

You should be able to discern what each of the following surgical terms means by looking at the root and the suffix, which either means to remove or to cut (as in an incision). Here's the short list:

- **Adrenalectomy:** Removal of an adrenal gland
- **Hypophysectomy:** Removal of the pituitary gland
- **Pancreatectomy:** Removal of a portion of the pancreas
- **Pancreatotomy:** Incision into the pancreas
- **Parathyroidectomy:** Surgical removal of parathyroid glands
- **Thyroidectomy:** Surgical removal of the thyroid

TECHNICAL STUFF

The adrenals, pituitary, thyroid, and parathyroid glands, along with the pancreas, can now be removed laparoscopically. A robotic thyroidectomy, using the da Vinci robotic machine, uses an under-the-arm approach, eliminating the neck scar associated with thyroid removal.

Terminology RX: Endocrine Pharmacology

Now, let's get to the good stuff — the drugs that can help treat conditions of the endocrine system.

One of the big daddy diseases of the endocrine system is diabetes, which affects millions of Americans. *Insulin* is administered via injection or subcutaneous pump to treat Type 1 diabetes. There are several types of insulin, including rapid acting, immediate acting, long acting, and even mixtures of more than one type. *Oral antidiabetics* (hypoglycemic drugs) are used to treat Type 2 diabetes. Insulin can also be administered in advanced cases.

Most diabetics have to perform a blood glucose test each day (sometimes multiple times per day) to help track their blood sugar levels. The good news is that diabetics having to finger-prick to check blood sugars can now make use of a newer device: a continuous blood sugar monitoring system. This system, a FreeStyle Libre Flash Glucose Monitoring System, by Abbott consists of a small sensor attached to the upper arm. The patient can wave a reader device over it to see the current blood sugar level or any change in levels over the past eight hours.

Thyroid diseases can seriously affect the body's growth, either in a meta or micro sort of way. Sources of drugs and supplements used to treat thyroid disease include desiccated beef or pork thyroid gland. Some are also made of synthetics. *Antithyroid drugs* are used to treat hyperthyroidism. They work by mimicking the thyroid hormone and inhibiting the production of T3 and T4.

Finally, there are drugs used to treat the pituitary gland, most notably *growth hormone therapy* and *hormone replacement therapy*.

IN THIS CHAPTER

- Finding out how your nervous system works
- Determining root words, prefixes, and suffixes appropriate to this system
- Using terminology of the nervous system to discuss common conditions and diseases
- Finding the right terms to use when diagnosing problems

Chapter 20

Calming Down: The Nervous System

Imagine that your body is a giant building filled with all sorts of workers. Blood cells, hormones, and all sorts of worker bees run around all day (and night!) making the company work better. At the center of this building is a huge computer system, upon which all the workers great and small depend. The computer is a lot like your nervous system — it's the hard-wiring that controls all the little activities your body performs. From the voluntary (raising your eyebrows) to the involuntary (the way your eyes dilate), the nervous system helps keep it all humming along better than the newest Mac or PC.

How the Nervous System Works

The nervous system is the body's built-in computer system, but it is far, far more complex than any state-of-the-art computer. With the brain acting as the CPU (central processing unit), messages are relayed via the spinal cord through nerve fibers, providing connections for incoming and outgoing data. The body has more than 10 billion nerve cells whose function is to coordinate its activities. We speak, hear, taste, see, think, move muscles, and our glands secrete hormones, all thanks to the nervous system. We respond to pain, danger, temperature, and touch as well, and we have memory, association, and discrimination. These functions are only a small part of what the nervous system controls.

The nervous system is made up of three subsystems.

- **The central nervous system (CNS)** includes the brain and spinal cord.
- **The peripheral nervous system (PNS)** is composed of cranial nerves that extend from the brain and spinal nerves that extend from the spinal cord.
- **The autonomic nervous system (ANS)** is a division of the peripheral nervous and controls and coordinates the functions of the body's vital organs, such as heartbeat and rate of breathing — functions we don't even think about.

The worker bees of the nervous system are called *neurons*. A neuron is microscopic, but a nerve is macroscopic, that is, it can be seen with the naked eye. A *nerve* consists of a bundle of dendrites and axons. *Dendrites* are the receptive branching fibers of neurons. *Axons* carry impulses away from the cell body. The dendrites and axons travel together like strands of rope.

Figure 20-1 illustrates the nervous system.

The Central Nervous System

The *central nervous system* consists of the brain and spinal cord. The *peripheral nervous system* consists of 12 pairs of cranial nerves and 31 pairs of spinal nerves. The *cranial nerves* carry or transmit impulses between the brain, the head, and the neck. The *spinal nerves* relay messages between the spinal cord, the chest, abdomen, and the extremities. The functions of the spinal and cranial nerves are mainly voluntary, involving smell, taste, sight, hearing, and muscle movement.

Brain

The *brain* is the central control center for regulating and coordinating body functions. It lies in the *cranial cavity* (within the skull). The *spinal cord*, continuous with the lower part of the brain, passes through the *foramen magnum*, an opening in the skull that allows the spinal cord to continue down through the vertebral column.

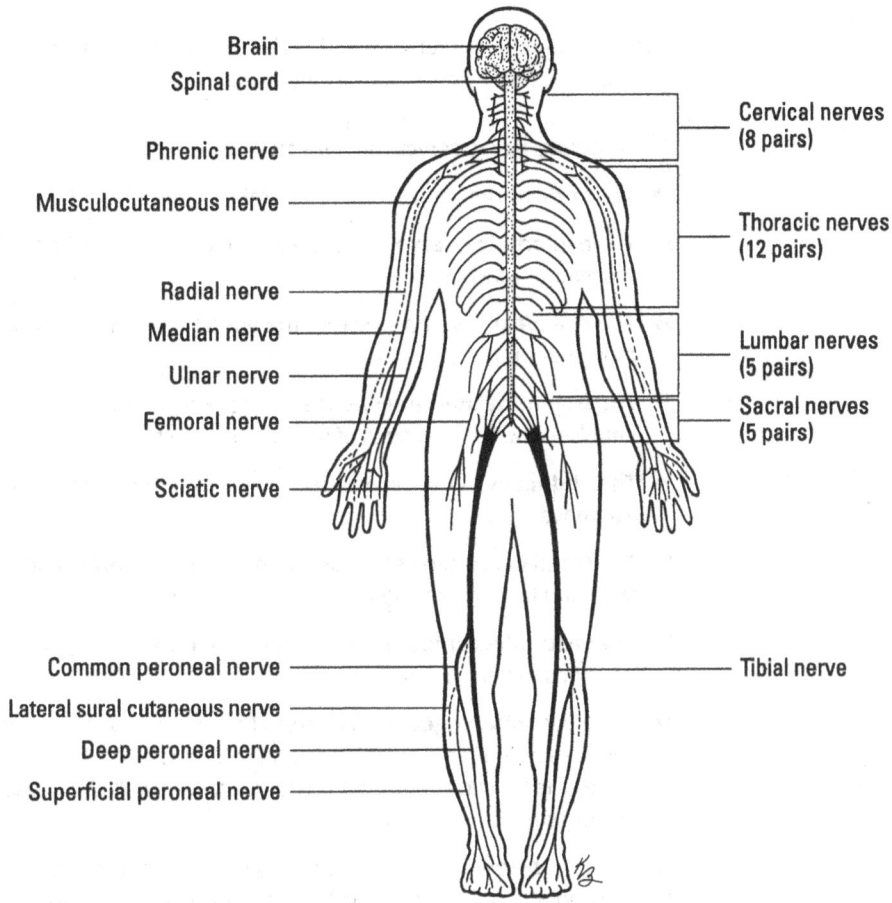

FIGURE 20-1: The nervous system.

Illustration by Kathryn Born

TECHNICAL STUFF

Most brains weigh between 2.5–4 pounds (40–60 ounces). The size of the skull offers only a general idea of the brain size, because the shape and thickness of the skull varies.

The brain's largest part is the *cerebrum*. Nervous tissue covering the cerebrum is called the *cerebral cortex*. The cortex is arranged in folds called *gyri* and depressions or grooves known as *fissures* or *sulci*.

TECHNICAL STUFF

Cerebral hemispheres are the paired right and left halves of the cerebrum that occupy most of the brain cavity. The left cerebral hemisphere controls the right side of the body, and the right hemisphere controls the left side.

Thought, memory, judgment, and association all take place in the cerebrum. *Efferent cranial nerves* carry motor impulses from the cerebrum to muscles and glands to produce movement and activity. There are 12 cranial nerves, and each addresses both an impulse and a function:

- **Olfactory nerve** serves the nose-to-brain impulses and the smell function.
- **The optic nerve** serves the eye-to-brain impulses and the vision function.
- **The oculomotor nerve** serves the brain-to-eye muscle impulse and the eye movement function.
- **The trochlear nerve** also serves the brain-to-eye muscle impulse and the eye movement function.
- **The trigeminal nerve** serves the head's skin and mucous membrane impulses and the functions of sensation in the face, scalp, teeth, and chin.
- **The abducens nerve** serves the brain-to-eyes impulse and the function of eye movement.
- **The facial nerve** serves the taste buds-to-brain impulse and the function of taste and facial expression.
- **The vestibulocochlear nerve** serves the ear-to-brain impulse and the functions of hearing and balance.
- **The glossopharyngeal nerve** serves the throat and taste buds-to-brain impulses as well as those of the brain-to-throat and salivary glands path. It serves the functions of throat sensation, taste, swallowing, and saliva production.
- **The vagus nerve** serves the impulses in the path from the throat, thoracic, and abdominal cavities to the brain and back. Functions include throat sensation, swallowing, and gut movement.
- **The accessory nerve** handles impulses going from the brain to the shoulder and neck muscles. It serves the functions of movement and head turning.
- **The hypoglossal nerve** takes care of impulses from the brain to tongue muscles and handles the function of tongue movement.

The outer surface of the cerebrum, the *cerebral cortex*, is made up of gray matter, and underneath this the *white matter* forms the central part of the brain. The cerebral cortex is the center that controls speech, vision, smell, movement, hearing, and thought processes and has four *lobes:*

- **The frontal lobe** is the center for voluntary movement, judgment, reasoning, and impulse inhibition.
- **The occipital lobe** (the back of each of the hemispheres) manages visual perception, association, and visual memory.

- **The parietal lobe** collects, recognizes, and organizes sensations of pain, touch, movement, and position.
- **The temporal lobe** correlates auditory and visual memory as well as language development.

In the middle of the cerebrum are spaces called *ventricles.* These spaces contain watery fluid that flows through the brain and around the spinal cord, called the *cerebrospinal fluid (CSF).* It protects the brain and spinal cord from shock, acting like a cushion. CSF can be withdrawn for diagnostic purposes or for relief of pressure on the brain.

The *cerebellum,* sometimes called the *hindbrain* because it is located under the back portion of the cerebrum, functions to assist in the coordination of voluntary body movement and maintaining body balance. The *brainstem* is a stemlike portion of the brain that connects the brain to the spinal cord. The *pons,* meaning "bridge," connects the cerebrum with the cerebellum and the brainstem. The *thalamus* acts as a relay station for body sensations such as pain, and the *hypothalamus* controls body temperature, sleep, appetite, and the pituitary gland.

The *medulla oblongata,* located between the pons and the spinal cord, regulates the centers that control respiration, heart rate, blood vessels, and the respiratory system. This is also sometimes known as the *reptilian brain.* It is the last part of the brain to shut down at death.

Spinal cord

The *spinal cord* passes through the vertebral canal from the medulla oblongata to the second *lumbar vertebra.* The spinal cord conducts nerve impulses to and from the brain. The cord carries all nerves that affect limbs and lower body and is a passageway for impulses getting to and from the brain.

A cross-section of the spinal cord shows an inner section of gray matter that contains cell bodies and dendrites of peripheral nerves, and an outer region of white matter that contains nerve fiber, surrounded by *myelin* sheaths, conducting impulses to and from the brain.

Meninges are three layers of connective tissue membrane surrounding the brain and spinal cord. The outer membrane, the *dura mater,* is a thick, tough membrane containing channels for blood to come into the brain tissue. The second layer around the brain and spinal cord, the *arachnoid membrane* (*arachnoid* meaning "spiderlike"), is loosely attached to other meninges. The *subdural space* is a potential space between the dura mater and the arachnoid that contains blood vessels. A space between the fibers and the third membrane is called the *subarachnoid space,* and it contains the *cerebrospinal fluid.* A third layer of meninges, closest to the brain and spinal cord, called the *pia mater,* is made up of delicate connective tissue with a rich supply of blood vessels.

TECHNICAL STUFF

The Latin translation of *dura mater* means "hard mother," whereas *pia mater* means "soft mother." *Meninges* were first named by a Persian doctor in the 10th century. When translated into Latin, that changes to *dura mater. Mater* was used because Persians thought that meninges were the mother of all other body membranes. Don't confuse your mater with your matter.

Peripheral Nervous System

It's worth mentioning here that the nervous system is one giant system that is subdivided into the central nervous system (which we just covered) and the peripheral nervous system. The peripheral nervous system then divides into two parts: the somatic system and the autonomic system. The autonomic system further divides to include sympathetic and parasympathetic systems. All subdivisions connect in some way to perform their functions, but they all remain part of the main nervous system.

The peripheral nervous system consists of the somatic system, or voluntary nervous system, whose actions we consciously control. Then there are groups of nerves that function involuntarily or automatically, without conscious control. These nerves compose the *autonomic nervous system.* This is system made up of nerve fibers and carries impulses from the central nervous system to glands, the heart, blood vessels, and the involuntary muscles, such as those found in the walls of the intestines and hollow organs — the stomach and urinary bladder, for example.

Peripheral nerves have different names, depending on the direction of the impulse they carry. *Afferent nerves* carry impulses to the brain and spinal cord from receptors like the skin, eyes, ears, and nose. *Efferent nerves* carry impulses from the central nervous system to organs that produce a response.

The automatic nervous system is further divided into the *sympathetic* and *parasympathetic systems.* Some of the autonomic nerves are called *sympathetic nerves.* The sympathetic nerves stimulate the body in times of stress and crisis by increasing the heart rate, dilating airways to supply more oxygen, and increasing blood pressure. Conversely, the parasympathetic nerves relax the involuntary nerves to calm you down.

Nervous Root Words

Now you know the major players in the nervous system. It's hard to believe the brain and spinal cord hold so much responsibility for the way your entire body functions. And like a supercomputer, one small glitch in how the neurons fire or how the messages are sent down the spinal cord can make the difference between, say, walking and being confined to a wheelchair.

Now let's start building some vocabulary. Table 20-1 lists prefixes and suffixes associated with the nervous system.

TABLE 20-1 **Relax with Nervous Prefixes and Suffixes**

Prefix	What It Means
Hemi-	Half
Hydr/o	Water, hydrogen
Hypn/o	Sleep
Pachy-	Thick
Para-	Beyond, around, beside
Polio-	Gray
Quadri-	Four
Sub-	Below, under
Suffix	**What It Means**
-algia	Pain
-itis	Inflammation
-lexia	Speech, word
-malacia	Softening
-mania	Obsessive, presumptive
-mnesia	Memory
-noia	Mind, will
-paresis	Partial paralysis
-phobia	Fear, aversion
-plegia	Paralysis
-schisis	Cleft or splitting
-thenia	Lack of strength or weakness
-us	Condition

Table 20-2 lists nervous root words and combining forms.

TABLE 20-2 **Nerve-Wracking Root Words**

Root Word	What It Means
Algesi/o	Excessive sensitivity to pain
Cephal/o	Head
Cerebell/o	Cerebellum
Cerebr/o	Brain, cerebrum
Crani/o	Cranium (skull)
Dur/o	Dura mater
Ech/o	Sound
Encephal/o	Brain
Esthesi/o	Feeling, nervous, sensation
Gangli/o, ganglion/o	Ganglion
Gli/o	Glue, supportive tissues of the nervous system
Hypothalam/o	Hypothalamus
Kinesi/o	Movement
Medull/o	Medulla
Mening/o	Membrane
Meningi/o	Meninges
Ment/o, phren/o	Mind
Myel/o	Spinal cord
My/o	Muscle
Narc/o	Numbness, stupor
Neur/o	Nerve
Phas/o	Speech
Pont/o	Pons
Psych/o	Mind
Radicul/o	Nerve root

Root Word	What It Means
Schiz/o	Split, division
Somn/l	Somnia, sleep
Thalam/o	Thalamus
Vag/o	Vagus nerve
Ventricul/o	Ventricle

It's All Related: More Nerve-Wracking Terms

So, here it is: The potpourri, the mish-mash, the great melting pot of nervous system terms. These are some of the most common phrases you'll hear in the doctor's office and hospital:

- **Anesthesia:** Without or loss of feeling or sensation
- **Anesthesiologist:** Physician who administers an *anesthetic* (a drug that reduces feeling)
- **Ataxia:** Lack of muscle coordination
- **Coma:** State of profound unconsciousness
- **Convulsion:** Sudden involuntary contractions of a group of muscles
- **Dementia:** Mental decline
- **Disorientation:** A state of confusion as to time, place, or identity
- **Gait:** A matter or style of walking
- **Monoplegia:** Paralysis of one limb
- **Neurologist:** Physician who specializes in *neurology,* the scientific study of the nervous system; does not perform surgery
- **Neurology:** The branch of medicine dealing with the study of the nervous system, functions and disorders
- **Neurosurgeon:** Physician who specializes in neurology and performs surgeries on the nervous system
- **Paraplegia:** Paralysis of the lower half of the body
- **Postictal:** Occurring after a seizure or attack

- **Psychiatrist:** Physician who treats mental disorders
- **Psychiatry:** Branch of medicine that deals with treatment of mental disorders (disorders often without any identifiable pathological cause)
- **Psychogenic:** Produced or caused by psychological factors
- **Psychogenetic:** Originating in the mind
- **Psychologist:** Specialist in psychology
- **Psychology:** The study of the mind, mental processes, and behavior
- **Psychosomatic:** Pertaining to the mind and the body
- **Quadriplegia:** Paralysis of all four limbs
- **Seizure:** Sudden involuntary contractions (convulsion)

Common Nervous Conditions

Because the nervous system is involved in so many aspects of your body's function, the conditions that affect it can have long-lasting implications on all bodily systems. Let's take a look at some of the pathological conditions pertaining to the central nervous system:

- **Aphasia** involves loss or impairment of the ability to speak.
- **Cerebrovascular accident (CVA)** is also known as a *stroke.* It can be a rupture *(hemorrhagic stroke)* or obstruction of an artery *(ischemic stroke),* producing headache, nausea, vomiting, possible coma, paralysis, and aphasia.
- **Coma** is a state of unconsciousness in which a person cannot be aroused.
- **Concussion** is a temporary dysfunction after injury, usually clearing within 24 hours. It's basically a bruise on the brain.
- **Dysphasia** is the condition of having difficulty speaking.
- **Epilepsy** refers to a sudden disturbance of the nervous system functioning due to abnormal electrical activity of the brain. It can manifest by a *grand mal seizure,* with loss of consciousness, limb contractions, and incontinence. It could also be as minor as an *absence seizure,* in which the person appears be "spaced out" for a moment.

  The Greek *epilepsia* means "seizure" and is derived from *epi* meaning "upon" and *lambancia* meaning "to seize." Officially, the term means "seized upon."

Grand mal (large) seizures (also called *tonic-clonic* seizures) are characterized by severe convulsions and unconsciousness. *Petit mal* (small) seizures (also called *absence seizures*) consist of momentary lapses of consciousness.

- **Hemiparesis** is slight paralysis of half (either right or left side) of the body.
- **Hemiplegia** is paralysis of the right or left side of body often occurring after a stroke.
- **Hydrocephalus** refers to an abnormal accumulation of fluid in the ventricles of the brain.
- **Irreversible coma** is a coma from which there is no response to stimuli, no spontaneous movement, and a flat or inactive *electroencephalogram* (a record of the brain's activity). This is what is known as a brain death.
- **Meningocele** is the protrusion of the meninges through a defect in the skull or vertebral column.
- **Myasthenia gravis** is muscle weakness marked by progressive paralysis that can affect any muscle in the body, but mainly those of the face, tongue, throat, and neck.
- **Neuralgia** means pain in a nerve.
- **Neuritis** is inflammation of a nerve.
- **Neuroma** is a tumor made up of nerve cells.
- **Neurosis** is an emotional disorder involving an ineffective way of coping with anxiety.
- **Palsy** means paralysis. One of the most common examples is *cerebral palsy,* a partial paralysis and lack of muscle coordination due to damage to the cerebrum of a fetus during pregnancy.
- **Paraplegia** comes from the Greek *para* meaning "beside" and *plegia*, meaning "paralysis." It is a paralysis of the lower body, usually due to a spinal injury or disease.
- **Polyneuritis** is the inflammation of many nerves.
- **Psychosis** refers to a major mental disorder characterized by extreme derangement, often accompanied by delusions and hallucinations.
- **Sciatica** is painful inflammation of the sciatic nerve in the thigh causing pain down the leg.
- **Shingles,** also known as *herpes zoster,* is a viral disease affecting peripheral nerves. Blisters and pain spread in a bandlike pattern following the route of peripheral nerves affected.

- **Subdural hematoma** is a blood tumor below the dura mater, produced by the collection of blood in tissue or a cavity.
- **Syncope** means fainting or sudden loss of consciousness.
- **Transient global amnesia** is an episode of short-term memory loss lasting a few hours, usually nonrecurring; the cause is not known, but may be ischemia or epileptic episode.
- **Trigeminal neuralgia (tic douloureux)** is a compression of the trigeminal nerve (cranial nerve V) causing stabbing or shock-like pain in the face.

TECHNICAL STUFF

Bell's palsy involves facial paralysis due to a disorder of the facial nerve; the cause is unknown, but complete recovery is possible.

Finding the Culprit: Nervous Diseases and Pathology

The diseases and more serious pathological conditions of the nervous system, again, have major implications for the way the rest of your body functions. From the way your muscles move to the coordination of involuntary reflexes, your nervous system can be subject to a wide range of serious pathological issues. Here are just a few of them:

- **Alzheimer's disease (AD):** Brain disorder marked by deterioration in mental capacity, caused by atrophy (wasting away) of the brain cells; develops gradually; early signs are loss of memory for recent events, and an impairment of judgment and comprehension
- **Amyotrophic lateral sclerosis (ALS):** Also called *Lou Gehrig disease,* a progressive muscular atrophy or wasting away, caused by hardening of nerve tissue in the spinal cord
- **Guillain-Barre syndrome:** Acute idiopathic polyneuritis, a rapid-in-onset, progressive motor neuron paralysis of unknown cause
- **Huntington's disease:** An inherited disease that causes progressive degeneration of the nerve cells in the brain resulting in physical, mental, and behavioral decline
- **Meningitis:** Inflammation of the meninges caused by bacteria *(bacterial meningitis)* or a virus *(viral meningitis),* an infection of subarachnoid spaces

- **Multiple sclerosis (MS):** Destruction of the myelin sheath around nerve fibers; scar tissue forms and prevents the conduction of nerve impulses, causing muscle weakness and paralysis
- **Parkinson's disease:** Degeneration of the nerves of the brain, occurring in later life, leading to tremors, weakness of muscles, and slowness of movement; a progressive condition that leads to muscle stiffness, shuffling gait (manner of walking), and forward-leaning posture

TECHNICAL STUFF

- James Parkinson, an English physician, described Parkinson's disease in 1817. It is also called *parkinsonism, paralysis agitans,* and *shaking palsy.*
- **Reye's syndrome:** Disease of the brain and other organs, such as the liver; affects children in adolescence; cause unknown but typically follows a viral infection; often combined with the administering of aspirin
- **Spina bifida:** Congenital defect of the spinal column due to malunion of the vertebral parts
- **Spina bifida occulta:** Vertebral lesion covered with skin and not seen; evident only on x-ray examination
- **Transient ischemic attack (TIA):** Sudden deficient supply of blood to the brain lasting a short time; sometimes called a "baby" stroke

TUMORS: UNWELCOME GUESTS

Tumors are another serious pathological issue affecting the nervous system. Working much the way a virus attacks a computer, tumors attach, grow, and wreak general havoc on anything they touch.

A *glioma* occurs in the brain tissue, whereas a *meningioma* arises from the meninges. Gliomas are highly malignant tumors that almost never metastasize or spread. Example of a glioma is an *astrocytoma,* a tumor composed of *astrocytes,* star-shaped brain cells. Gliomas are usually removed surgically. Meningiomas are most often benign and surrounded by a capsule, but may cause compression or distortion on the brain.

Another type of tumor is a *neuroblastoma.* This is a malignant tumor arising from nerve cells. It may be inherited and occurs most often in adrenal glands; it occurs in babies and early childhood and is treated with combined surgery and chemotherapy.

Testing, Testing: Nervous Radiology and Diagnostic Tests

Now that you've read about some of the nervous system's conditions and diseases, here's a bit about how to diagnose them. Because many of the following tests deal with delicate parts, such as the spinal cord and brain, physicians try to keep invasive measures to a minimum. It's certainly a good idea to find a solid, reputable facility you feel comfortable with instead of going to Joe Bob's House of MRIs.

And now, to the testing:

- **Cerebral angiography:** *Contrast medium* (such as dye) is injected into an artery, and images are taken of the blood vessel systems of the brain. This is also called *arteriography.*
- **Cerebrospinal fluid analysis** analyzes cell count, bacterial smears, and cultures of the CSF when disease of the meninges or the brain is suspected.
- **Computerized tomography (CT) scans** are performed on the brain to locate a tumor, foreign matter, or blocked vessel.
- **Electroencephalography (EEG)** is a recording of the electrical activity of the brain, performed to diagnose epilepsy, tumors, brain damage, and to determine brain death.
- **Electromyography (EMG)** is a record of the electrical activity of a muscle, performed to diagnose nerve and muscle dysfunction and spinal cord disease.
- **Electronystagmography (ENG)** is a group of tests to diagnose dizziness, balance disorders, and evaluate brain function.
- **Evoked potential test** is similar to the EEG but records the brain's electrical response to visual, auditory, and sensory stimuli.
- **Intrathecal contrast-enhanced CT scan (cisternography)** is a procedure when contrast dye is injected in the spinal sac to detect spinal and spinal nerve root abnormalities.
- **Lumbar or spinal puncture** is when cerebrospinal fluid is withdrawn for analysis from between two lumbar vertebrae. Contrast medium for x-ray studies such as a *myelogram* or *intrathecal medicine* may be administered via lumbar puncture procedure.
- **Magnetic resonance imaging (MRI)** is a noninvasive technique producing cross-sectional and vertical images of soft tissues of the brain by use of magnetic waves. Unlike a CT scan, the MRI produces images without the use

of radiation or contrast medium. It is used to visualize tumors, edema, and to confirm multiple sclerosis.

- **Myelogram** is a procedure in which contrast medium is injected into the CSF, and x-rays are taken of the spinal cord.
- **Neurosonography** uses ultra-high-frequency sound waves to evaluate the nervous system, including the brain and spinal cord.
- **Polysomnography** is a technique to measure brain and body activity during sleep.
- **Positron emission tomography (PET)** is a technique that permits viewing of a slice of the brain and gives information of brain function such as blood flow.
- **Single-photon emission computerized tomography (SPECT)** is a very sensitive nuclear method of detecting bone abnormalities and is also used to visualize blood flow patterns in the brain to diagnose CVA or a brain tumor.

Paging Dr. Terminology: Nervous Surgeries and Procedures

Most surgeries of this system involve removal of tumors in the brain itself, whether malignant or benign. Tumors of the spinal cord can also be removed surgically. Surgery on the brain and the spinal cord is, as you might imagine, *very* involved and detailed, due to the complexity of nerves and the tissue involved. So, again, think reputable institution and not Craniotomy Mart.

But, we digress. Let's start getting inside your head, literally:

- **Craniotomy:** Surgical cutting into and opening the skull to gain access to the brain tissue for surgery
- **Decompression craniectomy:** A portion of the cranium (skull) is removed to relieve brain swelling following traumatic brain injury or a stroke
- **Hypophysectomy:** Removal of the pituitary gland to treat tumors, specifically craniopharyngiomas
- **Laminectomy:** Excision of the posterior arch of a vertebra
- **Neurectomy:** Excision of a nerve

- **Neuroplasty:** Surgical repair of a nerve
- **Ventriculoperitoneal (VP) shunting:** Surgical procedure used primarily to treat hydrocephalus when cerebrospinal fluid (CSF) collects in the brain's ventricles. The shunt is inserted to relieve pressure on the brain caused by the excess fluid.

Terminology RX: Nervous Pharmacology

Now it's time to treat yourself to some drugs. Here are some common types of medications used to treat disorders and conditions of the nervous system:

- **Anticonvulsants, hypnotics, and sedatives** are used to treat various types of seizures.
- **CNS stimulants** are used to treat attention deficit disorders.
- **Cognition adjuvant therapy** is given to treat Alzheimer's disease.
- **Hypnotics** are used to treat sleeping disorders; examples include barbiturates and nonbarbiturates.

The Greek root of *hypnotics*, *hypnos*, means "to sleep."

5 Name That Plumbing

IN THIS PART . . .

Relieving yourself with terminology about how the body makes pee

Getting down with the male and female reproductive systems

IN THIS CHAPTER

- Figuring out how your urinary system works
- Checking out root words, prefixes, and suffixes appropriate to this system
- Using terminology of the urinary system to discuss common conditions and diseases
- Finding the right terms to use when diagnosing problems

Chapter 21

When You Gotta Go: The Urinary System

You probably don't give much thought to how your urinary plumbing works every time you use the restroom. However, it becomes a major concern the minute your, uh, output, isn't putting out like it should.

Welcome to the wonderful world of the urinary system! From kidneys to bladders, your body is full of all sorts of parts whose sole purpose is to clean your system of toxins by way of creating urine.

Believe it or not, a whole arm of the medical profession is dedicated to helping you add your contribution to the toilet bowl on a regular basis. So the next time you see someone with a license plate that reads, for example, 2PCME, you can bet it's a urologist on the way to work. Let's take a look at what takes up so much of his or her time.

How the Urinary System Works

The urinary system is made up of the *kidneys* (you have two), *ureters* (also two), *bladder* (one), and *urethra* (one). This system's main function is to remove urea, the waste product of metabolism, from the bloodstream and excrete the urea (in the urine) from the body.

So, how does that big steak dinner you ate last night turn into the next morning's output in the form of urine? Well, food and oxygen combine in cells to produce energy, a process called *catabolism.* In the process, food and oxygen are not destroyed, but small particles making up the food and oxygen are rearranged in new combinations, and part of the result is waste products. Waste products in the form of gases (carbon dioxide) are removed from the body by exhaling through the lungs. *Nitrogenous* waste (the by-product of protein food) is more difficult to excrete from the body than gases. This kind of waste is secreted as a soluble dissolved in water, a waste substance called urine. The main function of the urinary system is to remove urea from the bloodstream.

Urea is formed in the liver from *ammonia* (which is, believe it or not, basically the same stuff you use to clean the kitchen). The bloodstream carries it (in the same manner as hormones and lymph) to the kidneys, where it passes with water, salts, and acids out of the bloodstream into the kidneys. The kidneys remove waste products, producing urine that travels through each ureter into the bladder. Urine is then excreted from the bladder via the urethra. Magically (or so it might seem), your steak dinner has turned into pee!

Figure 21-1 shows the urinary system.

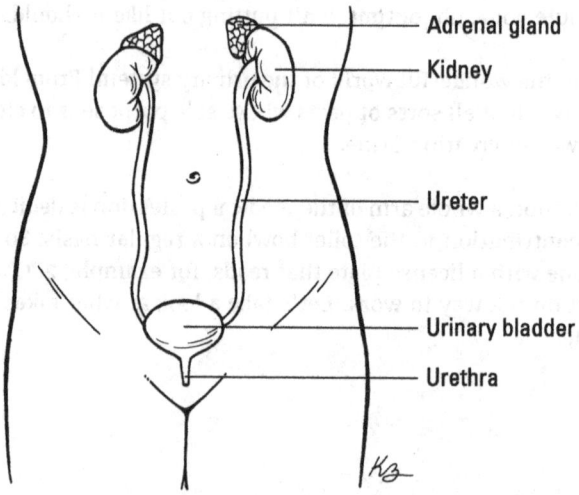

FIGURE 21-1: The urinary system.

Illustration by Kathryn Born

THE STORY BEHIND WHAT'S IN THE BOWL

Here are the vital stats of your wee-wee. Normal urine is translucent pale amber in color with the distinctive odor you are familiar with. It consists of 95 percent water with dissolved substances, nitrogenous waste, pigments, toxins, hormones, and sometimes abnormal substances like blood, glucose (sugar), and albumin. Of course, if your naked eye can see blood in your urine, it's time to call your physician.

Average urine output in a 24-hour period is approximately 1000–2000 mL (milliliters). Urine's normal *specific gravity* should be somewhere between 1.015 and 1.025. Specific gravity is the weight of a substance compared with the weight of some other substance taken as a standard. Water is the usual standard in liquids. The specific gravity of water is 1. If urine shows a specific gravity of 1.025, it means the urine is 1.025 times heavier than water.

Be on the lookout for dark yellow urine. This means your pee is overly concentrated, which may indicate a degree of dehydration.

Kidneys

You have two *kidneys*, unless you've had one removed. Kidneys are dark reddish brown, bean-shaped organs that are located behind the abdominal cavity on each side of the spine in the lumbar region. They are embedded in a cushion of *adipose* (fat) tissue and surrounded by connective tissue for support. Each kidney is about the size of a fist and weighs approximately 8 ounces. The left kidney is a little larger and sits a little higher than the right one.

Each kidney consists of an outer *cortex* and an inner *medulla* region. The cortex contains millions of nephrons, and the medulla contains the collecting *tubules* (small tubes). A segment on the medial border of each kidney, called the *hilum*, allows the blood vessels, nerves, and ureter to pass through. The *nephron* is the kidney's functional and structural unit, or the "brains" of the kidney. Each is a urine-producing microscopic structure, consisting of a *renal corpuscle* and *renal tubule*.

Hilum's Latin meaning is "a small thing or a trifle." This is a term for a depression or pit in an organ where vessels and nerves enter.

Glomeruli (singular *glomerulus*) are clusters of *capillaries* (small vessels) at the entrance of each nephron. They help filter the blood, beginning the process of urine production. In the blood-filtering process, water and solutes from the blood in the glomeruli pass through the capillaries and the walls that make up the glomeruli into the tubules. Tubules have the ability to remove substances your body needs and return them to the blood.

The Greek word *pyelos* means "tub-shaped vessel," which describes the shape of each kidney.

Ureters

You have two *ureters* (right and left). They are muscular tubes about 15–18 inches long, lined with mucous membrane, extending from the renal pelvis down to the bladder. The left ureter is longer because the left kidney sits higher in position. The urine enters the bladder in spurts via each ureter every 10–30 seconds.

At the bladder entrance is a *ureteral orifice* (opening) that opens to allow urine into the bladder from each ureter. The orifice works in sequence with the *peristaltic* (wavelike) action that propels the urine through the ureter. This action prevents urine from flowing back into the ureter when the bladder contracts.

Urinary bladder

The *urinary bladder* is a hollow, very elastic muscular sac in the pelvic cavity. It acts as a temporary reservoir or "holding tank" for urine. It has two openings to receive the urine coming from each ureter. Another opening, the urethra, provides an exit route for the urine out of the body. The *trigone* is a triangular space at the base of the bladder where the ureters enter the bladder.

TECHNICAL STUFF

An average bladder holds more than 250 ml of urine before producing the desire to urinate.

Contraction of the bladder and *internal sphincter* is an involuntary action, whereas the action of the *external sphincter* is controlled by you. The act of preventing or concluding *voiding* (urination) is learned and voluntary in a healthy body.

Urethra

The *urethra* is a membranous tube that carries urine from the bladder to the exterior of the body. The process of expelling or voiding urine is technically called *micturition*. The external opening of the urethra is the *urethral meatus* or *urinary meatus*. The female urethra is about 1½ inches long, and its only function is urination. In the male, it is approximately 8 inches long. It extends from the bladder neck through the prostate and through the penis. The male urethra carries both urine and reproductive organ secretions (see Chapter 22). Thanks to Mother Nature, the urethra can't mix sperm and urine, so it's difficult to pee with an erection. That sure prevents unwanted embarrassment during those tender moments.

Catheter comes from the Greek *catheter*, meaning "a thing let down." A catheter lets down urine from the bladder.

Micturate comes from the Latin *mictus*, which means "a making of water." From the verb *micturate* comes the noun *micturition*. Be sure to note the spelling: *Micturition* (expelling urine) is often misspelled as *micturation*.

WARNING

The *p* is silent in *pneumonia*, just as pee is silent in a swimming pool. That's why you probably should not frequent swim-up bars on vacation. You never know what is lurking in the water.

FILTRATION, REABSORPTION, AND SECRETION . . . OH, MY!

As blood passes through the glomeruli of each kidney, the process of forming urine begins. There are three steps to this process: filtration, reabsorption, and secretion. Glomerular walls are thin to permit water, salt, sugar, and nitrogenous waste such as urea, creatinine, and uric acid to filter out of the blood. Each kidney is surrounded by a cuplike structure that collects the substances filtering out of the blood. This cuplike structure is called *Bowman's capsule.*

If the process of forming urine stopped here, the body would lose a great deal of needed water, sugar, and salt that would be filtered out of the blood with the waste. Each Bowman's capsule is connected to a long twisted tube called a *renal tubule.* As the water, salt, and waste pass through this tubule, the materials that the body needs are able to reenter the bloodstream through tiny capillaries. By the time the filtrated material reaches the end of the renal tubule, the materials that the body needs to keep have been reabsorbed.

The waste, along with some water, salt, and acids, passes from the renal tubule into the central collecting area of the kidney. Thousands of tubules deposit urine into the *central renal pelvis,* a space that fills most of the medulla of the kidney. Cuplike divisions of the renal pelvis called *calyces* (singular *calyx*) receive the urine, which is (as we mention earlier) made up of 95 percent water, plus 5 percent urea, creatinine, acids, and salts. The renal pelvis narrows into the ureter that carries the urine to the urinary bladder, where it is temporarily stored. When the bladder reaches its capacity, the urge or need to void (urinate) is felt — then it's off to the bathroom you go, and urine is expelled from the bladder via the urethra.

Urinary Root Words

Now it's time to turn on the flow (pun *entirely* intended) of prefixes, suffixes, and root words. In the case of the prefixes and suffixes, you will find that these beginnings and endings of urinary words tend to allude to some sort of condition or state of the urinary system. Table 21-1 gets you started with prefixes and suffixes.

TABLE 21-1

Starting and Stopping the Flow: Urinary Prefixes and Suffixes

Prefix	What It Means
An- or a-	Without
Dys-	Difficult, painful
Poly	Many, much
Retro-	Backward
Trans-	Through or across
Suffix	**What It Means**
-continence	To stop
-ectasis, -ectasia	Dilation or expansion
-emia	A blood condition
-graphy	Process of recording
-iasis	Condition
-itis	Inflammation
-lysis	Loosening, separating
-megaly	Enlargement
-ptosis	Drooping, sagging, prolapse
-tripsy	Surgical crushing
-uria, -uresis	Urination, urine

Now that you know your urinary prefixes and suffixes coming and going, you can get to the heart of these wee words. Table 21-2 is a list of the most common root words and combining forms in the world of all things urinary.

TABLE 21-2

To Pee or Not to Pee: Urinary Root Words

Root Word	What It Means
Albumin/o	Albumin
Azot/o	Nitrogen
Bacteri/o	Bacteria
Cal/i – calic/o	Calyx or calix
Cortic/o	Cortex (the renal cortex is the outer section of the kidney)
Crypt/o	Hidden
Cyst/o	Urinary bladder
Dips/o	Thirst
Glomerul/o	Glomerulus (cluster of small vessels)
Glyc/o	Sugar
Hydr/o	Water
Keton/o	Ketones
Lith/o	Stone
Meat/o	Meatus
Medull/o	Medulla inner section of the kidney
Nephr/o	Kidney
Noct/i	Night
Olig/o	Scanty
Pyel/o	Renal pelvis
Py/o	Pus
Ren/o	Kidney
Trigon/o	Trigone
Ur/o, urin/o	Urine, urea, urinary tract
Ureter/o	Ureter (you have two)
Urethr/o	Urethra (you have one)
Vesic/o	Urinary bladder

TIP

To keep your urethra and ureters straight, remember that ureter has two *e*'s, and urethra has one *e*. You have two ureters and one urethra.

Common Urinary Conditions

Ah, your urinary system. So few parts, yet so many possible things that can go wrong. Who hasn't enjoyed a few days on the cranberry juice diet thanks to an inconvenient and painful bladder infection? And who could forget the joys of passing a good, old-fashioned kidney stone? Good times — not so much.

When you are dealing with common conditions, remember that inflammation is the arch nemesis of the urinary system. When your urinary parts are inflamed, bacteria have a perfect place to grow amidst a system transporting waste material. This results in infection and a great deal of discomfort. Here are some of the usual suspects:

- **Cystitis:** Inflammation of the bladder
- **Ureteritis:** Inflammation of a ureter
- **Urethritis:** Inflammation of the urethra
- **Urinary tract infection (UTI):** Infection of one or more organs of the urinary tract

Finding the Culprit: Urinary Diseases and Pathology

Although the typical urinary conditions can cause inconvenience and discomfort, they are sometimes signposts for more serious pathological conditions and diseases. These more serious issues range from diseases that affect kidney function to various varieties of cancer:

- **CRF (chronic renal failure):** When kidney function is not sufficient, leading to dialysis or transplantation
- **Cystocele:** Protrusion or sagging of the bladder
- **End-stage renal disease (ESRD):** Chronic irreversible renal (kidney) failure
- **Epispadias:** Congenital defect in which the urinary meatus is located on the upper surface of penis; usually corrected surgically shortly after birth

- **Essential hypertension:** High blood pressure without apparent cause
- **Glomerulonephritis:** Inflammation of kidney glomeruli caused by any number of things, including connective tissue diseases like *lupus,* endocrine diseases like diabetes, or bacterial infection like untreated *Group A Betahemolytic Streptococcus*
- **Hydronephrosis:** Water or fluid distention in the renal pelvis caused by obstruction of the ureter
- **Hydroureter:** Distention of ureter with urine due to blockage
- **Hypernephroma:** Renal carcinoma in adults
- **Hypospadias:** Congenital defect in which the urinary meatus is located on the under side of the penis; usually corrected surgically
- **Incontinence:** Inability to prevent voiding of urine
- **Nephritis:** Inflammation of the kidney
- **Nephroblastoma:** Kidney tumor containing developing cells *(Wilms' tumor)*
- **Nephrolith:** Kidney stone
- **Nephrolithiasis:** Kidney stones or renal calculi
- **Nephroma:** Tumor of the kidney
- **Nephromegaly:** Enlargement of the kidney
- **Nephroptosis:** Drooping or fallen kidney
- **Nephrotic syndrome:** Condition due to excessive protein loss in urine
- **Nephrosis:** Any disease of the kidney
- **Polycystic disease:** Multiple fluid-filled sacs (cysts) in the kidneys
- **Pyelitis:** Inflammation of the renal pelvis
- **Pyelonephritis:** Inflammation of renal pelvis
- **Renal calculi:** Stones in the kidney
- **Renal cell carcinoma:** Malignancy of kidney involving the *renal parenchyma* (all its essential parts)
- **Renal colic:** Pain due to blockage during passage of a kidney stone
- **Renal hypertension:** High blood pressure resulting from kidney disease (secondary hypertension)
- **Wilms' tumor:** Malignant kidney tumor, occurs in childhood; also known as adenomyosarcoma
- **Transitional cell carcinoma:** Malignancy affecting bladder, ureters, and renal pelvis

- **Urinary retention:** Blockage in passage of urine or muscle control problems leading to incomplete voiding with the same result
- **Urinary incontinence:** Inability to hold urine in the bladder

Testing, Testing: Urinary Radiology and Diagnostic Tests

Testing the urinary system for diseases and pathological conditions is a bit more involved than peeing in a cup and sending the sample off to the lab. Physicians can prescribe all kinds of tests to root out the problems that affect your plumbing.

First, let's start with some of the tests that do involve the old reliable urine sample. These tests are part of a total *urinalysis* (microscopic analysis of urine), also known as the *UA*, or blood screening process to evaluate adequate functioning of the urinary system:

- **Addis count:** Urine test to determine kidney disease; total volume measurement of urine output in 24-hour period is used to evaluate kidney function
- **BUN (blood, urea, nitrogen):** Measures amount of urea in the blood; when kidney is diseased or fails, urea accumulates, leading to unconsciousness and death
- **CCT (creatinine clearance test):** Measures the ability of the kidney to remove *creatinine,* a white crystallized compound, from the blood
- **Phenylketonuria (PKU):** Substance found in urine of newborns indicating congenital problems (routinely performed on newborns)

TECHNICAL STUFF

Excessive bilirubins can cause *jaundice* in newborns.

Physicians might also recommend diagnostic imaging or x-rays to be performed on the urinary system. These imaging procedures are, for the most part, non-invasive with the exception of having to add *contrast media* (often a dye) to the body so that problems show up on the x-ray. Some common diagnostic imaging procedures include the following:

- **CAT scan:** Stands for *Computerized Axial Tomography;* a transverse x-ray of kidneys to diagnosis tumors, cysts, abscesses, and hydronephrosis
- **Cystogram:** X-ray of bladder

- **Cystopyelogram:** X-ray of bladder and renal pelvis
- **Cystourethrogram:** X-ray of bladder and urethra
- **IVP (intravenous pyelogram):** Injection of contrast media into a vein that travels to the kidneys where it is filtered into the urine; x-rays show the dye filling the kidneys, ureters, bladder, and urethra to diagnose stones, tumors, and cysts
- **KUB (kidneys, ureters, bladder):** Demonstrates the size and location of kidneys in relationship to other organs in abdominal and pelvic regions
- **Nephrogram:** X-ray of kidney
- **Pyelogram:** X-ray of renal pelvis
- **Radioisotope scan:** Images of kidneys after injection of radioactive medium into the bloodstream
- **Renal angiography:** X-ray of blood vessels of kidneys to diagnose bleeding or renal artery stenosis
- **Retrograde pyelogram:** Contrast media is injected into the bladder and ureters through a cystoscope; x-rays are taken determine the presence of stones or obstruction
- **Ultrasonography (ultrasound):** Kidney size, tumors, hydronephrosis, polycystic kidney, and ureteral/bladder obstructions are some of conditions diagnosed by using sound waves
- **Voiding cystourethrogram (VCUG):** Bladder is filled with contrast media; x-rays are taken of bladder and urethra as urine is expelled

And now for the fun part — endoscopy! Though the following procedures might create some feelings of reservation, just remember that if your physician cannot properly diagnose it, he or she cannot treat it. So, buck up, put on your big girl/big boy pants, and get over your fear of the scope. Some of the most common urinary endoscopic procedures are these:

- **Cystoscope:** Instrument used to visually examine the bladder
- **Cystoscopy:** Visual examination of the bladder
- **Nephroscopy:** Visual examination of the kidney
- **Urethroscope:** Instrument used to visually examine the urethra
- **Urethroscopy:** Visual examination of the urethra
- **Ureteroscope:** Instrument used to visually examine the ureter
- **Ureteroscopy:** Visual examination of the ureter
- **Urinometer:** Instrument used to measure the specific gravity of urine

Paging Dr. Terminology: Urinary Surgeries and Procedures

A plethora of surgeries and procedures are available to help treat disorders and diseases. Like procedures for other body systems, these most often involve excisions, incisions, and repairs. Think of your surgeon as the master plumber of human pipes. These are some typical procedures used in fixing your peeing parts:

- **Cystectomy:** Surgical excision of the bladder
- **Cystoplasty:** Surgical repair of the bladder
- **Cystostomy:** Creation of an artificial opening to the bladder
- **Cystotomy:** Incision into the bladder
- **Dialysis:** A kidney machine does the work that a nonfunctioning kidney can't, removes waste material such as urea from the bloodstream
- **ESWL:** Extracorporeal (outside the body) shock wave lithotripsy
- **Fulguration:** Destruction of living tissue with an electric spark, used to remove bladder growth or small tumor
- **Hemodialysis:** Artificial kidney machine filters waste from blood
- **Lithotripsy:** Surgical or shock wave disintegration or crushing of kidney stones
- **Nephrectomy:** Surgical excision of a kidney
- **Nephrolysis:** Separation of the kidneys from other body structures
- **Nephrolithotomy:** Surgical removal of a kidney stone through incision into the kidney
- **Nephropexy:** Surgical fixation of a kidney
- **Peritoneal dialysis:** Waste removed from the blood via fluid exchange through the peritoneal cavity
- **Pyelolithotomy:** Incision into the renal pelvis to remove stones
- **Pyeloplasty:** Surgical repair of the renal pelvis
- **Renal angioplasty:** Dilatation of a stenosed or obstructed area in renal arteries with possible stent insertion to keep the vessel open
- **Renal biopsy:** Biopsy of a kidney performed at time of surgery or through the skin (subcutaneous or closed) in which a needle is inserted with ultrasound

guidance; tissue is obtained and later used to diagnose diseases from cancer to diabetes damage

- **Renal transplant:** Surgical implantation of a kidney to replace a nonfunctioning kidney; because each kidney performs the same function, the body can survive with only one kidney
- **Ureterectomy:** Surgical excision a ureter
- **Ureterostomy:** Creating an artificial opening into a ureter; usually used to create an opening from the ureter to the skin so urine can be collected in a bag
- **Ureterotomy:** Incision into a ureter
- **Urethropexy:** Surgical fixation of the urethra
- **Urethrovesical suspension:** Surgical suspension of the bladder and urethra
- **Urostomy (ileal conduit):** Following a cystectomy, this conduit redirects urine so it drains into a bag located on the abdomen

Terminology RX: Urinary Pharmacology

The medications used most often in the treatment of urinary conditions and diseases are used for lots of other bodily issues. You will no doubt recognize these drug families, as they are crossover drugs.

Traditional antibiotics are typically used to treat urinary tract infections. These drugs are most effective against gram-negative E. coli organisms, the common culprits in UTIs (urinary tract infections). *Gram-negative* is a negative response to a *Gram's stain*, a staining method to detect microorganisms. Though drinking a lot of cranberry juice is helpful when you have an uncomfortable UTI, it is not a panacea. Rely on prescription antibiotics to really wipe out the infection and get your pee flowing again. Another type of drug common in treating urinary tract infections is the family of *sulfonamides*.

Diuretics, often taken for hypertension, make the kidneys work overtime. A potassium (K) supplement is often given to maintain therapeutic potassium levels in the blood. A diuretic increases the excretion of urine, putting the entire urinary system into overdrive, which is not good for the kidneys or for sodium and potassium levels. This is why great caution is exercised when prescribing these drugs, and all drugs in this family are by prescription only. There are some common, everyday items that have diuretic effects, such as the caffeine in your coffee or soda.

URINARY ODDS AND ENDS: ADDITIONAL VOCABULARY

We couldn't leave this chapter without including some useful terms that don't necessarily fit into our usual categories. Commit these potpourri urinary words to memory, and you'll be the star of the doctor's office:

- **Anuria:** Absence of urine
- **Azotemia:** Excessive urea and nitrogen in the blood
- **Azoturia:** Excessive urea and nitrogen in urine
- **Catheter:** A flexible tubelike device for withdrawing or instilling fluid
- **Diuresis:** Increased excretion of urine
- **Diuretic:** An agent or medication used to increase the amount of urine production (water pill)
- **Dysuria:** Difficulty or painful urination
- **Enuresis:** Bedwetting
- **Glycosuria:** Sugar or glucose in urine
- **Hematuria:** Blood in urine
- **Nephrologist:** Physician who specializes in treating kidney disease
- **Nephrology:** The study of the kidney, its anatomy, and functions
- **Nocturia:** Night urination
- **Oliguria:** Scanty urination
- **Polyuria:** Excessive urination
- **Pyuria:** Pus in urine
- **Urinary:** Pertaining to urine
- **Urologist:** Physician who specializes in treating diseases of the male and female urinary system and male reproductive system
- **Urology:** The study of the male and female urinary system and male reproductive system
- **Urinary catheterization:** Passage of a catheter through the urethra into the bladder to withdraw urine

IN THIS CHAPTER

- Looking at how the male reproductive system works
- Rooting out root words, prefixes, and suffixes appropriate to this system
- Talking terminology of the male reproductive system and common conditions and diseases
- Diagnosing the right terms to use when diagnosing problems

Chapter 22

Check the Plumbing: The Male Reproductive System

They say it takes two to tango.

You can't create life without input from both the male and the female reproductive organs. Both are equally important to the process of babymaking, which is why they each get their own chapter in this book.

Normally, we would say, "Ladies first," but in this case, let's start our reproductive discussion with the guys, who donate the "little soldiers" responsible for egg fertilization.

How the Male Reproductive System Works

The reproductive system in the male has two main functions, to produce *spermatozoa* (singular: *spermatozoon*), the male reproductive cells, and to secrete *testosterone*, the male hormone. The male reproductive organs, or gonads, are the *testes*. They are supported by accessory organs, ducts, and glands. The ducts include the *epididymides* (singular: *epididymis*) *vas deferens*, *ejaculatory ducts*, and the *urethra*. Glands include *seminal vesicles*, *prostate*, and *bulbourethral glands* (or *Cowper's glands*). The supporting structures include the *penis*, *scrotum*, and *spermatic cords*.

The spermatozoon is called *sperm* for short. Each sperm is a microscopic cell, measuring less than 1/100,000th the size of the female *ovum*. Its structure is uncomplicated, composed of a head region that contains the hereditary material, or *chromosomes*, and a tail. This tail region, called the *flagellum*, is a hairlike structure that makes the sperm *motile* (able to move by itself), resembling a tadpole.

The sperm cell contains little food and cytoplasm, because a sperm only needs to live long enough to travel from its point of release in the male to where the ovum (egg cell) lies in the female in the *fallopian tube*. Only one spermatozoon can penetrate a single egg and achieve fertilization. Imagine, of the approximately 300–500 *million* spermatozoa that can be released in a single ejaculation, only one can complete the fertilization process.

TECHNICAL STUFF

The male reproductive system produces 100 million sperm per day (that's a rate of 1,000 for every heartbeat), from puberty until death! The organs of the male reproductive system are designed to produce and release billions of spermatozoa throughout the male's lifetime.

In addition, the male reproductive system secretes the male hormone (or *androgen*) testosterone. Testosterone is necessary for the proper development of the male gonads from the fetal stage through adulthood, the testes or testicles (singular: *testis*) and accessory organs of the testes, the prostate gland, and seminal vesicles. Testosterone is also responsible for the production of secondary body characteristics of the male, such as a facial hair and voice deepening. The prostate gland and seminal vesicles secrete fluid to ensure the sperm cells' lubrication and *viability* (the ability to live).

Figure 22-1 takes a look at this system's anatomy, and the organs and parts that make up the system.

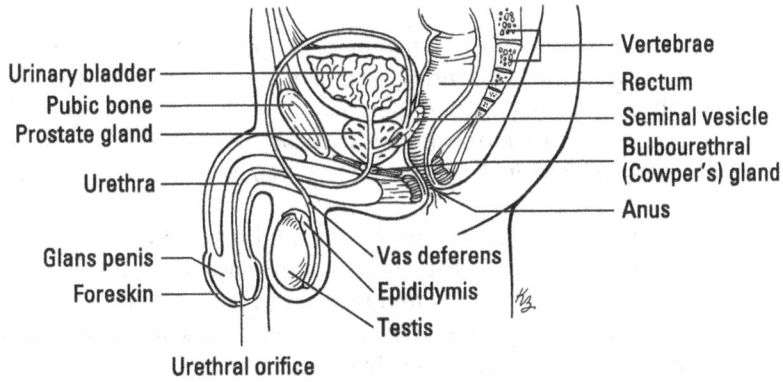

FIGURE 22-1: The male reproductive anatomy.

Illustration by Kathryn Born

Testes

The male *gonads* consist of two *testes* or *testicles*, which are egg-shaped glands that develop in the kidney region before descending into the scrotum before birth.

The interior of a testis is composed of a large mass of narrow coiled tubules called the *seminiferous tubules*. These contain cells that manufacture spermatozoa. These tubules are the *parenchymal tissue* of the testis, meaning they perform the essential work of the organ. Other cells in the testis, called *interstitial cells* (or *Leydig cells*), manufacture the male hormone testosterone. These tubules come together and enter the head of the *epididymis*.

The *scrotum* is a sac enclosing the testes on the outside of the body. The scrotum lies between the thighs in order to expose the testes to a lower temperature than if they were enclosed within the body. This lower temperature is necessary for the adequate maturing and development of sperm.

Between the anus and the scrotum, at the floor of the pelvic cavity in the male is the *perineum*, which is similar to the perineal region in the female.

Ducts

Once formed, sperm cells move through the seminiferous tubules and are collected in ducts that lead to a large tube at the upper part of each testis, the *epididymis*. The spermatozoa become motile and move into the epididymis, where they are stored.

The epididymis runs the length of each testicle, is about 20 feet long when uncoiled, and is the passageway for sperm from the testis to the body surface. It stores sperm before ejaculation and secretes a portion of the *seminal fluid* (semen).

The vasa deferentia are a pair of tubes approximately 0.3 cm in diameter and 2 feet long. The tubes, a continuation of the epididymis, carry the sperm up into the pelvic region and around the urinary bladder, where they connect with the seminal vesicle duct to form the ejaculatory duct. It is the vas deferens that is cut or tied off when a male sterilization procedure, called a *vasectomy,* is performed.

Ejaculatory ducts are formed by the joining of vas deferens with the ducts of the *seminal vesicles,* which are located at the base of the bladder and open into the vas deferens as it joins the urethra. These vesicles secrete a thick yellow substance, seminal fluid, which nourishes the sperm cells and forms much of the volume of the ejaculated semen or seminal fluid.

Urethra

Semen is a combination of fluid and spermatozoa, ejected from the body through the *urethra.* In the male, the *genital orifice* (opening) combines with the urinary urethral opening. The male urethra is part of the urinary system as well as the reproductive system because it aids in the output of both urine and semen.

Cowper's glands, or bulbourethral glands, are just below the prostate gland and also secrete fluid into the urethra. The urethra passes through the penis to exit the body.

Prostate

At the region where the vas deferens enters the urethra, and almost encircling the upper end of the urethra, is the *prostate gland.* This gland secretes a thick alkaline fluid which, as part of the seminal fluid, aids in the motility of the sperm. This gland is also supplied with muscular tissue that aids in the expulsion of sperm during ejaculation. The alkaline also protects the sperm from acid present in the male urethra and the vagina of the female.

Prostate comes from the Greek *pro* meaning "before." *Statis* means "standing"; by anatomy, it is the gland standing slightly before and below the bladder.

Penis

The penis is composed of three rounded masses of erectile tissue and at its tip expands to form a soft, sensitive region called the *glans penis.* The glans penis is covered with a retractable double fold of skin called the *prepuce* (foreskin). The penis contains the urethra that carries both seminal fluid and urine. It is the organ by means of which sperm is ejected into the female vagina.

Male Reproductive Root Words

To really stretch a metaphor, as the human race needs both male and female reproductive systems in order to survive by creating new life, the medical terms associated with the male reproductive system need both prefixes and suffixes to create new words.

Table 22-1 lists some prefixes and suffixes to know when it comes to male reproductive terminology.

TABLE 22-1

Making Word Babies: Male Reproductive Prefixes and Suffixes

Prefix or Suffix	What It Means
-cele	Hernia, swelling
-ectomy	Surgical removal of
-ism	State of
-itis	Inflammation
-megaly	Enlargement
-orrhea	Excessive discharge
-pexy	Surgical fixation
-plasty	Surgical repair of
Hydro-	Water, fluid
Trans-	Through, across, beyond

And now for the glue that holds these medical terms together. Take a look at the root words and combining forms that pertain to this system, shown in Table 22-2.

TABLE 22-2

Life Force: Male Reproductive System Root Words

Root Word	What It Means
Andr/o	Male
Balan/o	Glans penis
Cry/o	Cold
Crypt/o	Hidden

(continued)

TABLE 22-2 *(continued)*

Root Word	What It Means
Epididym/o	Epididymis
Genit/o	Genitals, reproductive organs
Gonad/o	Gonads
Olig/o	Scanty, few, little
Orch/o, orchi/o, orchid/o	Testis, testicle
Phall/o	Phallus, penis
Prostat/o	Prostate gland
Scrot/o	Scrotum
Sperm/o	Spermatozoon
Spermat/o	Spermatozoa
Test/o, testicul/o	Testis, testicle
Urethr/o	Urethra
Vas/o	Vessel or duct, vas deferens
Vesic/o	Bladder
Vesicul/o	Seminal vesicles

Pathological Male Reproductive Conditions

The makeup of the male reproductive system, with all its tubes and ducts, can be complicated and subject to several types of conditions. Here are some of the pathological conditions associated with the male reproductive system:

- **Adenocarcinoma of the prostate:** Malignant tumor of the prostate; second most common cause of cancer deaths in men over 50; radical (complete) prostatectomy along with radiation and chemotherapy is the most common treatment
- **Andropathy:** Diseases of the male
- **Anorchism:** The state of absence of a testicle, one or both

- **Aspermia:** Condition of absence of sperm
- **Balanocele:** Protrusion of glans penis (through rupture of prepuce)
- **Balanitis:** Inflammation of glans penis
- **Balanorrhea:** Excessive discharge from the glans penis, often the first symptom of a sexually transmitted disease
- **BPH (benign prostatic hypertrophy/hyperplasia):** Enlargement or excessive development of prostate gland in males over 60 years of age, can cause a urinary obstruction with inability to empty the bladder completely or all at once; surgical treatment is *prostatectomy*
- **Cryptorchidism:** Undescended testicle (*crypt* meaning "hidden"); two months before birth, testicles should descend into scrotal sac
- **Epididymitis:** Inflammation of the epididymis
- **Epispadias:** Congenital (present at birth) opening of the male urethra on the upper surface of penis
- **Erectile dysfunction:** Inability of male to attain or maintain an erection to perform sexual intercourse
- **Hydrocele:** Hernia or sac of fluid in the testis or in the tube leading from the testis, can occur in infancy and usually resolves during the first year of life
- **Hypospadias:** Congenital opening of the male urethra on the undersurface of the penis (present at birth)
- **Impotence:** Lack of power to obtain erection or to copulate
- **Oligospermia:** Condition of scanty sperm (in seminal fluid)
- **Orchitis/orchiditis:** Inflammation of testes or a testis
- **Phimosis:** Narrowing of the opening of the foreskin over the glans penis that does not allow the foreskin to retract, obstructing urination and causing secretions to accumulate under the prepuce, leading to infection
- **Priapism:** Prolonged abnormal erection of penis with pain and tenderness
- **Prostatitis:** Inflammation of the prostate gland
- **Prostatocystitis:** Inflammation of prostate gland and bladder
- **Prostatolith:** Stone in the prostate
- **Prostatorrhea:** Excessive discharge from the prostate
- **Testicular carcinoma:** Malignant tumor of the testis, classified according to type of tissue involved; examples: *seminoma, embryonal carcinoma,* and *teratocarcinoma* (a malignant *teratoma*); commonly treated with surgery: orchidectomy, radiation, and chemotherapy

- **Testicular torsion:** Twisting of spermatic cord causing decreased blood flow to testicle; occurs most often during puberty; considered a surgical emergency
- **Varicocele:** Large, herniated, swollen veins near the testis, associated with *oligospermia* (lower than normal amount of sperm) and infertility

Finding the Culprit: Male Reproductive Diseases and Pathology

Unfortunately, some of the most common diseases of the male reproductive system are the kind that make headlines, and not in a good way. Sexually transmitted diseases (STDs) are very serious, highly contagious, and can affect everything from your ability to conceive to your relationships with future sexual partners.

Also known as *venereal diseases*, the following conditions occur in both male and female and are among the most communicable diseases in the world, transmitted by unprotected sexual intercourse, via body fluids. Here are the usual suspects:

- **AIDS (acquired immunodeficiency syndrome)** is a sexually transmitted disease by exchange of body fluids during a sexual act or with use of contaminated needles and contaminated blood transfusion, affecting the body's immune system. It is caused by HIV (Human Immunodeficiency Virus).
- **Chlamydia,** the bacterium Chlamydia trachomatis, is the causative agent; includes diseases of the eye and genital tract. It causes discharge from the penis in males and genital itching, and vaginal discharge in females. It can cause infertility in women if it spreads to the ovaries and uterus and causes pelvic scarring secondary to the infection.
- **Genital herpes** is infection of the skin and mucous membranes of the genitals, caused by Herpes virus hominis type 2. Symptoms include reddening of the skin with small fluid-filled blisters and ulcers. Remission and relapse periods occur, and no drug is known to be effective as a cure.
- **Gonorrhea** is a contagious inflammation of the genital tract mucous membranes due to infection with bacteria known as Gonococcus. Other areas of the body such as the eye, mouth, rectum, and joints may be affected. Symptoms include *dysuria* (painful urination) and discharge from the urethra. Many women can carry this disease without symptoms, but others have pain, vaginal and urethral discharge. Penicillin is the method of treatment.

- **Human immunodeficiency virus (HIV)** is the retrovirus causing AIDS. HIV infects T-cell helpers of the immune system, allowing for opportunistic infections like *candidiasis, P. carinii, pneumonia, tuberculosis,* and *Kaposi's sarcoma.*
- **Human papilloma virus (HPV)** is a sexually transmitted disease causing benign or cancerous growths in male and female genitals (venereal warts). *Venereal warts* are also known as *condyloma acuminatum* (plural: *condylomata acuminata*).
- **Syphilis** is a chronic infectious disease affecting any organ of the body and is caused by a spiral-shaped bacteria known as *Treponema pallidum.* A *chancre,* or hard ulcer, usually appears a few weeks after infection, most often on external genitals but may also be on the lip, tongue, or anus with enlargement of lymph nodes. Infection can spread to internal organs, and later stages include damage to brain, spinal cord, and heart. Syphilis can be *congenital* (existing at birth) to a newborn if transmitted from the mother during pregnancy via the placenta. Penicillin is the method of treatment.
- **Trichomoniasis** means infection of the urinary tract of either sex and is caused by the one-cell organism *Trichomonas.* Males may have no symptoms or could develop *urethritis* (inflammation of the urethra), or prostate enlargement. Females develop itching, dysuria, and vaginal discharge.

TECHNICAL STUFF

Ongoing data from the CDC (Centers for Disease Control and Prevention) demonstrate that gonorrheal infections have become resistant to *fluoroquinolone* antibiotics such as *ciprofloxacin* and *ofloxacin.* As a consequence, as of 2007, this class of antibiotics is no longer recommended for the treatment of gonorrhea in the United States. The most commonly recommended treatment is an injection of a *cephalosporin* class of antibiotics called *ceftriaxone.*

Venereal is derived from Venus, the goddess of love. A venereal disease was thought in ancient times to be one of the misfortunes of love.

Testing, Testing: Male Reproductive Radiology and Diagnostic Tests

It's time to test those testes! Okay, bad pun, but you get the drift. Though there aren't tons of laboratory tests and diagnostic procedures used for this system, they remain important methods for helping men of all ages find peace when it comes to issues of concern related to sexual health.

One very common test is *semen analysis*. This test is performed as part of fertility studies and also to establishment fertility status. Sometimes the test is performed to determine sperm viability for couples having difficulty conceiving. It can also be performed following a vasectomy to assure that the procedure was successful. In this case, semen is collected in a sterile container and analyzed microscopically; sperm cells are counted and examined for motility and shape. Analysis is also done at six weeks following vasectomy and again at three months, to establish aspermia.

Another common test for men is the *GC/Chlamydia test*, performed by inserting a small cotton swab into the opening of the urethra to obtain a sample, which is then tested for gonorrhea and Chlamydia.

A general *viral culture* tests for herpes and HIV, and is performed simply by swabbing an open sore.

In *VDRL*, also known as the *Venereal Disease Research Laboratory test*, the blood is tested to diagnose syphilis. Because the syphilis antigen stays in the blood for a lifetime, it can have far-reaching effects.

The *PSA (prostate specific antigen test)* is a prescreening test that can be performed yearly on males over 50. This is a prescreening mechanism for precancerous conditions of the prostate gland. Any rise or elevation of PSA level is followed up by other investigations.

Prostate carcinoma is both serious and scary. Any time a disease, particularly cancer, is associated with a reproductive system, it can cause more than just physical symptoms. It can be emotionally and mentally devastating, because we associate our sexual identities with our sexual systems. Much as a woman feels devastated by breast cancer, a man can feel equally devastated by a cancer affecting his sexual health. Prostate cancer is one of the most common cancers associated with the male reproductive system.

Here are some typical prostate carcinoma investigations:

- **Digital rectal examination (DRE)** of prostate
- **Prostate specific antigen (PSA)** blood test
- **Transrectal ultrasound/ultrasound examination** of prostate through the rectum using sound waves

Paging Dr. Terminology: Male Reproductive Surgeries and Procedures

You've found the problem, now it's time to call the plumber, or, in this case, the urologist. Take a look at some of the procedural terms you'll need to know about all things male:

- **ART (Assisted reproductive techniques):** Includes procedures such as IUI (intrauterine insemination), IVF (in vitro fertilization), and ICSI (intracytoplasmic sperm injection)
- **Balanoplasty:** Surgical repair of the glans penis
- **Brachytherapy:** A form of radiation therapy to treat prostate cancer in which radioactive seeds are implanted directly into malignant prostate tissue
- **Circumcision:** Surgery to remove the foreskin (prepuce) from the penis; usually performed on newborn male but can be performed in adult males for *phimosis* (narrowing of the opening of the foreskin over the glans penis obstructing urination and causing secretions to accumulate under the foreskin, leading to infection)
- **Hydrocelectomy:** Surgical removal of a hydrocele
- **Microsurgical vasovasostomy:** Restoration of fertility following a vasectomy; a surgical re-joining of interrupted vasa deferentia
- **Orchidectomy:** Surgical removal of one or both testes (if both, called *castration*)
- **Orchidopexy:** Surgical fixation or "stitching in place" of a testicle
- **Orchioplasty:** Surgical repair of testis
- **Penile implant:** Surgical implanting of a penile prosthesis to correct erectile dysfunction (*prosthesis* means "artificial body part")
- **Prostatectomy:** Excision of prostate gland
- **Transrectal ultrasound prostate biopsy (TRUS):** Prostate biopsy that is taken under ultrasound control via the rectum.
- **TUMT (transurethral microwave thermotherapy):** A *prostatron* is used to deliver microwaves heating the area for one hour, to eliminate excessive tissue present in BPH; no anesthetic required

- **TUREP (transurethral resection of ejaculatory ducts):** Corrective procedure in treatment of infertility
- **TURP (transurethral resection of prostate):** *Resection* (removal of part or all of the gland) through the urethra; cutting back or removal of the prostate if enlargement of the prostate may interfere with urination
- **Varicocelectomy:** Surgical removal of a varicocele
- **Vasectomy:** Excision of a portion of the vas deferens to perform male sterilization; vas deferens on each side is cut, a portion removed, and the free ends are tied off or clipped, done through an incision in the scrotum; sterilizes the male in a way that sperm is not released with the seminal fluid; does not interfere with nerves or blood supply to the testis or penis; hormone secretions, sex drive, and potency not affected
- **Vasoepididymostomy:** Surgical joining of vas deferens and epididymis used in treatment of infertility as in postvasectomy (a.k.a. a vasectomy reversal)

TECHNICAL STUFF

The da Vinci surgical robot can remove the prostate, allowing a shorter hospital stay, fewer complications, and less postoperative pain.

Terminology RX: Male Reproductive Pharmacology

Believe it or not, there is more to male reproductive pharmacology than that infamous pill to aid in *erectile dysfunction (ED)*. However, that pill certainly is nice, and you will wow all your friends by knowing its official generic name, which is *sildenafil citrate.Vasodilators* like this keep things cooking in the bedroom for those who are experiencing difficulty.

The usual routine for any inflammations is antibiotics, and it's no different for the male reproductive system.

Finally, on a more serious note, *amebicides, antifungal agents,* as well as good old penicillin, are used to treat the STD family of bacteria. Amebicides treat amebal infections, almost always of the intestines; fungicides treat fungi, most commonly *tinea cruris,* or jock itch; penicillin is still the treatment for syphilis.

Say What? Male Terminology Tongue Twisters

Every now and then, you come across a medical term that leaves you saying, "Whaaat?!?" Let's face it: Some medical terms just sound plain strange and they can present a real challenge when it comes to pronouncing them. Lucky for you, most of these hard-to-say words and phrases are somewhat rare, so you won't likely encounter them on a daily basis. But if you want to impress your medical friends at the office holiday party, keep these tongue-twisting gems in your back pocket.

Here are some ouch-worthy procedures to know:

- **MESA (microsurgical epididymal sperm aspiration):** When a vas deferens is scarred from a previous surgery, sperm is directly collected from a single epididymal tubule. Once 10–20 million sperm have been collected, the semen is used for fertilization with the partner's egg.
- **Penile implant:** Surgical implantation of a penile *prosthesis* (artificial substitute for a missing body part) to correct erectile dysfunction.
- **Prostatolithotomy:** Incision into the prostate to facilitate removal of a stone or calculus.

And now for something completely, well, uncomfortable. Here are some conditions and disorders that will make the burliest of guys cringe:

- **Brodie:** Black spot on glans penis; an indication of gangrene.
- **Immobile cilia:** Sperm count is normal but sperm are non-mobile.
- **Pitres:** Hypoesthesia of the scrotum and testes in neurosyphilis.
- **Reifenstein:** Hereditary male pseudohermaphroditism, with hypogonadism, hypospadias, and gynecomastia.
- **Rocher:** In torsion of a testis. The epididymis cannot be distinguished from the body of the testis.

MORE MALE REPRODUCTIVE VOCABULARY

For the final push of this chapter, we spill some additional vocabulary words you may need to know to speak definitively about the male reproductive system, while refreshing your memory on a few others. Here is the crazy mix of words that help you understand this system:

- **Aspermia:** Absence of sperm
- **Artificial insemination:** Introduction of semen in to the vagina by artificial means
- **Coitus/copulation:** Sexual intercourse between male and female
- **Condom:** Protective covering for the penis, worn during coitus
- **Ejaculation:** Male orgasm, ejection of seminal fluid from the male urethra
- **Genitalia:** Reproductive organs
- **Gonads:** Male and female sex glands; in the male, testes; in the female, ovaries
- **Heterosexual:** A person who is attracted to the opposite sex
- **Homosexual:** A person who is attracted to the same sex
- **Impotence:** Inability to achieve or maintain an erection or to copulate
- **Oligospermia:** Scanty amount of sperm in seminal fluid
- **Orgasm:** Climax of sexual intercourse
- **Penis:** The male organ of copulation or sexual intercourse and the means by which sperm travels from the male to the female; considered an accessory organ of the reproductive system
- **Polyorchism:** Presence of more than two testes
- **Puberty:** Period when secondary sex characteristics develop and ability to reproduce sexually begins
- **Sterilization:** The process that renders person unable to produce offspring
- **Testalgia:** Pain in a testis, also called **orchialgia, orchidalgia,** and **orchiodynia.** No matter how you slice it, it all adds up to *ouch!*

IN THIS CHAPTER

- Checking out how the female reproductive system works
- Rooting out root words, prefixes, and suffixes appropriate to this system
- Using female reproductive system terminology to discuss common conditions and diseases
- Pinpointing the right terms to use when diagnosing problems

Chapter 23

A Life Force: The Female Reproductive System

If you thought the male reproductive system was complicated, you ain't seen nothin' yet, baby! Not only is the female system the other half of the reproductive puzzle that helps create a human life, it is also the vessel that helps sustain that little life in the nine months prior to birth. It's the docking station where sperm and egg meet and the storage facility for the end product. That's a lot of pressure to put on one system — create life, sustain new life, and nurture new life. Oh yeah, not to mention the business of squeezing something the size of a cantaloupe out of something the size of a mango.

How the Female Reproductive System Works

The female reproductive system produces the female reproductive cell, or sex cell, secretes the hormones estrogen and progesterone, and provides the conditions to establish a pregnancy, together with providing a safe place for the pregnancy to develop and grow.

The *gonads* (the *ovaries* in the female), together with the internal accessory organs consisting of the *fallopian (uterine) tubes, uterus, vagina, external genitalia,* and *breasts (mammary glands)* make up the reproductive system in the female. Reproduction is achieved by the union of the female reproductive cell, an *ovum,* and the male reproductive cell, a *spermatozoon* (or *sperm* for short), resulting in *fertilization.*

Gynecology is the study of the organs, hormones, and diseases of the female reproductive system. *Obstetrics* is the specialty dealing with care of the female during pregnancy and delivery of the newborn, including the 6–8-week period following delivery.

The female and male sex cells (ovum and sperm) differ from normal body cells. Each sex cell, also called a *gamete,* is a specialized cell, containing half the number of chromosomes (23) of a normal body cell (46). As the ovum and sperm cells unite, the resulting cell produced, called the *zygote,* contains half the genetic material from the female sex cell and half from the male sex cell. This combination provides a full normal complement of hereditary material.

Take a closer look now at the working parts of the female system in Figure 23-1.

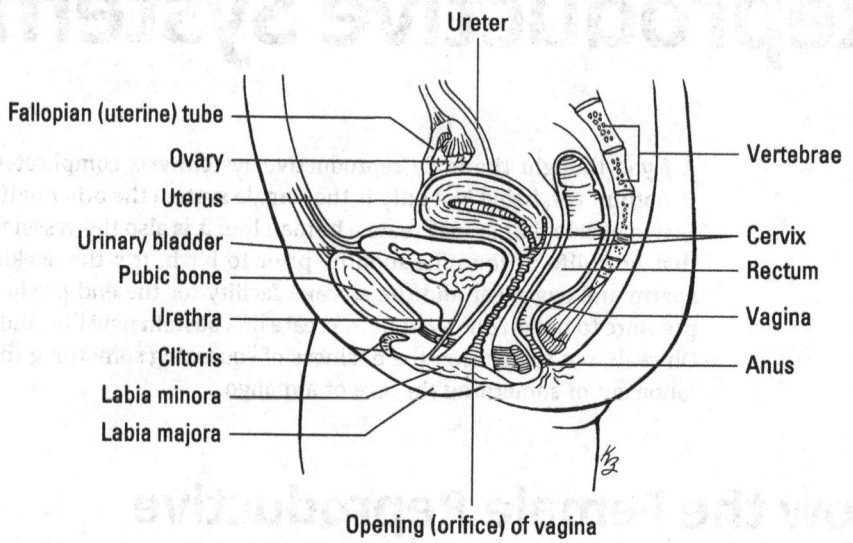

FIGURE 23-1: The female reproductive system.

Illustration by Kathryn Born

Ovaries

The *ovaries* are two almond-shaped glands, located on either side of the uterus in the pelvic cavity. They are held in place and connected to the uterus by the *broad* and *ovarian ligaments.* These organs have two functions: First, they release a mature ovum each month in a process known as ovulation. They also produce and secrete the sex hormones, estrogen and progesterone. *Estrogen* secretion begins development of female secondary sex characteristics, as well as manages the cyclic or menstrual changes in the uterus, preparing for a fertilized ovum. *Progesterone* is produced in the *corpus luteum* of the ovary and in the placenta in order to support and nurture a fertilized ovum.

Each ovary contains thousands of sacs called graafian follicles. Each of these follicles contains an ovum. As an ovum matures, the graafian follicle ruptures to the surface, and the ovum leaves the ovary. The ruptured follicle fills with blood and yellow material and becomes a *corpus luteum*. Near each ovary is a ductlike tube called the fallopian tube. The fallopian tubes and ovaries are called the *adnexa*, or accessory structures of the uterus.

The graafian follicle is named after Reinier de Graaf, a Dutch anatomist who discovered the graafin sac in 1672.

Fallopian tubes

The *fallopian tubes* lead from each ovary to the uterus.

The ovum, after its release, is caught up by *fimbriae*, the fingerlike projections at the end of the fallopian tube. The tube is lined with small hairs that, through their motion, sweep the ovum in a process that takes approximately five days to allow that ovum to pass through the fallopian tube. Fertilization takes place within the fallopian tube if spermatozoa are present. If intercourse has taken place near the time of ovulation, and no contraception is used, sperm cells will be in the fallopian tube when the ovum passes through. If intercourse has not taken place, and the ovum is not fertilized, and it will disintegrate.

Fallopian tubes are named after Italian anatomist Gabriele Falloppio (1523–1562). He was also responsible for naming the vagina and placenta. We sure wouldn't want to be his kid. Heaven only knows what he might name you.

Figure 23-2 shows the menstrual cycle.

Uterus

When fertilization occurs anytime between puberty and menopause, the fertilized ovum will grow and develop in the *uterus*. Hormones (estrogen and progesterone) are secreted from the ovary, and the hCG hormone is secreted from the placenta, the blood-vessel-filled organ that grows in the wall of the uterus during a pregnancy.

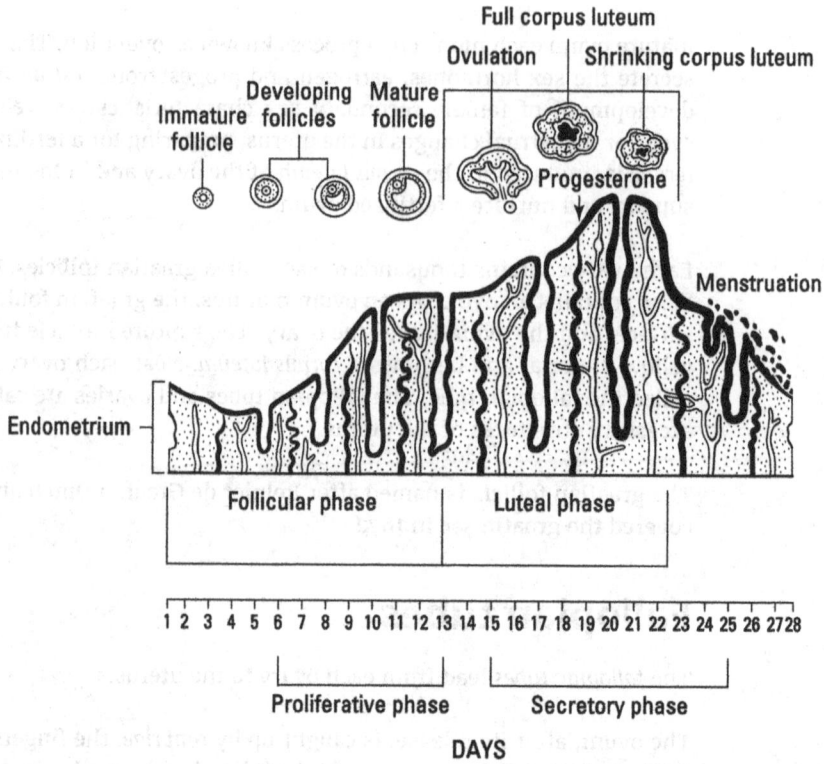

FIGURE 23-2: The menstrual cycle.

Illustration by Kathryn Born

The *uterus* is a muscular organ located between the bladder and the rectum. The uterus is pear-shaped, with muscular walls and a mucous membrane lining with a rich supply of blood vessels. The upper rounded portion of the uterus is called the *fundus*, and the large central portion is called the *corpus* or *body*. It is within the body and fundus of the uterus that a pregnancy grows. The *epithelial mucosa* of the uterus is more commonly called the *endometrium*. The muscular layer is the *myometrium* in the middle, and the outer membranous tissue layer is the *perimetrium*. The narrow lower portion of the uterus is called the *cervix*, meaning "neck." The cervix has an opening at its lower end, leading to the vagina (birth canal), which opens to the outside of the body.

Vagina

The *vagina* is a muscular tube approximately 6 inches long and lined with mucous membrane. The entrance to the vagina is called the *introitus*.

The *clitoris* is situated in front of the vaginal opening and the *urethral meatus.* The clitoris is similar in structure to the penis in the male, being an organ made up of sensitive, erectile tissue.

Bartholin's glands are two small glands on each side of the vaginal opening. They produce a mucous secretion that lubricates the vagina.

Bartholin's gland is named after Caspar Thomeson Bartholin, a Danish anatomist (1655–1738).

The region between the vaginal opening and the anus is called the *perineum.* This may be torn during the process of childbirth in a vaginal delivery. To avoid a perineal tear, the perineum may be cut prior to delivery. This incision is called an *episiotomy.*

The external genitalia (organs of reproduction) of the female are together called the *vulva.* The *labia majora* are the outer lips of the vagina, and the *labia minora* are the smaller inner lips. The *hymen* is a mucous membrane partially covering the entrance to the vagina. The clitoris and Bartholin's glands are also part of the vulva.

TIME TO ACCESSORIZE!

The *breasts* are considered accessory organs of the reproduction system. They are *mammary,* or milk-producing glands, composed of fatty tissue, *lactiferous* or *milk-carrying ducts,* and sinus cavities, which carry milk to the opening or nipple. The breast nipple is called the *mammary papilla,* and the dark pigmented area around the nipple is the *areola.*

During a pregnancy, hormones from the ovaries and placenta stimulate gland tissue in the breasts to their full development. After *parturition* (giving birth), hormones from the pituitary gland stimulate milk production in a process known as *lactation.*

There are two hormones involved in milk production: *oxytocin* and *prolactin.* These hormones also work to assist during labor, delivery, and the recovery of the mother. Oxytocin stimulates the uterus to contract, inducing parturition. Following delivery, oxytocin helps contract the uterus back to its normal size. It also reacts on the breasts to stimulate the release of milk. Prolactin stimulates breast development and the formation of milk in the postpartum period. The act of sucking promotes prolactin production, which in turn, promotes further milk production.

Female Reproductive Root Words

So, for lack of a better metaphor, prefixes and suffixes combined with root words are kind of like ova and sperm. Separately, they don't make much sense. But together, they produce a whole new being. In this case, of course, it's a word and not a baby. But they *are* cute, aren't they?

Table 23-1 lists some pertinent prefixes and suffixes.

TABLE 23-1

Half of the Puzzle: Female Reproductive Prefixes and Suffixes

Prefix	What It Means
Ante-	Before
Dys-	Painful, difficult
Endo-	Within
Hydro-	Water
Intra-	Within
Multi-	Many
Neo-	New
Nulli-	None
Peri-	Around
Primi-	First
Secundi-	Second
Suffix	**What It Means**
-algia	Pain
-arche	Beginning
-cyesis	Pregnancy
-ectomy	Surgical removal of
-itis	Inflammation
-lipsis	Omit or fail
-optosis	Sagging

Suffix	What It Means
-orrhaphy	Suture
-orrhea	Discharge, flow
-oscopy	Visual examination
-otomy	Incision into
-para, parous	Bearing, bringing forth
-plasty	Surgical repair
-rrhagia	Burst forth, excessive flow
-salpinx	Fallopian tube
-tocia	Labor

By adding in the root words and combining forms, you start to create your own little word babies. If you've ever spent any time at the OB-GYN's office, even as a patient, you will probably recognize many of the female-related roots shown in Table 23-2.

TABLE 23-2

Life-Giving Roots of the Female Reproductive System

Root Word	What It Means
Amni/o	Amnion
Cephal/o	Head
Cervic/o	Cervix/neck
Chori/o	Chorion
Colp/o	Vagina
Culd/o	Retrouterine pouch (cul-de-sac)
Cyes/o, cyes/i	Pregnancy
Embry/o	Embryo
Endometri/o	Endometrium
Episi/o	Vulva
Fet/o	Fetus
Fimbri/o	Fimbria

(continued)

TABLE 23-2 *(continued)*

Root Word	What It Means
Galact/o	Milk
Genit/o	Genitalia
Gonad/o	Ovaries
Gravida	Pregnancy
Gynec/o, gyn/o	Woman, female
Hymen/o	Hymen
Hyster/o	Uterus
Lact/o	Milk
Lapar/o	Abdomen
Mamm/o, mast/o	Breast
Men/o	Menstruation
Metr/o, metr/io	Uterus
Mult/i	Many
My/o	Muscle
Myometri/o	Myometrium
Nat/o, nat/i	Birth
Null/i	None
Obstetr/o	Midwife
Olig/o	Scanty
Omphal/o, umbilic/o	Umbilicus, navel
Oophor/o	Ovary
Ov/o, ov/i, ovul/o	Egg, ovum
Ovari/o	Ovary
Papill/o	Nipple
Pelv/i, pelv/o	Pelvis
Perine/o	Perineum
Prim/i	First
Pseud/o	False

Root Word	What It Means
Puerper/o	Childbirth
Salping/o	Fallopian tube
Thel/o	Nipple
Tub/o	Tube
Umbilic/o	Umbilicus, navel
Uter/o	Uterus
Vagin/o	Vagina
Vulv/o	Vulva

FULL CIRCLE: THE MYSTERIES OF THE 28-DAY MENSTRUAL CYCLE REVEALED

What actually happens on a monthly basis once menstruation begins?

At puberty the beginning of menstruation is called *menarche,* which can begin as early as age 9 or as late as 15 or 16. Every menstrual cycle is divided into approximately 28 days (give or take, depending on your body's makeup) that can be grouped into four time periods:

- **Days 1–5, menstrual period:** Bloody fluid containing disintegrated *endometrial* cells and blood cells is discharged through the vagina.
- **Days 6–13, postmenstrual period:** When the menstrual period has ended, the lining of the uterus begins to repair itself as the hormone *estrogen* is released by the maturing *graafian follicle (developing egg sac).*
- **Days 13–14, ovulation:** The graafian follicle ruptures, and the ovum leaves the ovary and is pulled into the fallopian tube.
- **Days 15–28, premenstrual period:** The empty graafian follicle fills with a yellow material and becomes known as a *corpus luteum.* The corpus luteum acts like an endocrine organ and secretes two hormones, estrogen and progesterone, into the bloodstream. The hormones stimulate buildup of the lining of the uterus in preparation for a fertilized ovum. If fertilization does not occur, the corpus luteum stops hormone production and regresses. The fall in hormonal levels leads to the breakdown of the *uterine endometrium,* and a new menstrual cycle begins, bringing the cycle back to day 1.

(continued)

(continued)

If fertilization does occur in the fallopian tube, the fertilized ovum moves into the uterus and implants in the *endometrium*. The corpus luteum continues to produce progesterone and estrogen, which supports the vascular and muscular development of the uterus lining. The *placenta*, the organ of communication between the mother and the embryo, now forms in the uterine wall. The placenta produces its own hormone as it develops in the uterus, called *human chorionic gonadotropin (hCG)*. hCG is the hormone tested for in the urine of women who suspect a pregnancy. When you pee on a pregnancy test stick, this is the hormone that makes that little plus sign appear. If you see it, pour yourself a champagne glass full of milk and celebrate — you're pregnant!

It's All Related: More Female Reproductive Anatomical Terms

There are so many medical terms associated with the female reproductive system that it's just not possible, especially in a book this size, to classify each and every one of them. In the following section, we provide a diverse array of both anatomical and clinical words that will keep you in the know regarding this system.

- **Adnexa:** Accessory parts of an organ
- **Anteversion:** Forward tipping of the uterus
- **Coitus/copulation:** Sexual intercourse
- **Estrogen:** Hormone produced by the ovaries responsible for female sex characteristics and building of uterine lining during the menstrual cycle
- **Gynopathic:** Pertaining to diseases of women
- **Hydrosalpinx:** Water in the fallopian tube
- **Leukorrhea:** White vaginal discharge, can sometimes contain white blood cells
- **Mastoptosis:** Sagging breasts
- **Menarche:** Beginning of menstruation
- **Myometrium:** Muscular layer lining the uterus
- **Oligomenorrhea:** Scanty menstrual flow
- **Orifice:** Opening
- **Progesterone:** Hormone produced by the corpus luteum in the ovary and by the placenta during pregnancy

- **Puberty:** Beginning of the fertile period when gametes are produced and secondary sex characteristics become evident
- **Retroversion:** Abnormal tipping backward of the uterus
- **Salpingitis:** Inflammation of fallopian tube

Some medical terms are specific to the *obstetrical* nature of this system. If you'll be spending any time in an OB's office, whether as an employee or patient, these are some handy terms to know:

- **Amnion:** Membrane enveloping the fetus
- **Antepartum:** Before birth, in relation to the mother
- **Chorion:** Outermost extraembryonic membrane enveloping the fetus
- **Congenital anomaly:** An abnormality or defect present at birth
- **Ectopic:** Occurring away from a normal position
- **Ectopic pregnancy:** Pregnancy occurring in the fallopian tube
- **Embryo:** The product of conception up to the eight-week period of gestation
- **Fetus:** The embryo from second month of pregnancy to delivery
- **Galactorrhea:** Discharge of milk from the breast
- **Gestation:** Period of time from fertilization to birth — in a human pregnancy, approximately 40 weeks
- **Gravida:** A pregnant female
- **Hyperemesis gravidarum:** Excessive vomiting during pregnancy
- **Intrapartum:** During labor and delivery, in relation to the mother
- **Lochia:** The vaginal discharge after childbirth
- **Meconium:** First stool of the newborn
- **Multigravida:** Female who has been pregnant two or more times
- **Multipara:** Female who has given birth to viable offspring two or more times
- **Neonate:** A newborn infant from birth to four weeks of age
- **Neonatologist:** A physician specializing in neonatology
- **Neonatology:** The study, diagnosis, and treatment of disorders of the newborn infant up to one month of age
- **Nulligravida:** Female who has never been pregnant

- **Nullipara:** Female who has never given birth
- **Parturition:** The act of giving birth
- **Postnatal:** Period after birth, referring to the newborn
- **Postpartum:** After delivery, in relation to the mother
- **Prenatal:** Period before birth, referring to the fetus

BABY STEPS: OB ABBREVIATIONS

Things happen fast in the birthing room, so OB physicians and their employees like to use abbreviations to keep the chatting to a minimum. Some abbreviations associated with obstetrics and neonatology are as follows:

AB: Abortion

CPD: Cephalopelvic disproportion; fetal head is too large to pass through the mother's pelvis

CS or C-section: Cesarean section

DOB: Date of birth

EDC: Expected date of confinement or delivery (due date)

FHS: Fetal heart sounds

L&D: Labor and delivery

LMP: Last menstrual period; date that last menstrual period began

NB: Newborn

OB: Obstetrics

RDS: Respiratory distress syndrome

SFH: Symphysis-fundus height, measurement taken from *symphysis pubis* (pubic bone) to *fundus* (highest level) of uterus; provides a growth record of the uterine fundus as a pregnancy progresses

SVD: Spontaneous vaginal delivery

- **Primigravida:** Female who is pregnant for the first time
- **Primipara:** Female who has given birth to viable offspring for the first time
- **Pseudocyesis:** False pregnancy
- **Puerpera:** Female who has just given birth
- **Puerperium:** Period after delivery until reproductive organs return to normal, about six to eight weeks
- **Quickening:** Female's first awareness of movement of fetus within the uterus, usually felt at 16–20 weeks' gestation
- **Secundigravida:** Female pregnant for the second time
- **Secundipara:** Female who has given birth to viable offspring for the second time

Common Female Reproductive Conditions

There's more to the female reproductive system than making babies. With all that equipment, there's bound to be a fair share of technical difficulties ranging from the downright annoying (yeast infections) to the long-lasting (loss of hormones due to menopause):

- **Amenorrhea:** Absence of menstrual period
- **Cervicitis:** Inflammation of the cervix
- **Dysmenorrhea:** Painful menstrual periods
- **Dyspareunia:** Painful or difficult intercourse
- **Endometritis:** Inflammation of endometrium
- **Gynatresia (atresia):** Absence of normal body opening (an *occlusion*); gynatresia usually refers to part of female genital tract, the vagina
- **HRT (hormone replacement therapy):** Replacement of hormones to treat menopausal symptoms (also called *ERT: estrogen replacement therapy*)
- **Hydrosalpinx:** Water in fallopian tube
- **Mastitis:** Inflammation of the breast occurring during breastfeeding, usually bacterial in nature
- **Menometrorrhagia:** Excessive menstrual flow both during and between menstrual periods

- **Menorrhagia:** Heavy menstrual period
- **Oophoritis:** Inflammation of ovary
- **PMD (premenstrual dysphoric syndrome):** Used to describe severe premenstrual syndrome, which results in a week or two of hormonally triggered clinical depression every month
- **PMS (premenstrual syndrome):** Cyclic disorder involving physical and emotional symptoms in the premenstrual phase (just before menses phase); symptoms include fatigue, bloating, tension, and irritability
- **Vaginitis:** Inflammation of the vagina

Some conditions of the female reproductive system are specifically related to pregnancy and childbirth:

- **Abruptio placentae:** Premature separation of placenta from the uterine wall causing bleeding and a rigid, painful abdomen and requiring emergency cesarean section
- **Dystocia:** Difficult or abnormal labor
- **Eclampsia:** Severe complication of pregnancy involving convulsions and/or coma in a pregnant female
- **Ectopic pregnancy:** Pregnancy occurring outside the uterus *(tubal pregnancy)* requiring emergency surgery
- **Intrauterine fetal death:** Fetal death occurring before expected date of birth
- **Missed abortion:** A fetal demise has occurred but miscarriage by expulsion has not taken place
- **Placenta previa:** Placenta develops in the lower uterine wall and may cover the cervix, blocking the birth canal and requiring a C-section; can be diagnosed by ultrasound
- **Preeclampsia:** Condition during pregnancy or shortly after delivery with high blood pressure, *edema* (swelling), and protein in the urine
- **Salpingocyesis:** Pregnancy occurring in fallopian tube or ectopic pregnancy
- **Spontaneous abortion:** A miscarriage, usually occurring before 12 weeks of gestation
- **Stillbirth:** Fetal death in utero, occurring before delivery

DEALING WITH INFERTILITY

Infertility affects roughly 12 to 13 out of every 100 couples in the United States, according to the Department of Human Health Services. As such, there are growing measures available to people who wish to pursue infertility treatment. Here are some common terms you may run into regarding this topic:

- **Intrauterine insemination (IUI):** Healthy sperm is collected and inserted into the uterus at ovulation time with the hope that Mother Nature will do the rest.
- **In vitro fertilization (IVF):** Eggs are retrieved from the ovary and fertilized with sperm in a laboratory setting (commonly in a Petri dish) where they develop into embryos and are then implanted into the uterus to continue maturation. This procedure is done after drug therapy to stimulate ovulation (oral chomiphene and/or injectable gonadotropins).
- **Petri dish:** Named after German bacteriologist Julius Richard Petri, this is a shallow cylindrical glass or plastic-lidded dish that biologists use to culture cells such as bacteria.
- **Gamete intrafallopian transfer (GIFT):** A modified version of IVF, where eggs and sperm (gametes) are placed into the fallopian tubes via laparoscopy with general anesthetic, with the hope that they are carried naturally to the uterus.
- **Zygote intrafallopian transfer (ZIFT):** Similar to the GIFT procedure, eggs are mixed with sperm in the lab, and fertilized eggs (zygotes) are placed into the fallopian tubes via laparoscopy with general anesthetic, with the hope that they are carried naturally to the uterus.

Finding the Culprit: Female Reproductive Diseases and Pathology

It's important to note that the following conditions not only influence the work of the body, but also the overall mental health of the women they affect. As with the male reproductive system, a woman's mental and sexual health are intricately interwoven with physical health. For many women, issues involving reproductive health often have long-lasting effects on feminine and sexual identity. This is especially true if it affects a woman's ability to conceive or involves loss of reproductive organs, so these diseases and pathological conditions should be addressed with the utmost care and sensitivity.

- **Adenomyosis** refers to endometrium growth in the myometrium of the uterus.
- **Breast carcinoma** is a malignant tumor of the breast. Tumors may spread to skin, chest wall, and lymph nodes located in axilla; they may metastasize (spread) to other parts of the body, including bones, lungs, liver, brain, and even ovaries. Breast carcinoma can be treated in a variety of ways, including *lumpectomy* (removal of cancerous lump only), removal of breast tissue but preserving skin and nipple for future reconstruction *(subcutaneous mastectomy),* removal of the entire breast (a simple or total mastectomy), or removal of breast, lymph nodes, and adjacent chest wall muscle in a single procedure (radical mastectomy).
- **Carcinoma of cervix** means malignant tumor of the cervix. *Papanicolaou (Pap) smear* detects early *cervical neoplasia* by microscopic examination of cells scraped from *cervical epithelium.*
- **Endometrial carcinoma** refers to malignant tumor of the uterus.
- **Endometriosis** involves endometrial tissue in an abnormal location, such as the ovaries or intestine, associated with dysmenorrhea, pelvic pain, and infertility.
- **Fibrocystic disease** is a disease of the breast. It is a benign condition involving one or more tumors of the breast.
- **Fibroid (leiomyoma)** is a benign tumor in the uterus composed of fibrous tissue and muscle, may cause pelvic pain or menorrhagia.
- **Ovarian carcinoma** means malignant tumor of the ovary *(adenocarcinoma).* It may be cystic or solid.
- **Ovarian cyst** is collections of fluid within a sac or cyst in the ovary.
- **PID (pelvic inflammatory disease)** refers to inflammation of female pelvic organs.
- **Prolapsed uterus** involves displacement of uterus down into the vagina.
- **Stein-Leventhal syndrome (polycystic ovary syndrome)** refers to adrenal gland malfunction resulting in facial hair *(hirsutism),* weight gain, and infrequent, abnormal, or absent menstrual periods.
- **TSS (toxic shock syndrome)** is a severe illness caused by bacterial infection, most often seen in menstruating women using tampons. Staphylococcus aureus is the bacterial culprit.
- **Vesicovaginal fistula** is when there is an opening between vagina and urinary bladder.

Testing, Testing: Female Reproductive Radiology and Diagnostic Tests

Thank goodness for modern medicine. It certainly helps ease the mind of many a woman by providing answers to the most pressing female reproductive questions. Most women will be familiar with some of these yearly (or more often for some) tests that, although causing a bit of discomfort at the time, give great comfort in the long run by offering diagnoses for many serious conditions.

- **ART (Assisted reproductive techniques):** Includes procedures such as IUI (intrauterine insemination), IVF (in vitro fertilization), and ICSI (intracytoplasmic sperm injection)
- **Chorionic villus sampling (CVS):** A prenatal test done early in pregnancy to detect congenital abnormalities in the fetus. A small tissue sample is taken from the villi of the chorion that forms from the fetal part of the placenta. This test can be done as early as 10 weeks into the pregnancy. It is similar to an amniocentesis procedure.
- **Hysterosalpingogram:** X-ray taken of the uterus and fallopian tubes after a dye is introduced in the uterus to see if it can move freely through the fallopian tubes and out to the ovaries; used to diagnose blockages in tubes that might lead to infertility
- **Mammogram:** X-ray film of the breast
- **Papanicolaou (Pap) smear:** Sample of cells of cervix are harvested and examined under microscopic analysis; the presence of cervical or vaginal carcinoma can be detected.
- **Pregnancy test:** Detects the presence of hCG in the urine or blood to diagnose pregnancy
- **Sonohysterography:** Recording uterus by sound waves (ultrasound)

Paging Dr. Terminology: Female Reproductive Surgeries and Procedures

Now that you're in tune with the working parts and possible issues involved with the female reproductive system, it's time to find out more about the things your physician can do to fix the feminine plumbing, so to speak. Obviously, many of these surgeries and procedures involve a woman's ability to conceive, whether it be putting an end to that ability through a hysterectomy or helping improve a woman's chances to get pregnant. First, let's talk about some general procedures.

- **Abortion** is the termination of a pregnancy before the embryo or the fetus is able to exist on its own. A spontaneous abortion may occur in a pregnancy up to and including 12 weeks, and is also known as a *miscarriage.* A therapeutic or induced abortion is a deliberate termination of pregnancy and is most commonly performed during the first trimester between 8 and 12 weeks.
- **Cervical cauterization** is a procedure performed following an abnormal Pap smear — with ablation of abnormal cervical tissue using an electric cautery.
- **Cervical conization** is a cone-shaped biopsy of tissue from the mouth of cervix for diagnostic purposes. This procedure often follows an abnormal Pap smear.
- **Colposcopy** is a magnified examination of the cervix, vagina, and vulva, using a colposcope used — to detect abnormalities.
- **Cryosurgery** refers to the use of cold or freezing temperature to destroy tissue, usually produced by a probe containing liquid nitrogen.
- **D & C** means dilatation and curettage. First, the *dilatation* (widening of the cervical opening) is accomplished. *Curettage* (scraping) is accomplished next by using a curette or metal loop to remove samples of the lining of the uterus for diagnostic purposes. Also performed to remove products of conception after an incomplete miscarriage or to reduce uterine bleeding.
- **Endometrial ablation** destroys (ablates) the endometrium (uterine lining) to treat dysfunctional or abnormal uterine bleeding.
- **Hysteroscopy** is visual examination of the uterus performed with a *hysteroscope.*

Many women opt for a permanent form of sterilization once they make the decision to not have more (or any) children. The procedures are very common, and each has its own set of pros and cons. Women are typically encouraged to choose the sterilization method best for their individual lifestyles and physical makeup. A very common sterilization method is *tubal ligation*, a procedure that involves cutting or interrupting and *ligating* (tying off) fallopian tubes to prevent passage of ovum. This procedure can be done laparoscopically or through an abdominal incision:

- **Laparoscopic method:** Laparoscope is inserted through the abdominal wall, and tubes can be sealed off with high-frequency spark *(cauterization)* or burning.
- **Tubal banding:** A band is wrapped around a section of each tube and tissue becomes *necrotic* (dies), providing a break between the two portions of tube.
- **Tubal clipping:** *Filshie clip* is used to clip off tubes, similar to banding method.

HAVING FUN WITH HORMONES: BEGINNING TO END AND BIRTH CONTROL IN BETWEEN

Menstruation and pregnancy not only depend on the hormones produced in the ovaries, but also on hormones secreted from the pituitary gland. *Follicle-stimulating hormones (FSH)* and *luteinizing hormones (LH)* help stimulate the development of the ovum and ovulation. After ovulation, LH influences the maintenance of the corpus luteum and its production of estrogen and progesterone.

During pregnancy the higher levels of estrogen and progesterone affect the pituitary gland itself, by shedding off its production of FSH and LH. When a woman is pregnant then, new ova do not mature, and ovulation cannot occur. This interaction, when hormones act to shut off the production of another group of hormones, is called *negative feedback*. This is the principle behind the action of birth control pills on the body. The *birth control pill* contains varying amounts of estrogen and progesterone, causing the hormone levels to rise in the blood. Negative feedback occurs, and the pituitary does not release FSH and LH. Ovulation cannot occur without these, and a woman cannot become pregnant.

Other female contraceptive measures include the IUD (intrauterine device) and the diaphragm. The *IUD* is a small coil placed inside the uterus by a physician. Its presence in the uterus (foreign body) irritates the uterine lining to prevent implantation of a fertilized ovum. A *diaphragm* is a rubber cup-shaped device inserted over the outside of the cervix before intercourse to prevent sperm from entering the cervix and moving into the uterus to the fallopian tubes.

The finale of this ongoing cycle occurs when the secretion of estrogen from the ovaries lessens, fewer eggs are produced, and menopause begins. *Menopause* is the gradual ending of the menstrual cycle and the natural process resulting from normal aging of the ovaries. Other names for menopause are "change of life" and "climacteric." Premature menopause can occur before age 35, whereas delayed menopause can occur after age 55. Artificial or "surgical" menopause occurs if the ovaries are removed or made nonfunctional by radiation therapy. Menopause is considered complete when menstrual periods have been absent for at least 12 months.

TECHNICAL STUFF

Laparoscopic tubal ligations were done in the 1970s, and the first *laparoscopic cholecystectomy* was performed in 1989.

Many surgical procedures for the female reproductive system require the repair or removal of some parts of the system. In the most serious cases (often involving cancer), the entire uterus and surrounding cervix are completely removed.

Keep in mind that breasts are considered part of this system as well, so in the following list you see terms referring to the surgical removal or repair of these body parts as well.

- **Abdominal hysterectomy:** Surgical removal of the uterus through the abdomen
- **Bilateral salpingo-oophorectomy:** Surgical removal of both tubes and both ovaries
- **Colpopexy:** Surgical fixation of the vagina to surrounding structures
- **Combination special (total hysterectomy and bilateral salpingooophorectomy):** Removal of uterus, cervix, both tubes, and ovaries; commonly referred to as *TAH-BSO (Total Abdominal Hysterectomy with Bilateral Salpingo-Oophorectomy)*
- **Hymenectomy:** Surgical removal of the hymen
- **Hysteropexy:** Surgical fixation of a misplaced or abnormally mobile uterus
- **Laparoscopic hysterectomy:** Surgical removal of the uterus using a laparoscope
- **Lumpectomy:** Removal of cancerous lump only in the breast
- **Mastectomy:** Surgical removal of a breast

  Subcutaneous mastectomy is removal of breast tissue that preserves skin and nipple for future reconstruction; simple or total mastectomy may involve removal of the entire breast; in a radical mastectomy, the breast is removed, along with the lymph nodes and adjacent chest wall muscle in a single procedure.
- **Myomectomy:** Surgical removal of a leiomyoma (fibroid) from the uterus
- **Oophorectomy:** Surgical removal of an ovary
- **Salpingectomy:** Surgical removal of a fallopian tube
- **Salpingo-oophorectomy (or oophoro-salpingectomy):** Removal of fallopian tube and ovary
- **Subtotal hysterectomy:** Surgical removal of uterus only (cervix left behind)
- **Total hysterectomy:** Surgical removal of uterus and cervix
- **Vaginal hysterectomy:** Uterus and cervix surgically removed via vagina
- **Vaginoplasty:** Surgical repair of the vagina
- **Vulvectomy:** Surgical removal of the vulva

TECHNICAL STUFF

The surgical robot can be used in procedures involving cervical and endometrial cancers, ovarian tumors, uterine fibroids, and pelvic prolapse. Robotics are used to perform laparoscopic-assisted vaginal hysterectomies, and total hysterectomies. The da Vinci robot can perform a robotic myomectomy, allowing a future pregnancy to follow the surgery.

Of course, because creating life and giving birth are two huge jobs of this system, you would be remiss to miss these obstetrical terms:

- **Amniotomy:** Incision into the amnion to induce labor. It's also referred to as *artificial rupture of membranes.*
- **Amniocentesis:** This involves surgical puncture to aspirate amniotic fluid via insertion of needle through the abdominal and uterine walls using ultrasound guidance. Fluid is used for the assessment of fetal health and maturity. This procedure is used to aid in diagnosis of fetal abnormalities. It is performed early in pregnancy at 16 weeks to determine fetal abnormalities such as *Down syndrome, spina bifida,* or to determine the sex of the fetus. It is done late in the pregnancy to determine lung maturity of the fetus.
- **Cesarean section:** This is surgical removal of the fetus through the abdominal and uterine walls. A *C-section* may be performed for a *breech* presentation (baby's head is not in downward position), multiple births, *placenta previa* (placenta develops in the lower uterine wall and may cover the cervix, blocking the birth canal), *abruptio placentae* (premature separation of placenta from uterine wall), *cephalopelvic disproportion* (when a baby's head or body is too large to fit through the mother's pelvis), failure to progress in labor, or any sign that the fetus is in distress.
- **Episiotomy:** Refers to incision of vulva or perineum. This is done during delivery to prevent tearing of the perineum.
- **Obstetrical ultrasound:** Ultrasound of the abdomen and pelvis determine fetal development, growth rate, and estimate fetal age, weight, and maturity.
- **Pelvimetry:** The measurement of the mother's pelvic to determine ability of fetus to pass through.
- **Salpingectomy:** Removal of a fallopian tube in order to remove an ectopic pregnancy.

Terminology RX: Female Reproductive Pharmacology

And now for a brief word about our friends, the drugs. Many women hoping to have children who are experiencing difficulties are very thankful to have drugs to treat fertility, such as *clomiphene citrate*. These little wonders work by stimulating the pituitary gland to release LH and FSH, thus increasing the body's ability to conceive. Though these drugs are not panaceas, they have helped countless women reach their goals of becoming mothers. On the other end of the conception spectrum, some babies want to make their appearance too early. In these cases, uterine relaxants are used to stop premature labor in pregnancy.

Analgesics are painkillers used to treat menstrual cramps and painful periods. Then there are the "antis." *Antifungal drugs* are used to treat vaginal yeast infections, whereas *anti-inflammatories* and *antibiotics* are used to treat some sexually transmitted diseases. (For more information about STDs that affect both woman and men, see Chapter 22.)

TECHNICAL STUFF

Your obstetrical history can be summed up in five letters coupled with five numbers: G-T-P-A-L.

G for Gravida: Number of pregnancies

T for Term: Number of pregnancies carried to term

P for Para: Number of pregnancies resulting in a liveborn infant

A for Abortus: Number of pregnancies ending in abortion, as the result of either a miscarriage or therapeutic abortion

L for Living: Number of living children

For example:

G3-T3-P3-A0-L3 means 3 pregnancies, carried to term, resulting in 3 live term infants who are still alive and well.

G3-T2-P2-A1-L2 means 3 pregnancies, 2 carried to term, resulting in 2 live term infants, one abortion or miscarriage, resulting in 2 living children.

G3-T3-P4-A0-L4 means 3 pregnancies, carried to term, resulting in 4 live term infants, who are still alive and well, indicating that one pregnancy resulted in twins.

TECHNICAL STUFF

The due date or EDC in a pregnancy is easily calculated by knowing the beginning date of last menstrual period (LMP). Count back three months and add seven days. Here's an example. LMP is March 25. Count back three months: February 25, January 25, December 25. Merry Christmas! Add seven days: Happy New Year!

6 The Part of Tens

IN THIS PART . . .

Checking out ten essential medical terminology references

Memorizing stuff with ten or so useful mnemonic devices

Twisting your tongue with ten sets of tough diseases

IN THIS CHAPTER

» Access the most widely used terminology references

» Find the type of reference that works best for your lifestyle

Chapter 24

Ten Essential Medical Terminology References

Oh, you know you want more. Medical terminology references, that is. What did you think we meant? Whether you are drawn to the stacks at your local library or prefer the click of the computer keyboard, here are ten terminology references that you can't live without.

Medterms.com

A subset site of MedicineNet.com, this medical reference includes over 16,000 terms. Via a simple search engine, the site can look for words of similar spelling and incorrect spelling — which is a boon for those of us who never won a spelling bee. The site also offers a word of the day and earns its street cred by the fact that its doctors authored the latest edition of the *Webster's New World Medical Dictionary*.

Medilexicon.com

This website is a good all-arounder, featuring a fully searchable list of medical abbreviations and a medical dictionary. It's a searchapalooza, offering search functions for drugs, medical instruments, and ICD-9 codes (codes used for medical charting and billing).

webMD.com

You can always count on webMD.com to provide the latest cutting-edge medical news and information. And, yes, you can also drive yourself insane using the Symptom Checker to pinpoint what ails you. (Once you start, you'll do it every time you feel a sniffle coming on.) In addition to the latest news, you can search for doctors, hospitals, drugs, and practically every medical topic known to man. Connect to blogs, message boards, expert forums, and even health quizzes, games, and slideshows.

Dorland's Illustrated Medical Dictionary, 32nd Edition

If you consider yourself a visual learner, consider Dorland's your new best friend. Not only does this dictionary have all the terms you need to know, it offers full illustrations to help get the point across. And, it's available both online at `www.dorlands.com` and in hardcopy format.

Mosby's Medical Dictionary, 10th Edition

This monster is well over 2,000 pages chocked full of medical terminology know-how. It includes a thumb-indexed dictionary and tons of illustrations to help you visualize the terms as actual body parts. Not exactly something you want to carry around in your book bag, but definitely handy to keep on your bookshelf. Plus, it makes a great doorstop or paperweight. Mosby's is famous for the number of colored pictures, which tends to be helpful for the novice medical terminology student.

Stedman's Medical Dictionary and Flashcards for Health Professionals and Nursing Illustrated, 7th Edition

This particular book is the major reference from this publisher, but the company also offers tons of smaller, more precise references if you want to narrow down your stack of books a bit. From illustrated flashcards and skill-building tools to guides to idioms, terms, and phrases, *Stedman's* is a one-stop shop for all things terminology. And, of course, it offers tons of online resources at www.stedmans.com as well if you want to travel light.

Taber's Cyclopedic Medical Dictionary, 23rd Edition

Taber's website at www.tabers.com says that it is the "world's best-selling health-sciences dictionary," offering over 56,000 terms. Like many of its competitors, *Taber's* offers not only the print version of its dictionary, but also a web component and terms sent directly to your PDA or wireless handheld device. *Taber's* other vital stats include: 700 full-color images, 2,500 audio pronunciations, customized bookmarking, "sounds like" search, and topic cross-linking. So, if you're checking out one particular part of a system, *Taber's* will point you in the direction of related information. That's a nice little bit of handholding.

Sloane's Medical Word Book, 5th Edition

This book, a spelling and vocabulary guide for medical transcription, is different from other medical reference books in that terms are organized by medical specialty: that is, obstetrics and gynecology, cardiology, and so forth. This book does not list definitions, just the words (thus the title), but this book is a savior when looking for a difficult or hard-to-spell term when looking in a standard medical dictionary could take hours if the spelling is not known. Searching by medical service narrows down the choices. Within each medical specialty are headings that further break down the choices and make the hunt easier.

Medicalmnemonics.com

This is a cool and fun website. If you need a little boost to help you remember words and terms, chances are you already use mnemonic devices. You know, like "I before E, except after C, or when sounding like A as in neighbor and weigh."

Mnemonics are often simple little phrases to help you recall what it is you're trying to learn and put on paper, into speech, or fill in on a standardized test. This is a whole website dedicated to the concept. Working much like a wiki, *you* can add your own devices to the database and help others. You can search the database (of course) or browse by systems and charts. You can even customize to fit your needs or set the site up to download to your smartphone or PDA. The coolest part is: It's totally free and not-for-profit. So thank your fellow medheads for sharing the love, and remember to share some yourself by adding your own useful mnemonics.

Medical Terminology Systems Quick Study Guide

The good folks at Bar Charts, Inc., figured, eh, why bother with all the pages and binding that ties down a traditional book! When you really want to know something, you want it to magically appear right before your eyes. Voila! Enter the *Quick Study Guide*, also known as the giant laminated poster. You've probably seen similar charts in the doctor's office showcasing your insides. This one is super handy and hits the terminology highlights. You can find all sorts of similar guides at `www.barcharts.com` for things like common abbreviations, individual systems terms (with illustrations), and even guides just for nurses. Who needs wallpaper when you can hang these babies up?

IN THIS CHAPTER

- Using simple phrasing devices to remember medical terms
- Discovering quick ways to recall simple system functions

Chapter 25
Ten or So Useful Mnemonic Devices

A *mnemonic device* is any kind of simple way to remember something, such as lists of terms, functions, or definitions. They are usually kind of silly, which makes them stand out in your mind. In fact, the sillier the better in most cases. After all, there is rarely anything memorable about the mundane. It's the weird and wacky that often stands out in our minds. In this chapter, we've compiled 11 great useful devices from one of our favorite websites, `www.medicalmnemonics.com`. (See Chapter 24 for more info on this cool site.)

Cranial Nerves

Don't strain your cranium to recall those cranial nerves. Just remember: "On Old Olympus Towering Top, A Finn And German Viewed Some Hops" to recall these nerves: olfactory, optic, oculomotor, trochlear, trigeminal, abducens, facial, auditory-vestibular, glossopharyngeal, vagus, spinal accessory, and hypoglossal.

Lung Lobe Numbers

To remember the location of the different sides of the lungs, think *tri* and *bi*. The tri-lobed lung lives on the right side, along with the tricuspid heart valve. The bicuspid and bi-lobed lung live on the left side of your body.

The Size of a Thyroid

Ever play that game where you look at the clouds and try to figure out what they look like? Well, you can do the same with the thyroid, which looks a little bit like a bra. To remember the size of the thyroid, just remember that breasts are bigger in women than men, so the thyroid is bigger in women. Even more, pregnant women have the largest breasts, and they also have the largest thyroids.

Scalp Layers

The layers of your scalp actually spell SCALP. Remember this easy formula:

Skin

Connective tissue

Aponeurosis

Loose Connective Tissue

Pericranium

SCALP!

Muscles of the Rotator Cuff

Rotator cuff injuries can be debilitating, especially for an athlete. You can remember the muscles of the rotator cuff by remembering SITS. These muscles are (clockwise from top): Supraspinatus, Infraspinatus, Teres minor, and Subscapularis.

Note: If a baseball pitcher injures these muscles, he SITS out for the rest of the game.

Radial Nerve

The muscles supplied by the radial nerve are the BEST! Remember:

Brachioradialis

Extensors

Supinator

Triceps

That's the BEST way to remember these muscles!

Face Nerves

You can recall what the major face muscles do by matching the action to the name. Think *M* and *facial*. The *mandibular* nerve is in charge of *mastication*. The *facial* nerve is in charge of *facial expression*.

Perineal versus Peroneal

Can't keep these two words straight? Just remember that perINeal is *in between* the legs. PerONeal is *on* the legs.

Sperm Path through Male Reproductive Tract

Poor Steve. He gets a tough break here, but he's the best candidate for remembering the path sperm takes to exit the male body. Meet Steve:

Seminiferous **T**ubules

Epididymis

Vas deferens

Ejaculatory duct

Carpal Bone Locations

Who knew the carpal bones could be so racy? This one is rated R, kids. When you're trying to think of these bones, consider that *Some Lovers Try Positions That They Can't Handle*:

Scaphoid

Lunate

Triquetrum

Pisiform

Trapezium

Trapezoid

Capitate

Hamate

Cranial Bones

Since cranial bones help make up your skull, keep skulls in mind to recall the bones and think "Old Parents Forget to Eat Spinach":

Occipital

Parietal

Frontal

Temporal

Ethmoid

Sphenoid

IN THIS CHAPTER

» Encountering some of the most challenging disease terms

» Practicing pronunciations to sound like a pro

Chapter 26

Ten Sets of Terminology Tongue-Twisting Diseases

Oh, you know you want more. Medical terminology terms, that is. Specifically, terms that twist the tongue and stand apart as some of the most challenging to write and pronounce.

Get to know these, and you'll be branded the resident expert in disease terminology. There is something for everyone here, from ten body system groups you've come to know and love.

Skeletal

These three diseases are named after the people who discovered them — and what tongue-twisting names they are! For example, *Kohler-Pellegrini-Stieda* is a condition with semilunar bony formation in the upper portion of the mediocollateral ligament of the knee due to trauma.

Then there's *Kummell-Verneuil*, which is compression fracture of vertebra occurring a few weeks after a spinal injury.

Moving south in the skeleton, you might encounter *Osgood-Schlatter*, which is osteochondrosis of the tuberosity of the tibia, usually occurring in adolescents. Kind of makes you wonder why there was no Dr. Smith or Jones involved, doesn't it?

Muscular

These muscular diseases sound like they were named on a dare. There is *de Quervain*, or painful synovitis caused by narrowing of the tendon sheath of the muscles in the thumb.

How about *Duchenne*? Do you know Duchenne? It's not a person, but rather spinal muscular dystrophy.

And taking the award for disease that sounds most like a character from Clue is *Munchmeyer*, also known as progressive ossifying polymyositis. Funny names, very unfunny diseases.

Integumentary

Your largest organ is a breeding ground for tongue-twisting diseases. There is *Lewandowsky-Lutz*, a rare hereditary skin disorder with macules and papules on hands and feet. Those who suffer from this are highly at risk for cancer or human papillomavirus (HPV). Males are at high risk for the very non-macho *Mucha-Habermann*, also known as acute parapsoriasis, a disease of the immune system characterized by rash and lesions on the skin. Going along with the two doctors for the price of one disease names, we also have:

- **Arndt-Gottron:** Skin condition with diffuse thickening of skin with underlying papules (scleromyxedema)
- **Hailey-Hailey (familial benign pemphigus):** Genetic disorder causing blisters to form on the skin
- **Oppenheim-Urbach:** Rare skin condition seen in diabetic patients and prevalent in families, presenting with red and yellow papules usually on lower limbs
- **Quinquaud (decalvaris folliculitis):** Inflammation of hair follicles, resulting in loss of hair, red scalp, and pustules around hair follicles

Sensory

These sensory disease names sound like they came straight out of an IKEA catalog. For example, *Pendred* is not a bookcase, but rather a genetic disorder that causes early hearing loss in children.

What about *Riga-Fede?* It's a rare oral (mouth) condition seen in newborns with ulceration of tongue and inner lower lip.

Finally, we have *Eales* (no, not eels), an ocular disease with inflammation and blockage of retinal blood vessels with recurrent retinal and vitreal hemorrhage. Fun, right?

Cardiovascular and Lymphatic

The heart is no stranger to oddly named diseases. Say these three times fast and you may have your own coronary:

- **Corvisart (Tetralogy of Fallot):** A congenital heart defect with coarctation of the aorta, a hole in the septum between ventricles, narrowing of the pulmonary outflow tract, and thickening of the right ventricular wall
- **Heller-Dohle:** Inflammation of the aorta that occurs in the late stages of syphilis
- **Rougnon-Heberden (Angina pectoris):** Severe pain in the chest associated with insufficient blood supply to the heart

Respiratory

These respiratory diseases aren't necessarily tongue-twisters, but they certainly do have odd names. There is *bird breeder's lung* (also called pigeon breeder's lung or bird fancier's lung), which is a type of hypersensitive pneumonitis (lung inflammation) caused by exposure to bird droppings. Then we have *Darlings*, which is caused by *Histoplasma* fungus in the lung. It is fatal if left untreated and is common in AIDS patients because of their suppressed immune systems.

Finally, there is *Bornholm*, which is caused by Coxsackie B virus. It is named after the Danish island where early cases occurred and is characterized by sharp chest pain and difficulty breathing. It's also known as Devil's grip because of the sudden onset and iron grip feeling around the rib cage.

Gastrointestinal

The names for these gastrointestinal diseases are almost as complicated as the diseases themselves. To be sure, none of these diseases is funny — but their names certainly are. Take *Cruveilhier*. Funny-sounding name for a not funny, very rare disease with patent paraumbilical vein due to portal hypertension with liver cirrhosis.

Another example is *Hirschsprung*, a congenital malformation of the enteric nervous system causing bowel obstruction in the newborn that is often associated with Trisomy 21 (Down syndrome).

Endocrine

In the endocrine system, the award for most oddly named disease goes (with much pomp and circumstance) to *Pompe*, an inherited disease caused by buildup of glycogen in body cells that impairs their ability to function normally. You can also blame MEN for what ails this system. Not human men, mind you, but *MEN*, which stands for multiple endocrine neoplasia. This is a group of disorders affecting the body's network of hormone-producing glands with tumors in parathyroid, pituitary, and pancreas. These growths can be benign or malignant.

Nervous

The nervous system brings even more wacky names to the tongue twister party. There is *Machado-Joseph-Azorean* (spinocerebellar ataxia), a rare inherited neurodegenerative disease which causes lack of muscle control and coordination of all extremities that progressively worsens with time.

Please also welcome *Spielmeyer-Vogt*, an inherited disorder that affects the nervous system in children with developing vision loss, motor disabilities, speech difficulties, and seizures.

Finally, direct from Germany is *Von Recklinghausen* (Neurofibromatosis), a genetic disorder characterized by tumor growth on nerves in tissues and organs. These tumors can become cancerous.

Urinary and Reproductive

The urinary and reproductive systems are, as you might expect, rife with off-color humor. Most of these diseases just sound funny. In reality, though, they can be quite serious. Take, for example, Munk. *Munk* is a kidney disease prevalent in children characterized by a buildup of fats in cells of the kidney tubules.

There is also *Marion's*, a congenital obstruction of the posterior urethra or bladder neck stenosis, and *Cacchi-Ricci* (medullary sponge kidney), a congenital disorder of kidneys characterized by cystic dilatation of collecting tubules in one or both kidneys.

On the reproductive side of things, one might suffer from *priapism*, a continuous painful erection. Named after Priapus, the Roman God of male potency, priapism is definitely a reason to call your doctor. So is *Peyronie*, which is a plaque or scar tissue that forms on the penis, causing reduced flexibility, pain, and a tendency for the penis to bend or arc during an erection. Ouch.

Lest you feel left out, ladies, there are some oddly named diseases for you as well. There is *Chiari-Frommel*, a rare endocrine disease affecting postpartum women featuring an overproduction of breast milk, lack of ovulation, and absence of menstrual period. Don't forget about *Schimmelbusch*, a benign breast disease with formation of numerous small cysts due to dilatation of the mammary ducts. Finally, there is *Breisky*, a progressive disease that involves wasting of the vulva (progressive weakness and deterioration) in postmenopausal women caused by hormone imbalance.

IN THIS CHAPTER

» Encountering some of the most difficult terms to spell

» Committing challenging spelling words to memory

Chapter 27

Top Ten Crazy-Hard-to-Spell Medical Terms

Even the most talented speller can get it wrong sometimes. Every day that you are working in the medical field and writing down or dictating terms, you are in a one-person spelling bee. So, it should come as no surprise to you that often the words and terms you need to spell are somewhat challenging. You're not in a smelly gym, fifth-grade bee anymore—this is the big time, baby!

Crazy-Hard-to-Spell Terms

Caput succedaneum: This is the term for face and head swelling of a newborn as result of trauma during delivery. One way to remember how to spell this term is to think of the word "succeed," which is similar to the succeed- at the beginning of the second word.

Stromuhr: This is a *rheometer*, which measures the amount and flow of blood through arteries. While not a long word, it's always a tricky one to remember because it looks and sounds nothing like what it actually is or does.

Sphenopalatine ganglioneuralgia: Also knows as an ice cream headache or brain freeze. Why is there a medical term for this condition in the first place? Who knows! But here's a really long, really hard-to-spell term for it!

Morsicatio linguarum: Is there a fancy way say "tongue biting"? Of course there is! And lucky for you, it's also hard to spell. This term looks like something from the world of Harry Potter, so perhaps you can create an incantation to help you spell it.

Sternutate: Why sneeze when you can sternutate? This is an odd word to spell because, though short, it doesn't follow the more traditional structure of many related medical terms. Best to just memorize it . . . or just say "sneeze" instead.

Horripilation: This is a hard-to-spell word for what is commonly known as goose bumps.

Veisalgia: A hangover. But harder to spell. Drink some hair of the dog and come up with a mnemonic device to remember this one.

Muscae volitantes: Spots before the eyes, also known as "eye floaters."

Obdormition: A limb falling asleep.

And finally . . . the big daddy . . .

Pneumonoultramicroscopic silicovolcanoconiosis: This term appears in most dictionaries as all one word, but to be correct in terminology, it should be broken after "microscopic." This is a lung condition caused by inhaling silica particles, specifically from a volcano; also commonly known as black sputum.

Appendix

Handy Study Guide

Here's a quick fix for you — a lot of quick fixes, in fact! Sometimes you just need a quick mental boost to help you study for a quiz, prepare for your first day as a med tech, or simply refresh your memory after a long week at work. That's why we've created this simple and quick reference known as the Handy Study Guide for your reading enjoyment.

This guide covers some of the top need-to-know info you might want to keep handy in a pinch. First up is a short list of the body systems along with a brief synopsis of each — in case you have a tendency to mix up your cranial nerves with your radial planes. Next, we give you a look into words that are commonly misspelled — because, hey, not everyone is a spelling bee champ. Then we give you a quick rundown of commonly used abbreviations, root words, prefixes, and suffixes. These are, according to our sources, some of the most-used words and word parts you'll run into on a day-to-day basis.

Synopsis of Body Systems and Their Parts

Skeletal System: bones, muscles, joints, ligaments and tendons

Muscular System: muscles, joints and tendons

Integumentary System: skin, glands, nails and hair

Sensory System: eyes, ears, nose, skin touch receptors

Cardiovascular and Lymphatic Systems: heart, blood vessels, blood and lymph nodes, vessels, lymph fluid, tonsils, spleen, thymus

Respiratory System: nose, pharynx, larynx, trachea, bronchi and lungs

Gastrointestinal System: mouth, pharynx, esophagus, stomach, small and large intestines, pancreas, liver and gallbladder

Endocrine System: hormones, pituitary gland, thyroid, pancreas, adrenal glands, and gonads

Nervous System: brain, spinal cord, hypothalamus, central nervous system and peripheral nervous system

Urinary System: kidneys, ureters, bladder and urethra

Male Reproductive System: testes, ducts, urethra, prostate and penis

Female Reproductive System: ovaries, fallopian tubes, uterus and vagina

Commonly Misspelled Medical Terms

Abdominoperineal, abduction, abscess, acapnia, access, accommodation, Achilles, adnexa, adolescence, adrenaline, afferent, alimentation, alopecia, Alzheimer, amenorrhea, analyze, aneurysm, anorexia, antepartum, antidote, aphthous, areola, arrhythmia, ascites, asphyxia, astigmatism, asystole, auricle, auscultation, biliary, borborygmus, brainstem, buccal, buttocks, cachexia, callous, callus, catheter, Caucasian, chickenpox, cirrhosis, curettage, cerumen, chancre, chlamydia, chyme, clitoris, cyanosis, decubitus, deoxyribonucleic, diabetes mellitus, diaphoresis, diaphragm, diarrhea, dilatation, diphtheria, distention, dyspareunia, eardrum, eczema, edentulous, effusion, elicit, empyema, epididymitis, eructation, erysipelas, ethanol, facelift, fascia, febrile, fibrillation, flaccid, foreskin, furuncle, gait, gallbladder, gamete, gangrene, gauge, gonorrhea, gyri, Helicobacter, hemoptysis, hemorrhoid, humerus, hirsutism, hygiene, icterus, inoculate, intraocular, introitus, intussusception, irradiate, ischemia, isthmus, joule, kyphosis, leukoplakia, lochia, lunula, melanin, menstruation, micturate, myasthenia, myxedema, nevus, nyctalopia, nystagmus, oophorectomy, ophthalmology, orifice, orthopnea, ossification, oxytocin, pacemaker, palliative, palpate, palpitation, Papanicolaou, patent, penicillin, perfusion, perineum, periosteum, peritoneum, pertussis, peroneal, phimosis, pons, prepuce, prosthesis, prostrate, protocol, pruritus, puerperium, rales, regurgitation, rhythm, saccule, sagittal, sedentary, sequela, sieve, splenectomy, sphincter, supersede, suppurative, syncope, syphilis, systole, tinnitus, tonsil, tonsillectomy, tricuspid, urticaria, uvula, venereal, ventricle, vertical, vesicle, vitiligo, wheal, xiphoid, zygote

Common Medical Abbreviations

ACL	anterior cruciate ligament
AIDS	acquired immune deficiency syndrome
AKA	above-knee amputation
ARDS	acute respiratory distress syndrome
ARF	acute renal (kidney) failure
BKA	below-knee amputation
BP	blood pressure
BSO	bilateral salpingo-oophorectomy
CABG	coronary artery bypass graft
COPD	chronic obstruction pulmonary disease
CVA	cerebrovascular accident (stroke)
DM	diabetes mellitus
D&C	dilatation and curettage
DNA	deoxyribonucleic acid
DNR	do not resuscitate
DTR	deep tendon reflexes
ECT	electroconvulsive therapy
FX	fracture
H&P	history and physical
HRT	hormone replacement therapy
I&D	incision and drainage
IBD	irritable bowel syndrome
IM	intramuscular
IV	intravenous
LBP	lower back pain
LLQ	left lower quadrant (abdomen)
LUQ	left upper quadrant (abdomen)
MCL	medial collateral ligament

MVP	mitral valve prolapse
O.D.	right eye
O.S.	left eye
ORIF	open reduction, internal fixation
PCL	posterior cruciate ligament
PERRLA	pupils equal, round, reactive to light/ accommodation
PFT	pulmonary function test
PMS	premenstrual syndrome
RLQ	right lower quadrant (abdomen)
RUQ	right upper quadrant (abdomen)
SOB	shortness of breath
T&A	tonsillectomy and adenoidectomy
TAH	total abdominal hysterectomy
THR	total hip replacement
TKR	total knee replacement
URI	upper respiratory (tract) infection
UTI	urinary tract infection

Common Root Words

Abdomin/o	abdomen
Aden/o	gland
Anter/o	front
Arteri/o	artery
Audi/o	hearing
Bronchi/o	bronchus
Carcin/o	cancer
Cardi/o	heart

Cephal/o	head
Cervic/o	neck or cervix
Cholecyst/o	gallbladder
Col/o	colon
Crani/o	skull
Cyt/o	cell
Derm/o, dermat/o	skin
Dors/i, dors/o	back
Duoden/o	duodenum
Encephal/o	brain
Enter/o	intestines
Gastr/o	stomach
Gynec/o	female
Hemat/o	blood
Hepat/o	liver
Hist/o	tissue
Intestin/o	intestines
Jejun/o	jejunum
Lapar/o	abdomen
Laryng/o	larynx
Lymph/o	lymph vessels
Mamm/o	breast
My/o	muscle
Myel/o	bone marrow
Nas/o	nose
Nephr/o	kidney
Neur/o	nerve
Ophthalm/o	eyes
Optic/o	seeing, sight

Or/o	mouth
Ot/o	ear
Path/o	disease
Pharmac/o	drug
Pneum/o	lungs
Pulmon/o	lungs
Rect/o	rectum
Rhin/o	nose
Sept/o	infection
Splen/o	spleen
Tend/o	tendon
Testicul/o	testicle, testis
Thorac/o	chest, thorax
Thyr/o	thyroid
Tonsil/o	tonsils
Ureter/o	ureter
Urethr/o	urethra
Uter/o	uterus
Ventr/o	front of body

Prefixes

A-/ or an-/	without or lack of
Ante-	before, in front of
Anti-	opposed, against
Bi- or bin-	two
Brady	slow
Dys-	difficult, painful, uncomfortable
Endo-	within

Epi-	on, over, upon
Eu-	normal
Ex-, exo-	outside, outward
Hemi-	half
Hydro-	water
Hyper-	excessive, above normal
Hypo-	below normal
Inter-	between
Intra-	within
Macro-	large
Micro-	small
Nulli-	none
Pan-	all
Para-	abnormal
Para-	beside, beyond, around
Per	through
Peri-	around
Polio-	gray
Poly	many, much
Post-	after or following
Pre-	before, in front of
Primi-	first
Quadri-	four
Re-	back
Retro-	backward, back
Secundi-	second
Semi-	half
Sub-	below, under
Tachy-	fast
Trans-	through, across, beyond

Suffixes

-algia	pain
-apheresis	removal
-ar, -ary	pertaining to
-ase	enzyme
-blast	immature
-capnia	carbon dioxide
-centesis	surgical puncture with needle to aspirate fluid
-chalasis	relaxation
-continence	to stop
-cusis	hearing
-cyesis	pregnancy
-cytosis	condition of cells
-desis	surgical fixation
-drome	run, running
-ectasis	stretching or expansion
-ectomy	surgical removal or excision
-emia	a blood condition
-flux	flow
-gen	producing
-genesis	production
-globin	protein
-globulin	protein
-gram	picture or finished record
-graph	instrument used to record
-graphy	process of recording
-iasis	abnormal condition
-ician	one who

-ism	state of or condition
-itis	inflammation
-lithiasis	calculus or stone
-lysis	loosening, separating
-lytic	destruction or breakdown
-malacia	softening
-megaly	enlargement
-metrist	specialist in the measurement of
-metry	process of measuring
-ologist	one who studies, a specialist
-ology	study of
-oma	tumor or mass
-opia	vision (condition)
-opsy	view of, viewing
-optosis	sagging
-orrhaphy	surgical fixation or suturing
-orrhea	flow, excessive discharge
-ory	pertaining to
-oscopy	visual examination of internal cavity using a scope
-ostomy	creation of an artificial opening
-otomy	process of cutting into
-oxia	oxygen
-para	to bear, live birth
-paresis	slight paralysis
-pathy	abnormality, disease
-pepsia	digestion
-pexy	surgical fixation
-phagia	eating or swallowing

-phonia	sound
-phoresis	carrying/transmission
-plasty	surgical repair or reconstruction
-plegia	paralysis
-pnea	breathing
-poiesis	formation
-prandial	meal
-ptosis	drooping, sagging, prolapse
-rrhagia	burst forth, excessive flow
-rrhaphy	suture repair
-rrhea	discharge or flow
-salpinx	fallopian tube
-schisis	cleft or splitting
-scope	instrument used to visually examine
-scopy	visual examination
-stasis	stop or control
-stenosis	narrowing or constricting
-thenia	lack of strength
-thorax	chest
-tocia	labor
-tresia	opening
-tripsy	surgical crushing
-tropia	to turn
-uria	urination, urine
-us	condition

Index

A

abdomen, 113, 116
abdominal area/cavity, 109, 113, 118, 226
abdominal hysterectomy, 344
abdominal ultrasound, 254
abdominocentesis, 61, 99, 256
abdominopelvic cavity, 109, 118
abdominoperineal resection, 257
abdominoplasty, 61, 84, 88, 176
abducens nerve, 282
abduction, 71, 158
abortion (AB), 336, 342
abrasion, 177
abruptio placentae, 338, 345
absence seizure, 288, 289
absorption, 242
acapnia, 231
accessory nerve, 282
accommodation, 182, 190
acetabulum, 137, 139, 147
Achilles tendon, 153
acid-fast bacilli, 235
acidosis, 23
acne, 171, 172
acne vulgaris, 171, 172
acoumeter, 191
acoustic neuroma, 193
acquired immunodeficiency syndrome (AIDS), 216, 318
acromegaly, 271
acromion, 136
acronyms, 19, 38–40
acrophobia, 83
activated charcoal, 259
acute lymphocytic leukemia (ALL), 215
acute myelogenous leukemia (AML), 215
acute parapsoriasis, 358
Adam's apple, 226
Addis count, 306
Addison, Thomas (pathologist), 266
Addison's disease, 266, 275
adduction, 71, 158
adductor magnus, 153
adenitis, 93
adenocarcinoma of prostate, 316
adenoidectomy, 238
adenoiditis, 234
adenoids, 225, 231
adenoma, 177, 213
adenomegaly, 93
adenomyosis, 340
adhesive capsulitis, 160
adipocyte cell, 106
adipose tissue, 177, 299
adnexa, 327, 334
adrenal cortex, 266
adrenal medulla, 126, 266
adrenal virilism, 23
adrenalectomy, 277
adrenaline, 126, 266, 270
adrenals, 125, 262, 266
adrenocorticotropic hormone (ACTH), 264
adrenopathy, 23
adult respiratory distress syndrome (ARDS), 227, 235
adult-onset diabetes, 274
aerochamber, 239
aerola, 329
afferent nerves, 284
ageusia, 192
air conduction (AC), 183
albinism/albino, 165, 177
albumin, 203
aldosterone, 264, 266
aldosterone antagonists, 221
alimentary tract, 11, 124–125, 241
alkaline phosphatase blood test, 255
alopecia, 172
alveolus/alveoli, 124, 135, 224, 226, 231
Alzheimer's disease, 40, 41, 290
amebicides, 322
amenorrhea, 70, 337
American Diabetes Association (ADA), 267
American Joint Committee on Cancer (AJCC), 175
amino acids, 242
ammonia, 298
amniocentesis, 84, 345
amnion, 335
amniotomy, 345
amylase/amylase blood test, 245, 255
amyotrophic lateral sclerosis (ALS), 159, 290
anabolic therapy, 148
anabolism, 106
anal fistula, 254
analgesics, 346
anastomosis, 257
anatomic positions/anatomical position, 112, 116
anatomical planes, 110–112
anatomy, 9–10, 102, 106, 119–121

androgens, 266, 312
andropathy, 316
anemia, 83, 212, 215
anesthesia/anesthesiologist, 287
aneurysm, 213
angina, 212
angina pectoris, 213, 359
angiocardiography, 219
angioplasty, 88, 220
angiotensin-converting enzyme (ACE) inhibitors, 221
anhidrosis, 178
ankylosing spondylitis, 144
ankylosis, 141
anoplasty, 257
anorchism, 316
anorectal manometry, 255
anosmia, 192
anovulatory, 70
anoxia, 231
antacids, 258
antepartum, 335
anterior, 111, 116
anteversion, 334
anthracosis, 233
antiarrhythmics, 221
antibiotics, 240, 259, 309, 319, 322, 346
anticholinergics, 259
anticoagulants, 210, 221
anticonvulsants, 294
antidiarrheals, 258
antidiuretic hormone (ADH), 265, 270
antiemetics, 259
antifungal agents/drugs, 322, 346
antigens, 206
antiglobulin test, 217
antihistamines, 240
antihypertensives, 222
anti-inflammatory, 72, 346
antiresorptive medications, 148
antithyroid drugs, 277
antitussives, 240
antonyms, 39–40
antrum, 244
anuria, 310
anus, 10
aorta, 122, 205, 210
aortic semilunar valve, 202
aortic stenosis, 212
apex, 231
Apgar score, 41
aphagia, 250
aphasia, 288
aphonia, 231
aphthous stomatitis, 250
apical, 231
apidose tissue, 107
aplastic anemia, 215
apnea, 83, 231
aponeurosis, 152
appendage, 137
appendectomy, 61, 85, 99, 257
appendicitis, 61, 253
appendicular skeleton, 137–138
appendix, 246
aqueous humor, 181
arachnoid membrane, 283
Aristotle (philosopher and physical scientist), 18
arrector pili, 166
arterial blood gases (ABG), 227, 237
arterial hypertension, 213
arteries/arterial system, 200, 202, 203
arteriogram, 100
arteriography, 100, 292
arterioles, 122, 203
arteriomalacia, 101
arterioplasty, 88
arthralgia, 100, 141
arthritis, 59, 80, 88, 101, 144, 148
arthrocentesis, 146
arthrodesis, 147
arthrogram, 146
arthroophthalmopathy, 102
arthropathy, 59
arthroplasty, 59, 88, 147
arthroscopy, 146
articular cartilage, 134, 138
articulations, 138, 141, 162
artificial insemination, 324
artificial rupture of membranes, 345
asbestosis, 233
ascites, 252
aspermia, 317, 324
aspirated, 221
assisted reproductive techniques (ART), 321, 341
asthma, 233
astigmatism, 190
astrocytes, 291
astrocytoma, 291
ataxia, 287
atelectasis, 227, 233, 234
atherosclerosis, 214
athlete's foot, 172
atlas, 135
atorvastatin, 222
atresia, 337
atrial fibrillation, 212
atriomegaly, 93
atrium/atria, 121–122, 202, 210
atrophy, 162
A-type natriuretic peptide (or polypeptide) (ANP), 262
atypical agents, 233
audiogram, 194
audiologist/audiology, 191
audiometry, 88, 194
auditory tube, 184
aural, 191
aures unitas (AU), 183

auricle, 184
auricular region, 114
auris dextra (AD), 183
auris sinistra (AS), 183
auscultation, 210, 227, 236–237
autologous, 71
autonomic nervous system (ANS), 11, 127, 280, 284
autopsy, 102
AV bundle/AV node, 205
axial skeleton, 134–137
axillae, 168
axillary lymph nodes, 206
axillary region, 114
axis, 134
axons, 280
azotemia, 310
azoturia, 310

B

baby teeth, 250
bacterial analysis, 175
bacterial endocarditis, 213
bacterial meningitis, 290
balanced salt solution (BSS), 196
balanitis, 317
balanocele, 317
balanoplasty, 321
balanorrhea, 317
balloon angioplasty, 220
bariatric surgery, 258
barium enema, 255
Bartholin's glands, 329
basal cell carcinoma, 174
basal layer, 165
basal metabolic rate (BMR), 265, 267
base, 231
belching, 251
Bell's palsy, 290
belly, 124
benign prostatic hypertrophy/hyperplasia (BPH), 317
bepridil hydrochloride, 222
BEST, mnemonic, 355
beta blockers, 196, 222
bicuspid valve, 202
bilateral, 70
bilateral salpingo-oophorectomy, 344
bile/bile pigments/biliary tract, 124, 245
biliary ducts, 245
bilirubins/bilirubin levels, 255, 306
bingo wings surgery, 176
binocular, 190
biology, 88, 102, 106
bird breeder's lung/bird fancier's lung, 359
birth canal, 328
birth control/birth control pill, 343
black lung disease, 233
bladder, 12, 298. *See also* urinary bladder
bleb, 171
bleeding time, 217
blepharitis, 190
blepharoplasty, 92, 176, 195
blind spot, 181
blood, 203–205
blood, urea, nitrogen (BUN) test, 306
blood cells, 10, 120
blood pressure (BP), 210, 218, 221
blood serum tests, 275
blood tests, 217
blood vessels, 10, 202–203
body (of stomach), 244
body cavities, 109–110, 118
body regions, 113–118
body systems, 106, 108–109, 365–366
bone conduction (BC), 183
bone densitometry (DEXA or DXA), 146
bone density, 146
bone marrow (BM), 39, 120, 132, 221
bone scan (scintigraphy), 146
bones, 107, 120, 132–134
bony tissue, 132
borborygmus, 252
Bornholm, 359–360
bowel preparations, 259
Bowman's capsule, 301
brachiocephalic, 139
brachioplasty, 176
brachytherapy, 321
bradyarrhythmia, 70
bradycardia, 70
bradykinesia, 141, 162
brain, 11, 280–283
brainstem, 283
breast carcinoma, 340
breasts, 12, 326, 329
Breisky, 361
Breslow's depth, 175
broad ligaments, 326
brodie, 323
bronchial washing, 237
bronchiectasis, 234
bronchioles, 124, 226, 231
bronchitis, 80, 88, 234
bronchoconstrictor, 232
bronchodilator, 232, 239
bronchogenic carcinoma, 235
bronchogram, 238
bronchoscope/bronchoscopy, 61, 85, 88, 237, 238
bronchospasm, 231
bronchus/bronchi, 124, 224, 226, 231
bruxism, 250
B-type natriuretic peptide (BNP), 262

buccal region, 114
buccinator, 153
buffalo hump, 275
bulbourethral glands, 12, 312, 314
bulla/bullae, 171
bullectomy, 239
bundle of His, 205
bunion, 144
Burkitt's lymphoma, 216
burns, 172
bursa/bursae, 138, 141
bursitis, 144, 158
buttocks, 153

C

C1-C7, 115, 135
calcaneus, 138, 139, 155
Calcilean, 221
calcitonin, 265
calcium, 141, 271
calcium channel blockers, 222
calculus/calculi, 252
calluses, 174
calyx/calyces, 301
cancellous bones, 134, 141
candidiasis, 319
canker sores, 250
capillaries, 122, 124, 202, 203, 210, 299
capnia, 224
capsule, 138
capsule endoscopy, 256
caput succedaneum, 363
carbon dioxide (CO_2), 12, 123, 124, 223–224, 230–231, 298
carbon monoxide, 10
carbuncle, 171
carcinogen/carcinogenic, 93, 110
carcinoma, 80
carcinoma of cervix, 340
Cardene, 222
cardiac, 88, 210
cardiac ablation, 219
cardiac arrest, 212
cardiac arrhythmia, 214
cardiac catheterization, 217, 219
cardiac cycle, 205
cardiac enzymes, 217
cardiac muscle, 120, 150, 151
cardiac pacemaker insertion, 220
cardiac scan, 219
cardiac sphincter, 244
cardiogram, 61, 85
cardiograph/cardiography, 61, 85
cardiologist/cardiology, 210
cardiomegaly, 60, 83, 88, 101, 212
cardiomyopathy, 80, 212
cardiopathy, 80, 99
cardiopulmonary resuscitation (CPR), 210, 227
cardiovascular system
  common conditions and terms, 212–213
  described, 108, 121–123, 199–207, 365
  diseases/pathology, 213–216
  pharmacology, 221–222
  tests/procedures, 217–218
  tongue twisters, 359
cardioversion, 219
carditis, 88
cardium, 200
Cardizem/Cardizem CD, 222
carpal bones/carpals, 137, 139, 356
carpal region, 114
carteolol hydrochloride, 222
cartilage, 107
Cartrol, 222
castration, 321
catabolism, 12, 106, 298
cataracts/cataract surgery, 182, 193, 195
catecholamines, 266
cathartic, 252
catheter, 301, 310
caudal, 111
cauterization, 342
cavities, 109–110, 118. *See also specific cavities*
cecum, 246
ceftriaxone, 319
celiac disease, 254
cells, 106–107. *See also specific cells*
cellular respiration, 224
cellulitis, 101
Centers for Disease Control and Prevention (CDC), 319
central glands, 262
central nervous system (CNS), 11, 126, 280–284
central renal pelvis, 301
cephalad, 111
cephalocentesis, 92
cephalomegaly, 92
cephalopelvic disproportion (CPD), 336, 345
cephalosporin, 319
cerebellum, 127
cerebral angiography, 292
cerebral cortex, 281, 282
cerebral hemispheres, 281
cerebral palsy, 289
cerebromalacia, 102
cerebrospinal fluid (CSF), 283–284, 292
cerebrovascular, 102
cerebrovascular accident (CVA), 288
cerebrum, 127, 281
cerumen, 168, 184
ceruminous glands, 168
cervical cauterization, 342
cervical conization, 342

cervical epithelium, 340
cervical lymph nodes, 206
cervical neoplasia, 340
cervical region, 114
cervical region (C), 114, 115
cervical vertebrae, 135
cervicitis, 92, 337
cervicodynia, 92
cervix, 328
Cesarean section (CS or C-section), 336, 345
chalazion, 192
chancre, 319
Cheat Sheet, 4
cheilophagia, 92
cheiromegaly, 93
chest cavity, 109, 226–227
chest CT, 238
chest x-ray (CXR), 237
chickenpox, 174
child onset diabetes, 274
chiropodist, 141
chiropractics/chiropractor, 142
chlamydia, 318
cholangiogram, 255
cholecystectomy, 88, 257
cholecystitis, 88, 253
cholecystogram, 255
choledocholithiasis, 93
choledocholithotomy, 257
choledocholithotripsy, 102
cholelithiasis, 93, 252
cholesteatoma, 193
cholesterol, 245
chondroma, 102
chondromalacia, 88, 102, 142
chorion, 335
chorionic villus sampling (CVS), 341
choroid, 181
chromosomes, 107, 312
chronic lymphocytic leukemia (CLL), 215
chronic myelogenous leukemia (CML), 215
chronic obstructive pulmonary disease (COPD), 38, 235, 237
chronic renal failure (CRF), 304
chyme, 244
cicatrix, 172
cilia, 225, 232
ciliary body, 181
ciprofloxacin, 319
circulatory system, 121–123
circumcision, 321
circumferential, 70
cirrhosis, 254
cisternography, 292
claustrophobia, 84
clavicle, 136, 140
cleft palate, 250
clitoris, 326, 329
clomiphene citrate, 346
closed fracture, 145
closed reduction, 145
clubfoot, 144
CNS stimulants, 294
coagulation time, 217
coarctation of the aorta, 214
coccygeal bones, 135
coccygeal region, 115
coccygodynia, 140
coccyx, 115
cochlea, 184
cochlear implants, 185
cognition adjuvant therapy, 294
coitus/copulation, 324, 334
colectomy, 257
colitis, 101
collagen, 166, 178
Colles' fracture, 132
colloid, 265
colon, 246
colonic polyposis, 252
colonoscope/colonoscopy, 88, 256
colostomy/colotomy, 61, 84, 100, 258
colpopexy, 344
colposcopy, 342
coma, 287
combination special, 344
combining forms, 8. *See also* root words
combining vowel, 57–58, 98
comedo/comedones, 171
comminuted fracture, 145
common bile duct, 245
compact bone, 134, 142
complete blood count (CBC), 218, 255
complete metabolic profile (CMP), 255
compound fracture, 145
compression fracture, 145
computerized axial tomography (CAT) scan, 38, 238, 306
computerized tomography (CT) scan, 146, 276, 292
concussion, 288
condom, 324
conductive hearing loss, 185
condyle, 142
condyloma acuminatum/ condylomata acuminata, 319
cones, 181
congenital heart disease, 214
congenital/congenital anomaly, 319, 335
congestive heart failure, 212, 214
conjunctival membrane, 182
conjunctivitis, 190
connective tissue, 107
constipation, 252
contraction, 150
contraindication, 72

contrast medium/media, 292, 306
convulsion, 287
CoolSculpting, 176
Coombs' test, 217
cor pulmonale, 235
core decompression, 147
Corgard, 222
corium, 166
cornea/corneal/corneal transplant, 180, 190, 195
corneal collagen cross-linking (CXL), 195
coronal plane, 111, 117
coronary arteries, 210
coronary artery bypass graft (CABG), 220
coronary artery disease (CAD), 214
corpus (body) (of uterus), 328
corpus luteum, 267, 327, 333
cortex, 125, 299
corticoids, 125
corticosteroids, 196, 239
cortisol, 264, 266, 270
corvisart, 359
cosmetic surgery, 176
costal, 140
costal cartilage, 136
costochondral, 102
Coumadin, 221
Cowper's glands, 12, 312, 314
cranial bones, mnemonic, 356
cranial cavity, 109, 116, 118, 280
cranial nerves, 11, 126, 280–281, 353
cranial sutures, 135
craniotomy, 102, 293
cranium, 134–135, 140
creatinine/creatinine clearance test (CCT), 306
cretinism, 272
Crohn's disease, 253
croup, 236
Cruveilhier, 360
cryobiology, 88
cryoextraction of cataract, 195
cryosurgery, 342
cryotherapy, 176
cryptorchidism, 317
Cushing's disease/syndrome, 275
Cushing's syndrome, 41
cuticle, 178
cutis laxa, 173
cyanosis, 94
cyanotic, 94
cystectomy, 88, 308
cystic duct, 245
cystic fibrosis, 236
cystitis, 88, 304
cystocele, 94, 304
cystogram, 88, 306
cystopexy, 88
cystoplasty, 308
cystopyelogram, 307
cystoscope/cystoscopy, 307
cystostomy/cystotomy, 308
cystourethrogram, 307
cysts, 171
cytologic studies, 237
cytologist/cytology, 89, 110
cytoplasm, 107
cytosis, 110

D

da Vinci (robot), 220, 277, 322, 345
Darlings, 359
date of birth (DOB), 336
de Quervain, 358
deafness, 185
debridement, 175
decalvaris folliculitis, 358
decompression craniectomy, 293
decongestants, 240
decortication of lung, 239
decubitus ulcer, 171
deep vein thrombosis (DVT), 218
defibrillation, 219
deglutition, 243, 250
deltoid, 152, 153, 154
dementia, 287
dendrites, 280
dense fibrous, 107
dental caries, 250
dentist, 250
deoxyribonucleic acid (DNA), 107
dermabrasion, 176
dermatitis, 92, 101, 102, 178
dermatologist/dermatology, 92, 178
dermatome, 92
dermatomyositis, 159
dermatoplasty, 102, 177
dermis, 165, 166, 186
developing egg sac, 333
Devil's grip, 359–360
diabetes insipidus (DI), 23, 267
diabetes mellitus (DM), 267, 274
diabetic ketoacidosis (DK), 267
diabetic nephropathy, 23
diabetic retinopathy, 193
dialysis, 308
diaper dermatitis, 173
diaper rash, 173
diaphoresis, 167, 178
diaphragm, 113, 118, 123, 153, 226–227, 343
diaphysis, 134, 137, 142
diarrhea, 84, 125, 252
diastole, 205, 211
diathermy, 162, 194
diet restriction, 258
digestion, 242
digestive system/digestive tract, 11, 108, 124–125, 241

digital rectal examination (DRE), 320
digital subtraction angiography, 219
digoxin, 221
dilatation and curettage (D & C), 342
dilation, 181
diltiazem hydrochloride, 222
diphtheria/diphtheria test, 175–176, 235
diplopia, 94, 190
directional planes, 115
directional terms, 110–112
diskectomy, 148
dislocation, 144
disorientation, 287
dissection, 71, 106
distal, 111, 116
distention, 214
diuresis, 310
diuretics, 239–240, 309, 310
diverticula, 252
diverticulitis, 253
diverticulosis, 101
doppler flow study, 219
dorsal, 111
dorsal body cavities, 109
dorsal region (D), 115
dorsalgia, 92
Down syndrome, 41, 345
dual-energy X-ray absorptiometry (Dexa), 146
Duchenne, 358
ductless (endocrine glands), 11, 262
duodenal ulcer, 252
duodenectomy, 89
duodenitis, 89
duodenotomy, 89
duodenum, 245–246
Dupuytren's contracture, 159
dura matter, 283, 284
dwarfism, 271
dypsnea, 231
dyscrasia, 212
dysfunctional, 70
dysgeusia, 192
dyskinesia, 142, 162
dysmenorrhea, 337
dysosmia, 192
dyspareunia, 337
dyspepsia, 251
dysphagia, 84, 250, 251
dysphasia, 250, 251, 288
dysphonia, 231
dyspnea, 84
dystocia, 338
dystrophy, 142, 162
dysuria, 310, 318

E

Eales, 359
ear, nose, and throat (ENT), 183, 227
eardrum, 184
ears, 182–185, 191
earwax, 184, 185
ecchymosis, 172
echocardiogram, 219
eclampsia, 338
ecthyma, 173
ectopic/ectopic pregnancy, 335, 338
eczema, 173
edema, 338
edentulous, 250
efferent cranial nerves, 281–282
efferent nerves, 284
ejaculation, 324
ejaculatory ducts, 12, 312, 314
elastography, 160
electrocardiography, 219
electroencephalogram/ electroencephalography (EEG), 289, 292
electrolysis, 177
electrolytes, 125, 271
electromyogram/ electromyography (EMG), 160, 292
electronic medical publishing, 18
electronystagmography (ENG), 292
elimination, 242
embolism, 212
embolus/emboli, 212
embryo, 335
embryology, 106
embryonal carcinoma, 317
embryonic stage, 106
emesis, 251
emetics, 259
emphysema, 233
empyema, 233–234
encephalitis, 89
encephalomegaly, 102
encephalopathy, 94, 102
endarterectomy, 220
endocarditis, 212
endocardium, 201, 211
endocervix, 70
endocrine glands, 11
endocrine system
  common conditions and terms, 270–274
  described, 108, 125–126, 261–268, 366
  diseases/pathology, 274–275
  pharmacology, 277
  tests/procedures, 275–277
  tongue twisters, 360
endocrinologist/ endocrinology, 270
endolymph, 184
endometrial ablation, 342
endometrial carcinoma, 340
endometrial cells, 333
endometriosis, 340
endometritis, 337

endometrium, 328, 334
endoscope/endoscopy, 61, 100, 256
endoscopic retrograde cholangiopancreatography (ERCP), 256
endoscopic surgery, 100
endotracheal intubation, 237
end-stage renal disease (ESRD), 304
end-to-end anastomosis, 214
enemas, 259
enteritis, 101, 253
enucleation, 195
enuresis, 310
enzymes, 124, 245, 246
epicardium, 201
epidermis, 165
epididymidis/epididymides, 12, 128, 312, 313
epididymitis, 317
epigastric region, 113
epiglottis, 224, 225, 244
epilepsy, 288
epinephrine, 126, 266, 270
epiphysis, 134, 142
episiotomy, 89, 329, 345
epispadias, 304, 317
epithelial cell, 106
epithelial mucosa, 328
epithelial tissue, 107
epithelioma, 110
epithelium, 165, 178, 226
eponyms, 18, 19, 40–41
equilibrium, 184
erect, 112
erectile dysfunction (ED), 317, 322
erthrocytes, 59
eructation, 251
erysipelas, 173
erythema, 89, 178
erythrocyte sedimentation rate (ESR), 218
erythrocytes, 84, 89, 110, 205, 211
erythrocytosis, 59
esophageal sphincter, 244
esophageal varices, 251
esophagitis, 89, 251
esophagogastroduodenoscopy (EGD), 89, 102, 256
esophagus, 124, 224, 225, 244, 251
esotropia, 192
essential hypertension, 213, 305
estrogen, 12, 128, 267, 327, 333, 334
estrogen receptor test, 276
estrogen replacement therapy (ERT), 337
ethmoid bone, 135, 225
etymology, 8, 19
eupnea, 231
eustachian tube, 184
euthyroid, 58, 272
eversion, 158
evoked potential test, 292
Ewing's sarcoma/tumor, 146
exanthema subitum, 173
exhalation, 227
exocervix, 70
exocrine glands, 262
exophthalmos, 272
exostoses, 144
exotropia, 192
expected date of confinement or delivery (EDC), 336
expectorants, 240
expiration, 122, 123, 227
extension, 158
extensor muscles, 153
external auditory meatus, 184
external genitalia, 12, 326
external oblique, 153, 154
external respiration, 224
external sphincter, 300
extracorporeal shock wave lithotripsy (ESWL), 308
eyes, 179–182, 190–191

F

face nerves, mnemonic, 355
facelift, 177
facial bones, 135
facial nerve, 282
fallopian tubes, 12, 128, 312, 326, 327
false ribs, 136
familial benign pemphigus, 358
fascia, 162
fasciectomy, 161
fasciitis, 162
fascinoma, 157
fasciodesis, 161
fasciotomy, 161
fasting blood sugar (FBS), 267
fat cell, 106
fatty acids, 242
febrile, 58
feces, 242
female reproductive cell, 12
female reproductive system, 325–329, 334–346, 366
female sterilizations, 100
femoropopliteal bypass, 220
femur, 132, 136, 137, 140
fenestration, 196
fertility, 320
fertilization, 12, 326, 334
fetal heart sounds (FHS), 336
fetus, 106, 335
fiberoptic endoscope, 256
fibrillation, 213–214
fibrinogen, 203
fibroblast cells, 166
fibrocystic disease, 340
fibroid, 340
fibromyalgia, 158

fibrosis, 110
fibula, 138, 140
Filshie clip, 342
filtration, 301
fimbriae, 327
first-degree burn, 172
fissures, 142, 171, 281
flagellum, 312
flat bones, 133
flatus, 252
flexion, 158
flexor muscles, 153
floppy valve, 214
flu, 235
fluoroquinolone, 319
fluroscopy, 146
flutter, 213–214
follicles, 168
follicular-stimulating hormone (FSH), 264, 343
fontanelle, 135, 142
foramen/foramen magnum, 135, 136, 280
forensic pathology, 94
foreskin, 313, 321
fossa, 142
fractures, 134, 143, 145
frontal bone, 134, 225
frontal lobe, 282
frontal plane, 111, 117
frontalis, 153
frozen shoulder, 160
fulguration, 308
fundus, 244, 328, 336
fungal testing, 175
furosemide, 222
furuncle, 171

G

gait, 287
galactorrhea, 89, 335
gallbladder, 124, 244, 245
gallbladder removal, 100
gallstones, 251, 252
gamete cell, 107, 267, 326
gamete intrafallopian transfer (GIFT), 339
gangrene, 173
gastrectomy, 89, 257
gastric emptying scan, 255
gastric juices, 244
gastric ulcer, 251
gastritis, 60, 89, 101, 251
gastrocnemius, 153, 155
gastrodynia, 60, 84, 89, 101, 251
gastroenteritis, 125, 253
gastroenterologist/gastroenterology, 251
gastroesophageal reflux disease (GERD), 254
gastrointestinal (GI) system
  common conditions and terms, 250–253
  described, 108, 124–125, 241–246, 365
  diseases/pathology, 253–254
  pharmacology, 258–259
  tests/procedures, 254–258
  tongue twisters, 360
gastrojejunostomy, 258
gastropathy, 60
gastroscopy, 256
gastrosis, 101
gastrostomy, 258
GC/Chlamydia test, 320
genes, 107
genital herpes, 318
genital orifice, 314
genitalia, 12, 324, 326. *See also* reproductive systems
genupectoral, 112
German measles, 174
gestation, 335
gigantism, 271
gingivitis, 92, 250
glans penis, 313
glaucoma, 181, 182, 192
Gleason grade, 41
glioma, 291
glomerulonephritis, 305
glomerulus/glomeruli, 299
glossopharyngeal nerve, 282
glottis, 225
glucagon, 126, 266, 270
glucocorticoids, 125
gluconeogenesis, 126, 266
glucose, 271, 275
glucose tolerance test (GTT), 267, 275–276
gluten enteropathy, 254
gluteus maximus/gluteus medius, 153, 155
glycemia, 102–103
glycogen, 271
glycosuria, 89, 310
Goetsch's skin reaction, 276
goiter, 272
gonadotropic hormone, 264
gonadotropins, 267
gonads, 12, 128, 267–268, 313, 324, 326
gonioscopy, 194
gonorrhea, 318
gouty arthritis (gout), 144
Graaf, Reinier de (anatomist), 327
graafian follicle, 327, 333
gracilis, 153
gram-negative, 309
Gram's stain, 309
grand mal seizure, 288–289
Graves' disease, 272
gravida, 335
Greek language, 8, 18, 19, 38, 87
greenstick fracture, 145
Group A Betahemolytic Streptococcus, 305

growth hormone (GH or hGH), 264, 270
growth hormone therapy, 277
growth plate, 134
Gullain-Barre syndrome, 290
gut, 124
gynatresia, 337
gynecologist/gynecology, 89, 326
gynecomastia, 23, 103
gynopathic, 334
gyri, 281

H

H2 blockers, 259
hair. *See* integumentary system
hair fiber, 168
hair follicle, 168
halitosis, 250
hallux valgus, 148
hard palate, 242
Hashimoto's thyroiditis, 272
hearing distance (HD), 183
heart, 200–202
heart arrhythmias, 219
heart attack, 212
heart block, 213
heart murmur, 214
heartburn, 251
helicobacter pylori antibody test, 255
helper T-cell lymphocytes, 216
hemangiomas, 174, 177
hematemesis, 94, 103, 251
hematocrit (Hct), 218
hematocyte, 89
hematologist/hematology, 211
hematopoiesis, 142
hematopoietic red bone marrow, 132
hematuria, 310
hemianopia (hemianopsia), 192
hemigastrectomy, 103
hemiparesis, 289
hemiplegia, 84, 289
hemochromatosis, 215
hemodialysis, 308
hemoglobin (Hgb or Hb), 205, 218
hemoglobin test, 218
hemolysis, 103, 211
hemolytic anemia, 215
hemophilia, 216
hemoptysis, 231
hemorrhage, 84, 212
hemorrhagic stroke, 288
hemorrhoids, 252
hemostasis, 211
hemothorax, 233–234
heparin calcium, 221
hepatic duct, 245
hepatitis, 89, 253
hepatoma, 252
hepatomegaly, 84, 94, 101, 252
hepatosplenomegaly, 60, 84, 101
hernia, 252
herniated disk, 144
herniorrhaphy, 85, 258
herpes, 170
herpes simplex, 250
herpes zoster, 289
heterosexual, 89, 324
hiatal hernia, 251
high-density lipoprotein (HDL), 217
hilum, 232, 299
hindbrain, 283
Hippocrates (father of medicine), 18, 19
Hippocratic Oath, 19
Hirschsprung's disease, 255, 360
hirsutism, 340
histiocytes, 166
histiotoma, 178
histologist/histology, 89, 106, 110
Histoplasma fungus, 359
Hodgkin's disease, 41, 216
Homan's sign, 41
homeostasis, 23, 125, 127, 265
homonyms, 42–43
homosexual, 89, 324
hordeolum, 192
hormone replacement therapy (HRT), 277, 337
hormones, 10–11, 12, 125, 128, 261, 263–268, 266, 312. *See also specific hormones*
horny cells, 165
horripilation, 364
human chorionic gonadotropin (HCG or hCG), 267, 334
human immunodeficiency virus (HIV), 216, 318, 319
human papilloma virus (HPV), 319
humerus, 132, 137, 140
Huntington's disease, 290
hydrocele, 317
hydrocelectomy, 321
hydrocephalus, 289
hydrocortisone, 266, 270
hydromassage, 89
hydronephrosis, 305
hydropenia, 94
hydrosalpinx, 94, 334, 337
hydroureter, 305
hymen/hymenectomy, 329, 344
hyperbilirubinemia, 212
hypercalcemia, 272
hypercholesterolemia, 103, 212
hyperchromia, 212
hyperemesis, 70, 84, 103, 251
hyperemesis gravidarum, 335
hypergeusia, 192
hyperglycemia, 23
hypergonadism, 23
hyperhidrosis, 103, 178

hyperkalemia, 274
hyperkeratosis, 178
hyperkinesia, 142, 162
hyperlipidemia, 212
hypernephroma, 305
hyperopia, 190
hyperparathyroidism, 274
hypertension, 58, 70, 212
hypertensive heart disease, 214
hyperthyroidism, 272
hypertrophy/hypertrophic, 61
hyperventilation, 231, 232
hyphens, use of, 97
hypnotics, 294
hypocalcemia, 272
hypochondriac regions, 113
hypodermic, 178
hypogastric region, 113, 114
hypoglossal nerve, 282
hypoglycemia, 23
hypoglycemic drugs, 274
hypogonadism, 23
hyponatremia, 274
hypoparathyroidism, 272
hypopharynx, 123, 124, 225, 242
hypophysectomy, 277, 293
hypophysitis, 271
hypospadias, 305, 317
hypotension/hypotensive, 58, 70, 212
hypothalamus, 125, 127, 262, 263–265, 283
hypothyroidism, 272
hypoxemia, 231
hypoxia, 231
hysterectomy, 85, 89, 100
hysterescope, 342
hysteropexy, 344
hysterosalpingogram, 103, 341

I

ichthyosis vulgaris, 173
ileal conduit, 309
ileitis, 89
ileocecal valve, 246
ileostomy, 84, 89, 258
ileum, 246
ileus, 252
iliac crests, 137
iliac regions, 113
ilioniguinal, 89
ilium, 13–1376, 140
immobile cilia, 323
immunity, 10
immunoglobulins, 203, 211
impacted fracture, 145
impetigo, 173
impotence, 317, 324
in vitro fertilization (IVF), 321, 339, 341
incidentaloma, 157
incision and drainage, 175
incontinence, 305
incus, 184
Inderal, 221
inferior, 111, 116
inferior vena cava, 122, 203, 205
infertility, 339
inflammation, 145, 216
influenza, 235
infraorbital region, 114
infrascapular region, 114
infraspinatus, 152, 153
infraumbilical, 70
inguinal hernia, 252
inguinal lymph nodes, 206
inguinodynia, 92
inhalers, 239
inspection, palpation, percussion, and auscultation (IPPA), 237
inspiration, 122, 225
insulin, 126, 245, 266, 270, 277
insulin-dependent diabetes mellitus (IDDM), 267, 274
integumentary system
  common conditions and terms, 171–172, 177–178
  described, 108, 120, 163–168, 365
  diseases/pathology, 172–175
  tests/procedures, 175–177
  tongue twisters, 358
integumentum, 164
interatrial septum, 202
intercostal, 142
intermitted claudication, 213
internal respiration, 224, 230
internal sphincter, 300
interscapular region, 114
interstitial cells, 313
interventricular septum, 202
intervertebral, 103
intestines, 124, 245–246
intracranial, 103, 142
intracytoplasmic sperm injection (ICSI), 321, 341
intradermal test, 175–176
intramuscular, 71
intraocular pressure, 181
intrapartum, 335
intrathecal contrast-enhanced CT scan (cisternography), 292
intrathecal medicine, 292
intrauterine, 71
intrauterine device (IUD), 343
intrauterine fetal death, 338
intrauterine insemination (IUI), 321, 339, 341

intravenous, 71
intravenous pyelogram (IVP), 307
introitus, 328
intussusception, 253
inversion, 158
involuntary muscles, 120, 150, 151
iodine, 271
ipsilateral, 111
iridectomy, 92
iris, 181
irregular bones, 133
irreverisble coma, 289
irritable bowel syndrome (IBS), 254
Isaacs syndrome, 159
ischemia, 219
ischemic stroke, 288
ischium, 13–1376, 140
islets of Langerhans, 126, 266, 270
isokinetic dynamometry, 160
isthmus, 265

J

jaundice, 306
jejunitis, 90
jejunolieostomy, 103
jejunostomy, 90, 258
jejunum, 246
jock itch, 322
joints, 120, 138, 144
juvenile diabetes, 274

K

Kaposi's sarcoma, 319
keloid, 172
keratin, 165, 168, 178
keratitis, 190
keratoconus, 190, 195
keratometer, 190
keratoplasty, 195
keratosis, 174
ketoacidosis, 274
kidneys, 12, 127, 298, 299–300
kidneys, ureters, bladder (KUB) procedure, 307
kinesiology, 162
kyphosis, 142

L

L1-L5, 115
labia majora/labia minora, 326, 329
labioglossopharyngeal, 103
labor and delivery (L&D), 336
labyrinth, 184
labyrinthectomy, 196
laciferous ducts, 329
lacrimal apparatus/ducts/glands, 182
lacrimatory, 90
lactation, 329
lamina, 136, 148
laminectomy, 293
Lanoxin, 221
laparoscope, 85
laparoscopic adjustable gastric band (LAGB), 257
laparoscopic cholecystectomy, 343
laparoscopic hysterectomy, 344
laparoscopic method, 342
laparoscopic tubal ligations, 343
laparoscopically, 100
laparoscopy, 92, 256
laparotomy, 85, 92, 257
large bowel, 246
large intestine, 124, 246
laryngectomy, 90, 238
laryngitis, 90, 101, 234
laryngoplasty, 238
laryngoscopy, 237
laryngotracheobronchitis, 103, 234
larynx, 224, 225, 244
laser angioplasty, 219
laser hair removal therapy, 177
laser photocoagulation, 194
laser therapy, 177
laser-assisted in situ keratomileusis (LASIK), 195
Lasix, 222
last menstrual period (LMP), 336, 346
lateral, 111, 116
lateral epicondylitis, 159
lateral recumbent, 112
lateromedial, 111
Latin language, 8, 18, 19, 38, 87
latissimus/latissimus dorsi, 152, 153
latrogenic, 85
latrophobia, 85
laxatives, 253
Legionnaires' disease, 235
leiomyoma, 80, 159, 340
leiomyosarcoma, 103, 159
lens, 180, 182
lesions, 146, 173
leukemia, 84, 215
leukocytes, 84, 90, 205, 211
leukocytosis, 213
leukopenia, 103
leukoplakia, 250
leukorrhea, 334
Leydig cells, 313
lichen planus, 171
ligament of Treitz, 41
ligaments, 120, 142, 162
ligating, 342
light pressure, 186
linea alba, 153
lipase, 245
lipid tests, 217
Lipitor, 222

lipocytes, 166, 178
lipoma, 178
lipoprotein electrophoresis, 217
lipoproteins, 217
liposuction, 110, 177
lipotripsy, 177
lithotripsy, 90, 308
liver, 113, 245
lobar pneumonia, 233, 235
lobectomy, 239
lobes, 232
lochia, 335
long acting beta-2 agonists (LABAs), 240
long acting muscarinic antagonists (LAMAs), 240
long bones, 132
longus, 153
loose, 107
Lopressor, 222
Lou Gehrig's disease, 159, 290
lovastatin, 222
low-density lipoprotein (LDL), 217
lower GI series, 255
lower respiratory infection (LRI), 236
lumbar puncture, 292
lumbar region (L), 113, 114, 115
lumbar vertebrae, 127, 135, 283
lumpectomy, 340, 344
lung biopsy, 237
lung plethysmography, 237
lung scan, 237
lung transplantation, 239
lung volume reduction surgery (LVRS), 239
lungs, 226–227, 232, 354
lunula, 178
lupus, 305
luteinizing hormone (LH), 264, 343
Lyme disease, 41
lymph nodes, 10, 122, 206
lymph vessels, 10
lymphadenitis, 213
lymphadenography, 221
lymphaedentitis, 216
lymphangiogram, 221
lymphatic system
  common conditions and terms, 212–213
  described, 108, 121–123, 206–207, 365
  diseases/pathology, 213–216
  pharmacology, 221–222
  tests/procedures, 217–218, 219–221
  tongue twisters, 359
lymphatic tissue, 123
lymphatic vessels, 206
lymphedema, 213
lymph/lymph fluid, 122, 200, 206
lymphocytes, 122, 174, 206
lymphosarcoma (lymphoma), 216

M

macroscopic, 71
macrotia, 192
macula lutea, 193
macular degeneration, 193
macule, 171
magnetic resonance cholangiopancreatography (MRCP), 256
magnetic resonance imaging (MRI), 38, 147, 160, 292–293
malabsorption, 258
malabsorption syndrome, 254
male reproductive cell, 12
male reproductive system, 311–314, 316–324, 366
malignant melanoma, 174
malleolus, 140
malleus, 184
maloccluded teeth, 250
mammary glands, 12, 326, 329
mammary papilla, 329
mammary region, 114
mammogram/mammography, 61, 85, 341
mammoplasty, 61, 92, 100
mandible, 135, 140
manometer, 211
Mantoux test, 175–176, 238
Marion's, 361
mask of pregnancy, 173
masseter, 153
mast cells, 166
mastectomy, 92, 344
master gland, 125, 262
mastication, 243
mastitis, 337
mastoid process, 134, 142
mastoidectomy, 196
mastoidotomy, 196
mastoptosis, 334
maxilla, 140
maxillary bones, 135, 225
maxillofacial surgeon, 250
measles, 174
meconium, 335
medial, 111, 116
medial epicondylitis, 159
mediastinal cavity, 123
mediastinum, 109, 123, 232
medical dictionary, 8, 59
medical terms, 363–364, 366
Medicalmnemonics.com, 352, 353
Medilexicon.com, 350
mediolateral, 111
Medterms.com, 349
medulla (kidney), 299
medulla oblongata, 127, 283
medullary sponge kidney, 361
melanin, 165, 178

melanocytes, 59, 165, 168
melanocyte-stimulating hormone (MSH), 264
melanocytic system, 80
melanoma, 80, 94
melanosis, 59
melasma, 173
melatonin, 264, 270
melena, 253
membrane, 107
menarche, 333, 334
Meniere's disease/syndrome, 193
meninges, 283, 284
meningioma, 291
meningitis, 290
meningocele, 289
meniscectomy, 148
meniscopexy, 148
menometrorrhagia, 337
menopause, 343
menorrhagia, 90, 338
menorrhea, 84, 90
menstrual cycle/menstrual period/menstruation, 128, 327, 328, 333–334
mental region, 114
mentalis, 153
Merkel cell carcinoma, 174
metabolic function/metabolism, 106, 125
metacarpal bones/metacarpals, 137, 140
metastasize, 235
metatarsal arthroplasty, 148
metatarsal bones/metatarsals, 138, 140
metoprolol tartrate, 222
Mevacor, 222
microdactyly, 103
microscopic, 72
microsurgical epididymal sperm aspiration (MESA), 323
microsurgical vasvasostomy, 321
microtia, 192
micturate, 301
micturition, 300
midsagittal plane, 111, 117
milk-carrying ducts, 329
mineral corticoids, 266
mineral salts, 125
mineralocorticoids, 125, 266
minimally invasive direct coronary artery bypass graft (MIDCAB), 220
Mirza technique, 161
miscarriage, 342
missed abortion, 338
mitochondrial myopathy, 159
mitral valve/mitral valve prolapse, 202, 211, 214
mnemonic devices, 353–356
mole, 174
molluscum contagiosum, 174
mongolism, 41
mononucleosis, 216
monoplegia, 287
morpheme, 32
morsicatio linguarum, 364
motile, 312
mouth, 11, 186, 224, 242–244
mucoid, 231
mucopurulent, 232
mucus/mucous, 231
multigravida, 335
multiloculated, 70
multipara, 335
multiparous, 71
multiple endocrine neoplasia (MEN), 360
multiple myeloma, 215
multiple sclerosis (MS), 291
Munchmeyer, 358
Munk, 361
muscaw volitantes, 364
muscle cell, 106
muscle tissue, 107
muscles, 120
muscular dystrophy, 160
muscular soft palate, 242
muscular system
  common conditions terms, 158–159, 161–162
  described, 149–155, 365
  diseases/pathology, 159–160
  tests/procedures, 160–161
  tongue twisters, 358
musculoskeletal system, 108, 120, 149. *See also* muscular system
myalgia, 84, 90, 100–101, 162
myasthenia, 162
myasthenia gravis, 159, 289
mycoplasma, 233
mycoses fungoides, 174
mydriatic drugs, 196
myelin sheaths, 283
myelogenous, 211
myelogram, 90, 292, 293
myocardial infarction, 212
myocarditis, 212
myocardium, 122, 201
myoclonus, 162
myofascial pain syndrome, 159
myology, 162
myolysis, 161
myoma, 110
myomectomy, 344
myometrium, 328, 334
myoparalysis, 158
myopathy, 162
myopia, 190
myoplasty, 161
myorrhaphy, 85, 161
myorrhexis, 85, 162
myosarcoma, 110, 160

myositis, 90, 110
myositis ossificans progressiva, 160
myotonia, 158
myringitis, 193
myringoplasty, 196
myringotomy, 196
myxedema, 272

N

nadolol, 222
nails. *See* integumentary system
naris/nares, 225
nasal bones, 135
nasal cavity/region, 114, 224
nasogastric, 251
nasogastric tube, 259
nasopharyngeal, 231
nasopharynx, 123, 224, 225, 242
nasoplasty, 85
nausea, 251
nebulizer, 232, 239
necrophobia, 90
necrosis, 90, 94
necrotic, 342
necrotizing fasciitis, 173
negative feedback, 343
neonate, 335
neonatologist/neonatalogy, 335
neoplasia, 72
neoplasm, 72, 110, 174
nephrectomy, 90, 308
nephritis, 213, 305
nephroblastoma, 305
nephrogram, 307
nephrolith, 305
nephrolithiasis, 94, 305
nephrolithotomy, 308
nephrologist/nephrology, 310
nephrolysis, 308
nephroma, 305
nephromegaly, 305
nephron, 299
nephropexy, 103, 308
nephroptosis, 305
nephroscopy, 307
nephrosis, 84, 305
nephrotic syndrome, 305
nerve ablation, 148
nerve cell, 107
nerve tissue, 107
nerves, 280
nervous system
  common conditions and terms, 287–290
  described, 126–127, 279–284, 366
  diseases/pathology, 290–291
  pharmacology, 294
  tests/procedures, 292–294
  tongue twisters, 360–361
neuralgia, 289
neurectomy, 293
neuritis, 59, 101, 104, 289
neuroblastoma, 291
neuroendocrine carcinoma, 174
neurofibromatosis, 361
neurologist/neurology, 90, 99, 287
neuroma, 289
neurons, 280
neuropathy, 59, 80, 99, 110
neuroplasty, 59, 294
neurosis, 289
neurosonography, 293
neurosurgeon, 287
nevus/nevi, 174
newborn (NB), 336
niacin, 222
nicardipine hydrochloride, 222
Nicobid, 222
nitrogenous waste, 298
nocturia, 310
nodes, 200
non-Hodgkin's lymphoma, 216
non-insulin-dependent diabetes mellitus (NIDDM), 267, 274
nonsteroidal anti-inflammatory drugs (NSAIDs), 148
nontropical sprue, 254
noradrenaline (norephinephrine), 126, 266
normal saline, 196
nose, 185, 224, 225
nuclear medicine test, 146
nucleotome, 148
nucleus, 107
nulligravida, 335
nullipara, 336
nyctalopia, 190
nystagmus, 192

O

obdormition, 364
obstetrical, 335
obstetrical ultrasound, 345
obstetrics (OB), 326, 336, 345
obstructive sleep apnea (OSA), 235
occipital bone, 135
occipital lobe, 121, 180, 282
occipital region, 114
occipitalis, 153
occlude, 211
occlusion, 337
occult blood test, 255
Occupress, 222
ocular muscles, 182
oculomotor nerve, 282
oculus dexter (OD), 181
oculus sinister (OS), 181
oculus uterque (OU), 181
odontalgia, 92
ofloxacin, 319
oil glands, 166

Old Lyme, Connecticut, 41
olecranon, 137, 140
olecranon bursa, 138
olfactory bulb, 185
olfactory epithelium, 185
olfactory nerve, 282
oligomenorrhea, 70, 334
oligospermia, 104, 317, 318, 324
oliguria, 59, 70, 310
online articles, 4
onychomalacia, 92
onychomycosis, 178
onychophagia, 92
oophorectomy, 61, 62, 90, 344
oophoritis, 61, 90, 338
oophorosalpingectomy, 62, 99
oophoro-salpingectomy, 344
open fracture, 145
open reduction, 145
ophthalmalgia, 190
ophthalmic antibiotics, 196
ophthalmologist/ophthalmology, 92, 190
ophthalmoscope/ophthalmoscopy, 190, 194
opththalmic, 190
optic disc, 181
optic nerve, 282
optician, 93, 190
optometer, 191
optometrist/optometry, 191
oral antidiabetics, 277
oral cavity, 242
oral surgeon, 250
orbicularis, 153
orbicularis oculi, 153
orbicularis oris, 153
orbital cavity/region, 114, 182
orchialgia, 90, 324
orchidalgia, 324
orchidectomy, 321
orchidopexy, 321
orchiectomy, 90
orchiodynia, 324
orchioplasty, 321
orchitis/orchiditis, 317
organ of Corti, 184
organomegaly, 110
organs, 106, 108
orgasm, 324
orifice, 334
orolingual, 93
oropharynx, 123, 224, 225, 242
orthodontist, 250
orthopedist/orthopedics, 142
orthopnea, 84, 231
orthotics, 142
Osgood-Schlatter, 358
osmesis, 192
osseous tissue, 132, 142
ossification, 142
ostealgia, 148
osteoarthopathy, 104
osteoarthritis, 144
osteoblasts, 134, 142
osteoclasis, 148
osteoclast, 142
osteodynia, 148
osteogenic sarcoma, 145–146
osteology, 132–134
osteomalacia, 146
osteomyelitis, 145
osteopath/osteopathy, 80, 142–143
osteopenia, 84
osteoplasty, 148
osteoporosis, 132, 145
osteosarcoma, 143
osteotomy, 85, 148
otalgia, 193
otitis externa, 193
otitis media (OM), 93, 183, 193
otodynia, 93
otologist/otology, 191
otorhinolaryngologist/otorhinolaryngology (ENT), 104, 191
otorrhea, 191
otosclerosis, 193
otoscope/otoscopy, 191, 194
oval window, 184
ovarian carcinoma, 340
ovarian cyst, 340
ovarian ligaments, 326
ovaries, 12, 128, 264, 326–327
over-the-counter (OTC), 240
ovulation, 333
ovum, 12, 128, 312
oximeter, 232
oxygen, 11, 123, 224, 230, 298
oxygenated, 205
oxytocin, 270, 329

P

P. carinii, 319
Paget's disease, 146
palatoplasty, 257
palmar fascia, 159
Palmar uniportal endoscopic carpal tunnel release, 161
palsy, 289
pancreas, 125, 245, 262, 266
pancreatectomy, 277
pancreatic duct, 245
pancreatitis, 23, 254
pancreatotomy, 277
panhypopituitarism, 271
Papanicolaou (Pap) smear, 340, 341
papillae, 186, 243
papillomas, 177
papule, 171
paracentesis, 256
paralysis agitans, 291
paranasal/paranasal sinuses, 104, 225

paraovarian, 70
paraplegia, 287, 289
parasympathetic systems, 284
parathyroid, 125, 262, 265
parathyroid hormone (PTH), 265
parathyroidectomy, 277
parenchymal tissue, 313
parietal bone, 134
parietal lobe, 283
parietal pleura, 109, 226
parkinsonism, 291
Parkinson's disease, 18, 41, 291
parotid, 243
paroxysm, 232
paroxysmal dyspnea, 233
partial thickness burn, 172
parturition, 329, 336
patch skin test, 176
patella, 137–138, 140
patellar bursa, 138
patellectomy, 148
patent, 232
pathological conditions, 93–94, 145
pathologist/pathology, 85, 94, 106, 121, 213
pathophysiology, 121
pectoral region, 114
pectoralis major, 152, 153, 154
pelvic cavity, 109, 118, 137
pelvic girdle, 136
pelvic inflammatory disease (PID), 340
pelvimetry, 93, 345
pelvis, 116, 136–137
pemphigoid, 173
Pendred, 359
penicillin, 318, 322
penile implant, 321, 323
penis, 12, 312, 314, 324
percussion, 211, 237
percutaneous diskectomy, 148
percutaneous transluminal coronary angioplasty (PTCA), 220
pericardial, 70
pericarditis, 212
pericardium, 201
perimetrium, 328
perineal, 313, 355
perineum, 116, 313, 329
perineuritis, 104
periodontal disease, 254
periodontist, 250
perioperative, 71
periosteum, 134
peripheral glands, 11, 262
peripheral nervous system (PNS), 11, 126, 280, 284
peristalsis, 125, 244, 300
peritoneal, 90
peritoneal dialysis, 308
peritonitis, 90
periurethral, 70
pernicious anemia, 215
peroneal, 355
peroneus brevis/longus, 153, 155
pertussis, 236
petechia, 172
petit mal seizures, 289
petri dish, 339
Peyer's patches, 211
Peyronie's disease, 41, 361
phacoemulsification, 195
phagocytosis, 207
phalangectomy, 148
phalanx/phalanges, 137, 140
pharmacology, 85
pharyngitis, 90
pharynx, 123, 124, 225, 242–244
phelbotomy, 220
phenylketonuria (PKU), 306
pheochromocytoma, 213
phimosis, 317, 321
phonics, 53–54
photophobia, 84
photoreactive keratectomy (PRK), 195
physiology, 10–11, 106, 121–128
physis, 134
pia mater, 284
pigeon breeder's lung, 359
pineal, 126, 262, 264
pinna, 184
pitres, 323
pituitary, 125, 262, 263–265
pityriasis rosea, 173
placenta, 334
placenta previa, 338, 345
planes (of body), 117
plasma, 203
platelets/platelet count, 203, 205, 218
pleura, 109, 226
pleural cavity, 109, 123
pleural effusion, 233
pleurisy, 90, 233
pleurocentesis, 239
pleurolysis, 90
pluralization, 38, 43–52
pneumoconiosis, 94, 104, 233
pneumocystis carinii pneumonia (PCP), 233
pneumonectomy, 239
pneumonia, 233, 319
pneumonitis, 91
pneumonoultramicroscopic silicovolcanoconiosis, 364
pneumothorax, 234
podarthritis, 93
podiatrist, 143
point of insertion, 151–152
point of origin, 151–152
polycystic disease, 305
polycystic ovary syndrome, 340

polycythemia vera, 215
polydipsia, 70, 274
polymyalgia rheumatica, 160
polymyositis, 158
polyneuritis, 289
polyorchism, 324
polyp, 171
polypectomy, 257
polyposis, 253
polysomnography, 293
polyuria, 59, 70, 274, 310
Pompe, 360
pons, 283
popliteal region, 114
pores, 167
portals, 100
positron emission tomography (PET), 147, 292
posterior, 111, 116
postictal, 287
postmenstrual period, 333
postmortem, 104
postnatal, 71, 90, 336
postoperative, 71
postpartum, 336
potassium (K) supplement, 309
preeclampsia, 338
prefixes. *See also specific body systems*
common, 33–34, 65–69, 370–371
copycats/kissing cousins, 27, 67
defining of, 96–97
in general, 8, 16, 17, 18, 23
matching of to situations, 69–72
not always part of medical terms, 98
as often mistaken for one another, 97
opposites, 27, 68
pronunciation, 54–59
pregnancy, 334, 338, 345
pregnancy test, 341
premenstrual, 71
premenstrual dysphoric syndrome (PMD), 338
premenstrual period, 333
premenstrual syndrome (PMS), 338
prenatal, 71, 90, 336
preoperative, 71
prepuce, 314
presbycusis, 104, 121, 193
presbyopia, 104, 121, 191
priapism, 317, 361
primary teeth, 250
primigravida, 337
primipara, 337
proctologist, 91
proctoscopy, 256
proetz test, 194
progesterone, 12, 128, 264, 267, 327, 334
progressive ossifying polymyositis, 358
prolactin (PRL), 264, 267, 329
prolapsed uterus, 340
pronation, 158
prone, 112
pronunciation, 54–59
propranolol hydrochloride, 221
prostaglandin analogs, 196
prostate, 12, 128, 312, 314
prostate carcinoma, 320
prostate specific antigen (PSA) test, 320
prostatectomy, 61, 317, 321
prostatitis, 317
prostatocystitis, 317
prostatolith, 317
prostatolithotomy, 323
prostatomegaly, 61
prostatron, 321
prosthesis, 143, 321
protatorrhea, 317
protein, 271
protein blood test, 255
protein pump inhibitors, 259
prothrombin time (PT), 218
protrusion of an intervertebral disk, 144
proximal, 111, 116
pruritus/pruritus ani, 172, 253
pseudocyesis, 337
pseudocyst, 70
pseudopregnancy, 71
psoriasis, 173
psoriatric arthritis, 144
psychiatrist/psychiatry, 288
psychogenetic, 288
psychogenic, 288
psychologist/psychology, 85, 288
psychosis, 101, 289
psychosomatic, 288
puberty, 324, 335
pubic region, 114
pubic symphysis, 137
pubis, 13–1376, 140
puerpera, 337
puerperium, 337
pulmonary, 91, 232
pulmonary abscesses, 234
pulmonary angiography, 237
pulmonary arteries, 203, 211
pulmonary circulation, 211
pulmonary edema, 214, 234, 235
pulmonary embolism, 234, 236
pulmonary embolus (PE), 227
pulmonary function tests (PFT), 237
pulmonary neoplasm, 234
pulmonary semilunar valve, 202
pulmonary veins, 211
punch biopsy, 176
punctae, 182

pupils equal, round, and reactive to light and accommodation (PERRLA), 181
purified protein derivative (PPD) test, 175–176
Purkinje fibers, 205
purpura, 172, 216
purulent otitis media, 191
pustule, 171
pyelitis, 305
pyelogram, 307
pyelography, 91
pyelolithotomy, 91, 308
pyelonephritis, 305
pyeloplasty, 308
pyloric sphincter, 244
pyloroplasty, 257
pyogenic, 178
pyuria, 310

Q

quadriceps, 153
quadriplegia, 84, 288
quantitative computerized tomography (QCT), 147
quickening, 337
quinquaud, 358

R

radial nerve, 281, 355
radical mastectomy, 340
radioactive iodine uptake, 276
radiography, 100
radioisotope/radioisotope scan, 255, 307
radius, 137, 140
rales, 232
Raynaud's phenomenon, 214
reabsorption, 301
rectosigmoid, 91
rectum, 246
rectus/rectus abdominis/rectus femoris, 153, 154, 155
red blood cells/red blood cell count (RBC), 205, 218
red bone marrow, 132, 143
reduction, 145
reduction mammoplasty, 100
references, 349–352
refraction, 182
regurgitation, 251
Reifenstein, 323
relapse, 215
remission, 215
renal angiography, 307
renal angioplasty, 308
renal biopsy, 308–309
renal calculi, 305
renal cell carcinoma, 305
renal colic, 305
renal corpuscle, 299
renal failure, 271
renal hypertension, 305
renal parenchyma, 305
renal pelvis, 127
renal transplant, 309
renal tubule, 299, 301
renin, 270
reproduction, 12
reproductive cell, 107
reproductive systems
  defined, 108
  female, 325–329, 334–346, 366
  male, 311–314, 316–324, 366
  overview, 127–128
  tongue twisters, 361
reptilian brain, 283
resection, 322
respiratory distress syndrome (RDS), 336
respiratory rate, 224
respiratory system
  common conditions and terms, 230–234
  described, 108, 123–124, 223–227, 365
  diseases/pathology, 235–236
  pharmacology, 239–240
  tests/procedures, 236–239
  tongue twisters, 359–360
respirologist/respirology, 230
respirometer, 104
retina, 180, 181
retinal detachment, 192
retinitis pigmentosa, 193
retrograde pyelogram, 307
retroversion, 335
Reye's syndrome, 291
rhabdomyosarcoma, 104
rheometer, 363
rheumatic heart disease, 214
rheumatoid arthritis, 144
rhinitis, 234
rhinokyphosis, 104
rhinoplasty, 85, 93, 238
rhinorrhea, 93, 231
rhomboid major, 153
rhytidectomy, 177
ribs, 136
rickets, 146
ringworm, 173
Rocher, 323
rods, 181
root words. *See also specific body systems*
  alphabetized list, 72–78
  common, 368–370
  defining of, 97–98
  directional, 112
  exterior of body, 24–26, 92–93
  in general, 8–9, 16, 17, 18, 23
  interior of body, 27–32, 87–91
  pathological conditions, 93–94

rosacea, 173
roseola, 173
rotation, 158
rotator cuff, 160, 354
rubella, 174
rubeola, 174
rugae, 244
rule of two, 204

S

saccule, 184
sacral region (S), 114, 115
sacroiliac, 137
sacrum, 135, 136, 140
sagittal plane, 111, 117
saliva, 243
salivary ducts, 243
salivary glands, 124, 243
salpingectomy, 62, 91, 344, 345
salpingitis, 335
salpingocyesis, 338
salpingogram, 62
salpingography, 62
salpingo-oophorectomy, 62, 99, 344
Salter-Harris system, 134
sarciodosis, 216
sarcoid, 91
scabies, 173, 174
SCALP, mnemonic, 354
scapula, 114, 136, 140
Schick test, 175–176
Schimmelbusch, 361
sciatica, 289
sclera, 180
scleroderma, 173
scleroplasty, 195
sclerosing solution, 176
sclerotherapy, 176
scoliosis, 101, 143
scrotum, 12, 128, 312, 313
sebaceous glands, 120, 167
seborrhea, 178
seborrheic keratosis, 174
sebum, 167
secondary hypertension, 213
second-degree burn, 172
secondigravida, 337
secretion, 301
secundipara, 337
sedatives, 294
seizure, 288
semantics, 32
semen, 314
semen analysis, 320
semicircular canals, 184
semimembranosus, 153, 155
seminal fluid, 128, 313
seminal vesicles, 12, 128, 312, 314
seminiferous tubules, 313
seminoma, 317
semitendinosus, 153
sensorineural deafness, 185
sensory system
  common conditions and terms, 192–193
  described, 108, 121, 179–189, 365
  diseases/pathology, 193
  pharmacology, 196
  tests/procedures, 194–196
  tongue twisters, 359
septa/septum, 202
septicemia, 94
septoplasty, 238
sequestrum, 145–146
serous otitis media, 191, 193
serratus/serratus anterior, 154
serum enzyme test/studies, 217
sesamoid bones, 133
SEVE, mnemonic, 355
seventh cervical vertebral muscle, 153
seven-year itch, 173
sex cell, 12, 107, 267, 326
sexually transmitted diseases (STDs), 318, 322
shaking palsy, 291
shingles, 289
short bones, 133
shortness of breath (SOB), 227
sialolithotomy, 104
sickle-cell anemia, 215
sigmoid colon, 246
sigmoidoscopy, 256
sildenafil citrate, 322
silent letters, 54–55
silicosis, 233
silver nitrate, 196, 240
simethicone, 258
single-photon emission computerized tomography (SPECT), 147, 293
sinoatrial (SA) node, 205, 211
sinuses, 207
SITS, mnemonic, 354
sixth disease, 173
skeletal muscle, 151
skeletal system
  common conditions and terms, 141–145
  described, 131–138, 365
  diseases/pathology, 145–146
  tests/procedures, 146–147
  tongue twisters, 357–358
skin. *See* integumentary system
skin biopsy, 176
skin cell, 106
skin scratch test, 176
skull, 132, 134–135
slipped disk, 144
slit lamp biomicroscopy, 194
small bowel, 245
small incision lenticule extraction (SMILE), 195
small intestine, 124, 245
smooth muscle, 151

soleus, 153
somatic system, 284
somatotropin, 264, 270
somnambulism, 104
sonohysterography, 341
soundalikes, 49–52
spastic colon, 254
special senses system, 108
specific gravity, 299
spelling, ways to practice, 17
spermatic cords, 12, 312
sperm/spermatozoon/spermatozoa, 12, 128, 264, 312, 313, 326
sphenoid bone, 135, 225
sphenopalatine ganglioneuralgia, 364
sphincters, 127, 244
sphygmomanometer, 211
spina bifida/spina bifida occulta, 291, 345
spinal cavity, 109, 118
spinal column, 115, 135–136
spinal cord, 11, 115, 127, 280, 281, 283–284
spinal nerves, 11, 126, 280
spinal puncture, 292
spine, 140
spinocerebellar ataxia, 360
spinous processes, 136
spirometer, 237
spleen, 123, 207
splenectomy, 91
splenomegaly, 60, 84, 91, 101, 213
spondylosyndesis, 148
spongy bone, 134
spontaneous abortion, 338
spontaneous vaginal delivery (SVD), 336
sprain, 144
sputum/sputum culture, 232, 237
squamous cell carcinoma, 174
squamous epithelial cells, 174
stapedectomy, 196
stapes, 184
steatorrhea, 253
Stein-Leventhal syndrome, 340
stent insertion, 220
sterilization, 324, 342
sternal region, 114
sternocleidomastoid, 152, 153
sternum, 136, 140
sternutate, 364
steroids, 125, 266, 270
stethoscope, 236–237
stillbirth, 338
stimulating hormones, 264
stomach, 124, 244, 251
stomatitis, 93
stool softeners, 258
strabismus, 192
stress test, 219
striated muscle, 151
stroke, 288
stromuhr, 363
sty/stye, 192
subarachnoid space, 283–284
subcostal, 70, 143
subcutaneous mastectomy, 340
subcutaneous tissue/layer, 166
subdural hematoma, 290
subdural space, 283
sublingual, 92, 250
sublingual gland, 243
submandibular gland, 243
submental region, 114
subtotal hysterectomy, 344
subumbilical, 70
sudden infant death syndrome (SIDS), 227
sudoriferous glands, 120, 167
suffixes. *See also specific body systems*
alphabetized list, 83–85, 99–101
common, 34–35, 79–83, 372–374
defining of, 98–99
in general, 16, 17, 18, 23
matching of to situations, 83–85
as part of every medical term, 96
pronunciation, 56–57
sulci, 281
sulfonamides, 309
superficial muscles, 152–155
superior, meaning above, 111, 116
superior vena cava, 122, 203, 205
supination, 158
supine, 112
suppurative otitis media, 193
supraclavicular region, 114
supraspinatus, 153
suture/suture joints, 135, 138
sweat, 167
sweat glands, 168
sympathetic nerves/systems, 284
symphysis pubis, 153, 336
symphysis-fundus height (SFH), 336
syncope, 290
synovectomy, 148
synovial cavity, 138
synovial joints, 138
synovial membrane, 138
syphilis, 319
systemic circulation, 211
systems. *See* body systems
systole, 205, 211. *See also specific systems*

T

T1-T12, 135
tachyarrhythmia, 71
tachycardia, 71
talipes, 144
target tissue, 270
tarsal bones/tarsals, 138, 140
taste buds, 186
teeth, 250
telangiectasis, 173
temporal bones, 134
temporal lobe, 121, 283
temporalis, 153
temporomandibular joint, 135
tendinitis/tendonitis, 91, 143, 158
tendinopathy, 159
tendons, 120, 143, 151–152, 162
tennis elbow, 159
tenodesis, 161
tenodynia, 143, 162
tenomyoplasty, 161
tenorrhaphy, 148, 161
tenosynovitis, 143, 159, 162
tenotomy, 148, 161
tensor fascia lata, 153, 155
teratocarcinoma, 317
teratoma, 317
testalgia, 324
testicles, 128, 312, 313
testicular, 91
testicular carcinoma, 317
testicular torsion, 318
testis/testes, 12, 128, 264, 312, 313
testitis, 91
testosterone, 12, 128, 264, 268, 312
tetany, 272
tetralogy of Fallot, 359
thalamus, 283
thalassemia, 215
thermoregulation, 164
third-degree burn, 172
thoracentesis, 91, 93, 238
thoracic cavity, 109, 118, 123, 226–227
thoracic duct, 207
thoracic processes, 136
thoracic region (T), 115
thoracic vertebrae, 135
thoracocentesis, 239
thoracomyodynia, 104
thoracotomy, 91, 93, 239
thorax, 116, 136
thrombocyte, 211
thrombolysis, 213
thrombophlebitis, 104
thymus, 123, 207
thyroid, 125, 262, 265, 354
thyroid carcinoma, 275
thyroid cartilage, 224, 265
thyroid scan, 276
thyroidectomy, 277
thyroiditis, 101, 272
thyroid-stimulating hormone (TSH), 264, 267, 270
thyromegaly, 101, 272
thyrotrophin, 264
thyroxine (T4), 264, 265
tibia, 138, 140
tibialis anterior, 153, 155
tinea, 173
tinea cruris, 322
tinea pedis, 172
tinnitus, 193
tissues, 106, 107–108
tonic-clonic seizures, 288–289
tonometry, 194
tonsillitis/tonsillectomy, 98–99
tonsils/tonsillitis/tonsillectomy, 80, 91, 98–99, 101, 123, 207, 225, 234, 238
topical drugs, 196
torticollis, 104, 160
total abdominal hysterectomy with bilateral salpingo-oophorectomy (TAH-BSO), 344
total hip replacement arthroplasty, 147
total knee joint replacement arthroplasty, 147
totally endoscopic coronary artery bypass graft (TECAB), 220
touch receptor, 186
toxic shock syndrome (TSS), 340
trabeculae, 143
trabecular carcinoma, 174
trachea, 100, 224, 225–226, 244
tracheitis, 234
tracheoplasty, 239
tracheostomy/tracheotomy, 84, 85, 237, 238
tragus, 184
transient global amnesia, 290
transient ischemic attack (TIA), 291
transitional cell carcinoma, 305
transplantations, 257
transrectal ultrasound prostate biopsy (TRUS), 321
transrectal ultrasound/ultrasound examination, 320
transurethral microwave thermotherapy (TUMT), 321
transurethral resection of ejaculatory ducts (TUREP), 322
transurethral resection of prostate (TURP), 322
transverse plane, 111, 117
transverse processes, 136
trapezius, 152, 153
Treitz, Wenzel (physician), 41
Treponema pallidum, 319
triceps brachii, 153
Trichomonas, 319

trichomoniasis, 319
tricuspid valve, 202
trigeminal nerve, 282
trigeminal neuralgia (tic douloureux), 290
triglycerides, 242
trigone, 300
triiodothyronine (T3), 264, 265
trisomy 21, 41
trochanter, 143
trochlear nerve, 282
trophic hormones, 264
true ribs, 136
tubal banding/clipping/ ligation, 342
tubal pregnancy, 338
tubercle, 143
tuberculin test, 238
tuberculosis (TB), 175–176, 235, 237, 319
tuberosity, 143
tubules, 127, 299
tummy-tuck, 176
tumors, 291
tuning fork test, 194
tympanectomy, 196
tympanic membrane, 184
tympanitis, 193
tympanometer/ tympanometry, 191
tympanoplasty, 196
Type 1/Type2 diabetes, 274

U

ulcer, 172, 251
ulcerative colitis, 254
ulna, 137, 140
ultrasonogram, 85
ultrasonography/ultrasound, 276, 307
ultrasound, 160
umbilical region, 113
unicomparmental hip/knee resurfacing, 147
unossified tissue, 135
upper extremities, 116, 137
upper GI series, 255
upper respiratory infection (URI), 227, 236
urea, 12, 298
ureteral orifice, 300
ureterectomy, 309
ureteritis, 304
ureterolith, 94
ureterolithotomy, 91
ureteropelvic/ureteropelvic junction (UPJ), 91
ureteroscope/ureteroscopy, 307
ureterostomy, 309
ureterotomy, 309
ureters, 12, 298, 300
urethra, 12, 128, 298, 300–301, 312, 314
urethral meatus, 300, 329
urethritis, 91, 304, 319
urethropexy, 85, 91, 309
urethrorrhea, 94
urethroscope/urethroscopy, 307
urethrovesical suspension, 309
urinalysis (UA), 306
urinary, 310
urinary bladder, 127, 300
urinary catheterization, 310
urinary incontinence, 306
urinary meatus, 300
urinary retention, 306
urinary system
  common conditions and terms, 304, 310
  described, 108, 127–128, 297–301, 366
  diseases/pathology, 304–306
  pharmacology, 309
  tests/procedures, 306–309
  tongue twisters, 361
urinary tract infection (UTI), 304
urination, 127, 274
urine, 12, 127, 299, 301
urinometer, 307
urologist/urology, 310
urostomy, 309
urticaria, 172
uterine endometrium, 333
uterine relaxants, 346
uterine tubes, 326
uterus, 12, 128, 326, 327–328
utricle, 184
uvea, 181
uvula, 243
uvulectomy, 257
uvulopalatopharyngoplasty (UPPP), 257

V

vagina, 12, 128, 326, 328–329
vaginal hysterectomy, 344
vaginitis, 338
vaginoplasty, 344
vagotomy, 257
vagus nerve, 282
valve surgery, 239
valves, 202
varicella, 174
varicose veins, 214
variocele, 318
variocelectomy, 322
vas deferens, 12, 128, 312
Vascor, 222
vasectomy, 91, 314, 322
vasodilators, 322
vasoepididymostomy, 322
vasopressin, 265, 270
vastus, 153
vastus lateralis/vastus medialis, 153, 155
veins, 122, 200, 202
veisalgia, 364
venae cavae, 211
Veneral Disease Research Laboratory (VDRL) test, 320
venereal, 319

venereal diseases, 318
venereal warts, 319
venipuncture, 220
venogram, 220
venous system, 203
ventilation, 123
ventilation perfusion scan (VPS), 227
ventilator, 232
ventral, 111, 116
ventricles, 122, 202, 283
ventriculoperitoneal (VP) shunting, 294
venules, 203
verruca, 174
vertebrae, 115, 134, 135
vertebral body, 136
vertebral canal, 127
vertebral column/disks, 135–136
vertigo, 193
vesicle, 172
vesicovaginal fistula, 340
vessels, 200
vestibulocochlear nerve, 282
viability, 312
villi, 246, 254
viral culture, 320
viral meningitis, 290
virtual colonoscopy, 256
viscera, 110
visceral muscle, 150, 151
visceral pleura, 109
viscerography, 91
visceromegaly, 94
visual acuity (VA), 181, 194
visual field (VF), 181
visual field test, 194
vitiligo, 172
vitrectomy, 195
vitreous body/vitreous humor, 181
vocabulary, building foundation of, 9
voice box, 244
voiding, 300
voiding cystourethrogram (VCUG), 307
voluntary nervous system, 284
voluntary striated muscle, 151
volvulus, 253
vomiting, 251
Von Recklighausen, 361
vulva/vulvectomy, 329, 344

W

warfarin sodium, 221
warts, 174
waste products, 12
water pills, 239–240
water warts, 174
Weber's test, 194
webMD.com, 350
wheal, 172
white blood cell differential count, 218
white blood cells/white blood cell count (WBC), 205, 218
white matter, 282
whooping cough, 236
Wilms' tumor, 305
windpipe, 225–226, 244
word elements, 96

X

xiphoid process, 136, 153
x-ray, 146

Y

yeast infections, 337, 346
yellow bone marrow, 143

Z

Zenker's diverticulum, 253
zygoma, 135
zygomatic bones, 135
zygomatic major/zygomatic minor, 153
zygote, 326
zygote intrafallopian transfer (ZIFT), 339

About the Authors

Beverley Henderson, CMT-R, HRT, has enjoyed a lifelong career in the medical field. Working in Ontario hospitals for 45 years, she also has more than 40 years' experience in medical terminology and transcription. She has managed the medical transcription unit of a large acute-care hospital and has taught medical terminology to adult learners at the university level. Beverley is a Certified Medical Transcriptionist with the Association for Healthcare Documentation Integrity (AHDI), formerly American Association for Medical Transcription. She was Director of Health Sciences Faculty and MT Course Coordinator at an online medical terminology and transcription school, where she developed course curricula and helped write and produce a series of medical terminology teaching videos. Now an empty-nester, she lives in Cayuga, Ontario in the summer and winters in Ajijic, Mexico, with her husband of 46 years.

Jennifer L. Dorsey, PhD, has been a writer and editor for more than 20 years. She has worked for publishers both large and small, mainly focusing her efforts on development editing, writing, and acquisitions. She has coauthored, revised, and ghostwritten titles in the business, medical, lifestyle, and personal growth categories. She received her B.A. in journalism from Saint Mary-of-the-Woods College, and her master's and Ph.D. from Saint Louis University. She lives in Illinois with her husband and three children.

Dedication

This book is dedicated to my family and friends. To the coworkers who have become my friends, gathered over a 45-year span while working at the Henderson Hospital, St. Joseph's Hospital, and McMaster University Medical Centre.

To my parents, Mary and Bill Hunter, I am only sorry they are not here to read this. To my daughter Michele, who showed me it's never too late to change careers. To my son Ian, living proof that intelligence, good looks, and respect do exist in one man. To my husband Richard, whose steadfast love and patience has allowed me to follow my career dreams down whatever road I wanted. To the new love of my life, my beautiful 2-year-old grandson, Axl Henderson, a clone of his father, who is a delight and a challenge all in the same minute.

—Beverley Henderson

To my husband Mike, for sharing the load, encouraging me to persevere, and always asking my "Should I do this?" question with "Why wouldn't you?"

—Jennifer L. Dorsey

Authors' Acknowledgments

My sincere thanks to Lindsay Lefevere, our acquisitions editor, for having the faith and trust in my medical knowledge to keep me on board the Wiley bandwagon as the old "new kid on the block." Never in my wildest dreams did I imagine myself accomplishing a feat of this magnitude. I thank Lindsay for giving me the opportunity to write about a subject that has been a large part of my career for many years. I am truly honored to be included in the accomplishments of Wiley publications.

To my "partner in crime" in this endeavor, Jen Dorsey. I could not have done this without her. With her expertise in writing, Jen has coached me through this experience. Her patience and understanding, not to mention her answers to my never-ending questions, went above and beyond the call of duty. Working with Jennifer again has been an absolute pleasure.

—Beverley Henderson

Thank you to my coauthor Beverly Henderson. Her medical knowledge is the heart of this book, and her passion really shows.

Big thanks go out to our talented acquisitions editor, Lindsay Lefevere, for having faith that we could pull this off. She's an editorial guardian angel. Thank you to Tim Gallan, Dummies editor extraordinaire. Thanks to our gifted technical editor, Gallaudet Howard, for pointing out ways to improve and update our terminology information. Innumerable thanks go out to all of the editorial and production folks, graphic artists, proofreaders, and indexers who make us look pretty darn good. You guys rock!

Thanks to my awesome, funny, delightfully precocious children, who keep me laughing and remind me of what is most precious in life. Most importantly, thank you so much to my wonderful husband, Mike, who loves me no matter what crazy project I sign up for and who has always believed this is the right path from the start.

—Jennifer L. Dorsey

Publisher's Acknowledgments

Executive Editor: Lindsay Sandman Lefevere
Project Editor: Tim Gallan
Technical Reviewer: Gallaudet Howard (previous edition)
Production Editor: Siddique Shaik
Illustrator: Kathryn Born
Cover Image: © Science Photo Library - PIXOLOGICSTUDIO/Getty Images